DIABETES
CASE STUDIES
Real Problems, Practical Solutions

—— **Boris Draznin,** MD, PhD, *Editor* ——

Cecilia C. Low Wang, MD, FACP, *Associate Editor*
Daniel J. Rubin, MD, MSc, FACE, *Associate Editor*

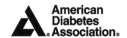

American Diabetes Association®

Director, Book Publishing, Abe Ogden; *Managing Editor*, Greg Guthrie; *Acquisitions Editor*, Victor Van Beuren; *Production Manager*, Melissa Sprott; *Production Services*, Cenveo Publisher Services; *Cover Design*, Lawrence Marie, Inc.; *Printer*, Data Reproductions.

Printed in the United States of America
1 3 5 7 9 10 8 6 4 2

The suggestions and information contained in this publication are generally consistent with the *Standards of Medical Care in Diabetes* and other policies of the American Diabetes Association, but they do not represent the policy or position of the Association or any of its boards or committees. Reasonable steps have been taken to ensure the accuracy of the information presented. However, the American Diabetes Association cannot ensure the safety or efficacy of any product or service described in this publication. Individuals are advised to consult a physician or other appropriate health care professional before undertaking any diet or exercise program or taking any medication referred to in this publication. Professionals must use and apply their own professional judgment, experience, and training and should not rely solely on the information contained in this publication before prescribing any diet, exercise, or medication. The American Diabetes Association—its officers, directors, employees, volunteers, and members—assumes no responsibility or liability for personal or other injury, loss, or damage that may result from the suggestions or information in this publication.

♾ The paper in this publication meets the requirements of the ANSI Standard Z39.48-1992 (permanence of paper).

Jane Chiang, MD, conducted the internal review of this book to ensure that it meets American Diabetes Association guidelines.

ADA titles may be purchased for business or promotional use or for special sales. To purchase more than 50 copies of this book at a discount, or for custom editions of this book with your logo, contact the American Diabetes Association at the address below or at booksales@diabetes.org.

American Diabetes Association
1701 North Beauregard Street
Alexandria, Virginia 22311

DOI: 10.2337/9781580405713

Library of Congress Cataloging-in-Publication Data
Diabetes case studies / [edited by] Boris Draznin.
    p. ; cm.
Includes bibliographical references and index.
ISBN 978-1-58040-571-3 (alk. paper)
I. Draznin, Boris, editor. II. American Diabetes Association, publisher.
[DNLM: 1. Diabetes Mellitus--Case Reports. WK 810]
RC660
616.4'62—dc23
                    2014042723

Contents

Preface   xiii
Introduction   xv

1. **DIAGNOSTIC DILEMMAS AND PROBLEMS WITH CLASSIFICATION**

Case 1: Maturity-Onset Diabetes of the Young (MODY) as a Diagnostic Possibility   1
S. Kochar and J.L. Gilden

Case 2: Diagnosis of Coexistent Maturity-Onset Diabetes of the Young in a Patient with Type 1 Diabetes   5
S. Azmi and R.A. Malik

Case 3: An Unusual Clinical Presentation of Diabetes Eventually Diagnosed as a Monogenic Form   8
V.N. Montes, A. Chait, and C.E. Taplin

Case 4: A Case of Monogenic Diabetes   12
R.H. Slover

Case 5: Recurrent Ketoacidosis: Lessons from Multiple Clinical Presentations   15
E. Ipp and K. Djekic

Case 6: Ketoacidosis in a Patient with Type 1 Diabetes on a Low-Calorie Meal Replacement Diet   19
K. Brown and D. Bessesen

Case 7: Reevaluation After Ketoacidosis Presentation   23
P. Cruz-Bravo and J.B. McGill

Case 8: Metabolic Syndrome-Related Comorbidities Typical of Older Adulthood Complicate Diabetic Ketoacidosis in a Youth with Type 2 Diabetes   26
K. Nadeau

Case 9: Not Your Usual Diabetic Ketoacidosis   32
R. Gaba, S.L. Samson, and A.J. Garber

Case 10: Ketosis-Prone Diabetes   36
          D. Saxon and N. Rasouli

Case 11: From a Total Daily Dose of Insulin of 415 Units to
          No Insulin: A Case of Ketosis-Prone Diabetes   39
          C.T. Nguyen and J.H. Mestman

Case 12: The Worst Case Scenario: Severe HHS in a Relatively
          Young Man   43
          E. Herman and M.E. McDonnell

Case 13: Unusual Cause of New-Onset Diabetes   49
          K.M. Shikuma and J.H. Mestman

Case 14: What Type of Diabetes?   53
          A.L. McCall

Case 15: Type 1 Diabetes versus LADA in a Patient Misdiagnosed
          with Type 2 Diabetes   58
          C.C. Low Wang

Case 16: Type 1 Diabetes Can Present at Any Age   61
          D.S.H. Bell

Case 17: Is This Type 2 Diabetes, Type 1 Diabetes, or
          Late Autoimmune Diabetes in Adults?   64
          D. Tripathy, S. Pinkson, M. Koops, and R.A. DeFronzo

Case 18: A Common Misdiagnosis   67
          I.E. Schauer

Case 19: Almost All Nonobese Young People with an Acute
          Onset of Diabetes Have Type 1 Diabetes   70
          D.S.H. Bell

Case 20: Symptomatic Postprandial Hyperglycemia   73
          A. Maturu and M. McDermott

Case 21: A Patient with Newly Diagnosed, Asymptomatic
          Hyperglycemia   77
          A. McElduff

Case 22: Glucokinase Maturity-Onset Diabetes of the
          Young and Pregnancy   80
          J. Apel and Ch-K. Koh

Case 23: Latent Autoimmune Diabetes of the Adult (LADA) in an
          Elderly Patient   83
          M. Shah, M. Sohrevardi, and D. Baldwin

2. HbA₁c DILEMMAS

**Case 24: A Diagnostic Dilemma in a Patient with Elevated
Glycosylated Hemoglobin**   86
S. Paturi and J.L. Gilden

**Case 25: An Unexplained Decline in HbA₁c in Spite of
Persistent Hyperglycemia**   90
D.S.H. Bell

**Case 26: What to Do with Discrepant HbA₁c and SMBG Results?
The Utility of Fructosamine and Glycated Albumin**   92
T. Gandrabura and D. J. Rubin

Case 27: A "Tricky" Low HbA₁c   95
C. Mazzucchelli, C. Bordone, D. Maggi, and R. Cordera

3. MORE INSULIN IS NOT ALWAYS THE SOLUTION: CASES OF SEVERE INSULIN RESISTANCE

**Case 28: Use of Insulin U-500 in a Patient with Severe
Insulin Resistance**   98
H. Mahmud and M.T. Korytkowski

**Case 29: Effective Use of U-500 Insulin via Insulin Pump in a
Type 2 Diabetes Patient with Severe Insulin Resistance**   102
V.B. Balakrishnan and E.S. Siraj

Case 30: U-500 Insulin Pump Case   105
A.L. McCall

**Case 31: Difficulties in Managing Patients with Insulin Resistance:
Alternatives to U-500 Insulin**   109
N. Movva, B.G. Theckedath, and J.L. Gilden

**Case 32: Management Issues in the Syndrome of Autoantibodies to
the Insulin Receptor (Type B Insulin Resistance)**   115
E. Cochran, R. Brown, and P. Gorden

Case 33: Type B Insulin Resistance   118
N.B. Jacob, H. Trevino, and C. Rhee

**Case 34: Adhering or Not? That Is the Question: A Case of
Glucolipotoxicity and Concentrated Insulin**   121
S. Deshmukh, R. Buzzola, M. Touza, M. Gardner,
and J.R. Sowers

**Case 35: Cosecreting Adrenal Tumor Causing Severe
Insulin Resistance**   124
K. Rivera, K. Cusi, and C. Edwards

Case 36: Management of Severe Insulin Resistance in a Pregnant
          Patient with Type 2 Diabetes: The Use of U-500 Regular
          Insulin via Continuous Subcutaneous Infusion   130
          T. Hor and D. Baldwin

4. UNUSUAL FORMS AND PRESENTATIONS OF DIABETES
Case 37: Diabetes in Hereditary Hemochromatosis   133
          D.A. McClain

Case 38: Challenging Insights from Albuminuria Early in the
          Course of Disease   137
          C. Demirci, V. Lewy-Weiss, and M.A. Sperling

Case 39: Copresentation of Addison's Disease and Type 1
          Diabetes in a 9-Year-Old Boy   141
          S. Majidi and J. Raymond

Case 40: Diagnosis of Addison's Disease and Type 1 Diabetes
          in Twin Boys   145
          A.D. Urban and W.V. Tamborlane

Case 41: New-Onset Type 1 Diabetes, Addison's Disease, and
          Hypothyroidism: A Case of Autoimmune Polyendocrine
          Syndrome Type 2   149
          L. Golden and R. Goland

Case 42: The Slow Progression of Type 1 Diabetes as
          Part of Autoimmune Polyendocrine Syndrome Type 2   153
          N. Pertzeva and B. Mankovsky

Case 43: Atypical Type 2 Diabetes with Profound Dyslipidemia 156
          J.H. Pettus and R.R. Henry

Case 44: Patient with Diabetes Who Has Hemiballismus   160
          M. Padilla and J. Mestman

Case 45: A Case of Diabetic Myonecrosis   164
          U. Azmat, J.E. Payne, K. Dungan, and S.W. Ing

Case 46: A Case of Stiff Person Syndrome in a Patient with
          Type 1 Diabetes   169
          M.P. Gilbert and M.H. Nathan

Case 47: Stiff Person Syndrome in a Patient with Multiple
          Autoimmune Diseases   172
          J. Hughes and J.B. McGill

Case 48: Glycogenic Hepatopathy in an Adolescent with
Type 1 Diabetes 175
N. Zuckerman-Levin, O. Mordechai, and N. Shehadeh

Case 49: Glycemic Control in a Child with Type 1 Diabetes
and Autoimmune Hepatitis 180
S. Muntoni and M. Congia

Case 50: Dizziness, Lightheadedness, and Syncope in a Patient with
Type 2 Diabetes 184
S. Paturi and J.L. Gilden

Case 51: Growth Hormone Excess-Induced Diabetic Ketoacidosis ... 189
A.P. Demidowich, M. Lodish, and K.I. Rother

Case 52: Refractory Angina in a Patient with Type 2 Diabetes 192
M. Kosiborod

5. DIABETES IN THE HOSPITAL SETTING

Case 53: Glycemic Control in a Patient with Type 2 Diabetes
Undergoing Cardiac Surgery 196
M.K. Figaro

Case 54: Inpatient Insulin Management for Complex Enteral Feedings 200
A.B. Barton, K.J. Evans, and L.F. Lien

Case 55: Glycemic Control in a Patient with Type 1 Diabetes
and Severe Burns 204
R.M. Hawkins and B. Draznin

Case 56: Combined Effect of Intravenous Insulin Infusion and
Subcutaneous Rapid-Acting Insulin for Glycemic Control in
Severe Insulin Resistance 208
M. Szkudlinska and I.B. Hirsch

Case 57: Therapeutic Hypothermia and Severe Insulin Resistance
in Patients with Diabetes and Cardiac Arrest 211
S. Seggelke and B. Draznin

Case 58: Extreme Insulin Resistance Following Heart Transplant 214
S. Gupta, D.J. Oakes, A. Therasse, A. Wallia, and M.E. Molitch

Case 59: Glycemic Control after Left Ventricular Assist Device
Placement in a Patient with Type 2 Diabetes 218
G. Staskus

Case 60: Management of Diabetic Ketoacidosis in a Patient
on Hemodialysis   222
R. Prabhushankar, S. Syed, and J.R. Sowers

Case 61: New Diabetes Emergency: Acute Rhabdomyolysis
Complicating Hyperglycemic Hyperosmolar Coma   226
C. Vaz and A. Chaudhuri

Case 62: Transitioning from Intravenous to Subcutaneous Insulin
in a Complicated Patient   232
K.J. Evans and L.F. Lien

Case 63: Failure to Coordinate Diabetes Care between Hospital and
Ambulatory Settings: A Threat to Safe and Quality Patient Care   237
S. Peavie and M. Falciglia

Case 64: Preventing Readmission: Translating the Hospital Diabetes
Regimen into a Home Regimen that Is Safe, Effective, and
Easy to Follow   240
J.J. Seley

6.   DIABETES MANAGEMENT PEARLS

Case 65: Novel Combination Therapy for Type 2 Diabetes   244
D. White and S. Goldman

Case 66: Do Many People with Type 2 Diabetes *Really* Need Insulin? 247
S.S. Schwartz

Case 67: Glycemic Control in a Patient with Type 1 Diabetes and
Peritoneal Dialysis   250
N. Khir, S. Brietzke, and J.R. Sowers

Case 68: Insulin Allergy in an Insulin-Requiring Patient   253
N. Mathioudakis

Case 69: Use of 3-Day Continuous Glucose Monitoring to Investigate
Persistent Fasting Hyperglycemia in Type 2 Diabetes   257
M. Griffith and M. Korytkowski

Case 70: Insulin Injections: What You "See" May Not Be
What You Get   261
R.J. Rushakoff, M.M. Sullivan, A. Shah,
and H.W. MacMaster

Case 71: Prolonged Insulin-Free Management of Type 1 Diabetes   265
D. Castillo and J. Aloi

Case 72: **Delayed Response to NPH Insulin**   267
M.B. Davidson

Case 73: **Reversal of Type 2 Diabetes by Weight Loss Despite Presence of Macro- and Microvascular Complications**   271
C. Peters, S. Steven, and R. Taylor

Case 74: **Glycemic Control in Older Adults with Diabetes and Use of New SGLT2 Inhibitors**   275
C. Horney and J. Wallace

Case 75: **Blood Glucose Control of Patients with Hypertriglyceridemia**   278
H. Beck-Nielsen

Case 76: **No Effect of Gluten-Free Diet in Prevention of Autoimmune Type 1 Diabetes and Other Autoimmune Disorders in a Child with Celiac Disease**   281
S. Muntoni and M. Congia

Case 77: **What Does It Take to Keep Glucose Normal?**   284
L.S. Phillips

Case 78: **Psychosocial Stressors and Management in an Adolescent with Type 2 Diabetes**   290
R. Nandagopal and K.I. Rother

7.   THE LIMITING FACTOR: ISSUES IN HYPOGLYCEMIA
Case 79: **Suicide, Homicide, or Diabetes-Related Incident?**   293
J.N. Carter

Case 80: **The Case of an Older Woman with Diabetes on Insulin Pump Therapy, Struggling with Cognitive Decline, Hypoglycemia, and Loss of Autonomy**   296
J.M. Hackel, L. Douyon, and J.B. Halter

Case 81: **Somnambulism (Sleepwalking) Caused by Nocturnal Hypoglycemia**   301
D.S.H. Bell

Case 82: **Hypoglycemic Unawareness**   304
A. Maturu and N. Rasouli

Case 83: **Successful Use of Plasmapheresis in the Treatment of Hypoglycemia Due to Insulin Antibody Syndrome**   307
P. Sharda, T. Gopan, R. Zimmerman, and E.S. Siraj

Case 84: Postprandial Hypoglycemia, an Uncommon Presentation
of Type 2 Diabetes   311
M.W. Salam and J.R. Sowers

Case 85: Factitious Hypoglycemia in a Type 2 Diabetic Patient   314
S.A. Seggelke

Case 86: Recurrent Hypoglycemia in a Patient with
Type 2 Diabetes   317
P. Srimatkandada, M.E. McDonnell, and S. Ananthakrishnan

Case 87: Munchausen Syndrome: Hypoglycemia in an Obese
Woman with Type 2 Diabetes   321
R.P. Robertson

Case 88: The Use of Medical Technologies for the Reduction of
Hypoglycemia in Type 1 Diabetes: Technology for
Hypoglycemia Reduction   324
V.N. Shah, A.W. Michels, and S.K. Garg

Case 89: Reversal of Insulin-Requiring Type 2 Diabetes and
Development of Hypoglycemia in a Morbidly
Obese Patient   329
D.S.H. Bell

Case 90: Munchausen-by-Proxy: Hypoglycemia in an Islet
Autotransplantation Recipient   332
R.P. Robertson

Case 91: Treatment of a Patient with Diabetes and Severe
Hypoglycemia   335
H. Beck-Nielson

Case 92: Hypoglycemia with Use of Glargine Insulin in the
Management of Type 2 Diabetes, Occurring with
Titration Aimed at Achieving Prebreakfast Glucose
Levels <100 mg/dL (5.6 mmol/L)   339
S. Adeel and L.S. Phillips

Case 93: Progressive Hypoglycemia Due to Insulinoma in a
Patient with Type 2 Diabetes: Treatment with Image-Guided
Minimally Invasive Pancreas-Sparing Surgery   345
M.-E. Patti, M.P. Callery, R.M. Najarian, M.S. Sawhney,
L. Mitzner, A.B. Goldfine, and A.J. Moser

8. NEUROPATHY IN DIABETES

Case 94: Managing Pain and Paralysis in Chronic Inflammatory
Demyelinating Polyneuropathy in Diabetes   351
A.I. Vinik

Case 95: Neuropathy in Metformin-Treated Type 2 Diabetes   354
A.I. Vinik

Case 96: A Case of Acute Sensory Neuropathy in Type 1 Diabetes   357
A.J.M. Boulton

Case 97: Nondiabetic Neuropathy in a Patient with Type 2 Diabetes   361
D.S.H. Bell

Case 98: Severe Distal Symmetrical and Autonomic Neuropathy
in a Patient with a Short Duration of Type 1 Diabetes   364
D.S.H. Bell

Case 99: Diabetic Amyotrophy and Neuropathic Cachexia   367
D.S.H. Bell

Case 100: High GAD Antibody Levels and Cerebellar Atrophy in a
Patient with Type 1 Diabetes   369
D.S.H. Bell

9. DIABETES IN PREGNANCY AND REPRODUCTIVE ISSUES

Case 101: Resolution of Infertility with Diabetes Therapy   372
D.S.H. Bell

Case 102: The Initial Pregnancy Visit of a Woman with Type 1
Diabetes and Diabetes Complications   375
A. McElduff

Case 103: Gastroparesis and Pregnancy   378
C. Peters and R. Taylor

Index   383

Preface

Medicine is said to exemplify a wholesome mixture of art and science through which scientific knowledge and discovery create a foundation for the art of deduction and application to arrive at the correct diagnosis and to select appropriate therapy.

Although the science is universal and the knowledge base is assumed to be similar, the art of practicing medicine is frequently different among practitioners. Thus, learning from many masters becomes an essential component of clinical and bedside education for younger clinicians. Furthermore, lifelong learning is a quintessential quality of excellent clinical skills. Knowing how our esteemed colleagues approach difficult cases as well as diagnostic and therapeutic dilemmas is a vital element of learning.

This is why we believe it is so important to present the original voices of leading diabetologists discussing their most challenging cases and explaining the underlying principles they use to solve diagnostic and therapeutic puzzles.

The cases presented in this volume do this by allowing each author or group of authors to demonstrate their own art of reasoning and their own style of problem solving. We sincerely hope this compilation of distinct voices adds value to the reader's learning. Like students of classical art who spend countless hours copying works of distinguished masters, we hope our readers will adopt the logic of distinguished diabetologists and use it to guide them while solving their own challenging cases that might resemble the ones presented in this anthology.

The authors and the editors are eager to present these challenging cases to the readers. If indeed our readers find these cases and discussions helpful to their practice, we will be deeply gratified.

Boris Draznin, MD, PhD, Editor
Director, Adult Diabetes Program
Division of Endocrinology, Metabolism, and Diabetes
University of Colorado Denver, School of Medicine

Cecilia C. Low Wang, MD, FACP, Associate Editor
Associate Professor of Medicine
Department of Medicine, University of Colorado
Anschutz Medical Campus/School of Medicine

Daniel J. Rubin, MD, MSc, FACE, Associate Editor
Assistant Professor of Medicine, Division of Endocrinology
Temple University School of Medicine

Introduction

Diabetes is an umbrella term for a heterogeneous group of disorders that meet a single criterion for diagnosis: hyperglycemia. The etiologic classification of diabetes ranges from the most commonly encountered, type 2 diabetes, to the less common, including maturity-onset diabetes of the young, and everything in between. Although type 2 diabetes makes up a significant proportion of all patients with diabetes, classifying a particular patient's disease accurately may be problematic; occasionally, even differentiating between type 1 and type 2 diabetes can present a challenge. Diabetes may come to clinical attention in conjunction with diseases of the exocrine pancreas, such as cystic fibrosis or hemochromatosis; in association with drugs or chemicals. such as glucocorticoids or phenytoin; other endocrinopathies, such as acromegaly or pheochromocytoma; uncommon forms of immune-mediated diabetes, such as Stiff-Person Syndrome; or genetic defects of insulin action, such as Leprechaunism.

Not uncommonly, the interpretation of hemoglobin A1C results can be affected by a number of factors, presenting a clinical dilemma to a practitioner, even though the diagnosis of diabetes itself may not often present a significant challenge.

Furthermore, the clinical presentations and complexities of diabetes management often present difficulties to the practicing clinician. The safe and effective use of insulin and other agents to lower glucose may require "thinking-outside-of-the-box" even for experienced clinicians. In addition, there is a rapidly growing array of medications available for treating diabetes. Additional considerations include the limitation to management by hypoglycemia, complications such as chronic kidney disease, and comorbidities such as obesity with concomitant worsening of insulin resistance. These are just a few of the factors that require a thoughtful approach to the management of individual patients. Patients with recurrent diabetic ketoacidosis or hyperglycemic hyperosmolar syndrome, ketosis-prone diabetes, and severe insulin resistance continue to challenge our clinical abilities.

Diabetes in the hospital setting presents a unique set of intricacies, including renal failure and dialysis, need for enteral or parenteral nutrition, severe burns or trauma, organ transplantation, and surgery. Transitions within and between the hospital and outpatient settings often raise the risk of worsening clinical outcomes resulting from gaps and miscommunications in management.

Last, the use of technology has improved the lives of many people living with diabetes, but the practical and effective use of continuous subcutaneous insulin infusions (insulin pumps) and continuous glucose monitors requires significant training, education, and ability to troubleshoot and sometimes to generate creative solutions to manage diabetes optimally in an individual patient.

One of the best ways to learn about these numerous complex issues related to diabetes diagnosis, classification, and management, is by pooling together the expertise of clinicians taking care of patients with diabetes, and by exploring these topics through case presentations and discussions. The aim of this casebook, *Diabetes Case Studies: Real Problems, Practical Solutions*, is to do exactly that. This casebook includes contributions from many leading diabetologists from around the world who take care of patients with diabetes and, through deliberate practice, have compiled their thoughts and insights from their experience and inquiry into the specific topics discussed. We have tried to maintain the individual "voices" of the contributing authors as much as possible. We felt this was important to preserve the integrity of their contributions while upholding a high standard for each case presentation and discussion.

This book is divided into nine sections detailed as follows:

1. Cases 1–23: Diagnostic Dilemmas and Problems with Classification
2. Cases 24–27: HbA$_{1c}$ Dilemmas
3. Cases 28–36: More Insulin Is Not Always the Solution: Cases of Severe Insulin Resistance
4. Cases 37–52: Unusual Forms and Presentations of Diabetes
5. Cases 53–64: Diabetes in the Hospital Setting
6. Cases 65–78: Diabetes Management Pearls
7. Cases 79–93: The Limiting Factor: Issues in Hypoglycemia
8. Cases 94–100: Neuropathy in Diabetes
9. Cases 101–103: Diabetes in Pregnancy and Reproductive Issues

We hope the reader with a specific clinical question in mind will use this list of topics or the index to go straight to the cases that will be most likely to address his or her clinical question. If the reader has a few spare minutes and would like to learn something surprising or new, flipping to any page and perusing a few cases may open a world of complex and intriguing cases with clinical reasoning outlined and discussed by "master clinicians" from many parts of the world. If the reader has more time and does not have a specific clinical question, he or she might consider taking the time to browse through this book, and even read a few sections, to gain insight into the art of clinical deduction from the leading diabetologists who submitted their challenging cases to this anthology. We hope that the reader will find this to be a useful collection of clinical cases and gain as much from reading and using it as we have from assembling and editing it.

Finally, for additional information, the reader is referred to the *American Diabetes Association Standards of Medical Care in Diabetes*, which are updated yearly and provide a comprehensive resource for many diabetes-related questions.

Case 1

Maturity-Onset Diabetes of the Young (MODY) as a Diagnostic Possibility

Suzi Kochar, MD,[1,2] and Janice L. Gilden, MS, MD, FCP, FACE[1,2]

A 19-year-old man (mother: African American; father: Caucasian) was referred for evaluation of incidentally elevated A1C (HbA$_{1c}$ = 8.3%; normal: 4.0–6.0) and fasting blood glucose (FBG = 172 mg/dL; 9.5 mmol/L). He denied symptoms of hyperglycemia or complications suggestive of diabetes.

Past medical history is unremarkable, including no use of tobacco, alcohol, or recreational drugs. Previous blood glucose tests completed last year reportedly were normal.

His father is thin, was diagnosed with diabetes at age 17 years, has been taking a single oral antihyperglycemic tablet (unknown name), and is thought to maintain good control without complications of diabetes; maternal grandmother has diabetes (therapy unknown). There is no family history of obesity.

Physical examination was normal without acanthosis nigricans, skin tags, xanthomata, abdominal striae, muscle wasting, or peripheral neuropathy. BMI was 19.3 kg/m².

Results of prior laboratory testing were as follows:

Urine ketones	negative
Thyroid-stimulating hormone (TSH)	1.14 µIU/mL (0.34–4.82)
Alanine aminotransferase (ALT)	16 units/L (10–65)
Alkaline phosphatase	114 units/L (50–136)
Sickledex	negative
Glucose-6-phosphate dehydrogenase (G6PD)	normal
Insulin antibody	<0.4 units/mL (0–1)
Fasting C-peptide	0.86 ng/mL (0.8–3.85)
Antinuclear antibody (ANA)	negative
Hemoglobin	15.2 g/dL

Repeat post-prandial blood glucose (BG) on the day of initial consultation was 201 mg/dL (11.1 mmol/L).

[1]Endocrinology Division, Department of Medicine, Rosalind Franklin University of Medicine and Science/Chicago Medical School, North Chicago, IL. [2]Endocrinology Section, Department of Medicine, Captain James A. Lovell Health Care Center, North Chicago, IL.

DOI: 10.2337/9781580405713.01

According to the American Diabetes Association, either HbA$_{1c}$ ≥6.5%, or FPG ≥126 mg/dL (7.0 mmol/L), or 2-h plasma glucose ≥200 mg/dL (11.1 mmol/L) during an oral glucose tolerance test, or a random plasma glucose ≥200 mg/dL (11.1 mmol/L) with classic symptoms is sufficient for a diagnosis of diabetes.[1] If a patient meets the criterion for HbA$_{1c}$ (two results ≥6.5%) but not FPG (<126 mg/dL or 7.0 mmol/L), or vice versa, that person should still be considered to have diabetes.[1]

The diagnosis of diabetes was made in our patient. The type of diabetes in this young patient was unclear, however. We ordered further testing, which included GAD antibody, anti-islet cell antibody (ICA), fasting insulin and C-peptide levels, TSH, and antithyroid antibodies. Zinc transporter antibodies were not available.

Diabetes can be divided into four clinical categories: *1)* type 1 diabetes (β-cell destruction, usually leading to absolute insulin deficiency); *2)* type 2 diabetes (progressive insulin secretory defects with insulin resistance); *3)* other types due to genetic defects in β-cell function, genetic defects in insulin action, diseases of the exocrine pancreas (e.g., cystic fibrosis), and drug- or chemical-induced diabetes; and *4)* gestational diabetes mellitus.[1]

Maturity-onset diabetes of the young (MODY) was considered due to the onset of non-obese diabetes occurring in both the patient and his father at a young age. It is also to be noted that his father has been controlled with one oral antihyperglycemic agent. MODY, a heterogeneous disorder, is characterized by diagnosis at a young age (<25 years of age), with autosomal dominant transmission, and lack of autoantibodies.[2] There was no evidence for hereditary hemochromatosis.

The patient returned to the clinic 2 weeks later. He remained asymptomatic and had not tested his blood glucose at home.
Laboratory tests from the first visit were as follows:

Glucose	154 mg/dL (8.5 mmol/L)
Fasting C-peptide	2.37 ng/mL (0.8–3.85)
Fasting insulin	18.90 mIU/L (0.0–24.9)

Antibodies were negative for ICA, GAD, thyroid, rheumatoid factor, and ANA. Hepatitis serology tests were negative, and the lipid profile was normal.

Studies report that only 6% of patients diagnosed with MODY are identified correctly by their providers. Most MODY patients are diagnosed as having type 1 diabetes (36%) or type 2 diabetes (51%). MODY, however, is responsible for 2.4% of diabetes in children younger than 15 years of age.[3,4]

MODY often presents without signs or symptoms of hyperglycemia and is diagnosed when a high glucose is discovered incidentally. Some forms of MODY, however, can cause significant hyperglycemia with typical symptoms.

MODY can result from mutations in one of at least six different genes that encode the glycolytic enzyme glucokinase (GCK) and five transcription factors: hepatocyte nuclear factor (HNF)-1α, HNF-1β, HNF-4α, insulin promoter factor-1, and neurogenic differentiation 1/β-cell E-box transactivator 2. These genes control pancreatic β-cell development, function, and regulation, and mutations can result in impaired glucose sensing and insulin secretion with minimal or no defect in insulin action.

Patients with HNF-1α- and HNF-4α-MODY usually present with signs and symptoms of hyperglycemia, including polyuria, polydipsia, and nocturia.[2] GCK-MODY often is diagnosed with incidental mild hyperglycemia.

Some members of families who have the genetic defect do not develop diabetes. Other patients can have classic MODY phenotypes without an identifiable mutation in MODY genes.

It is important to distinguish MODY from type 1 and type 2 diabetes because optimal treatment and risk for diabetes complications differ. Although sulfonylureas are usually effective for treatment of MODY type 1, 3, and 4, about 30% to 40% of patients need insulin therapy to control blood glucose. MODY type 2 can usually be managed by exercise and diet alone. In addition, distinguishing MODY from type 1 or type 2 diabetes allows earlier identification of at-risk family members.[5]

A random blood glucose of 423 mg/dL (23.4 mmol/L) was obtained on the day of the return outpatient visit. He was admitted to the hospital for management of hyperglycemia.

Blood tests obtained during hospital admission showed the following:

Fructosamine	458 μmol/L (normal = 190–270)
Iron	142 μg/dL (65–175)
Ferritin	207 ng/mL (26–388)
β-Hydroxybutyrate	0.06 mmol/L (≤0.28 or less)
Glucose	300 mg/dL (16.6 mmol/L)

There was no evidence of pancreatitis.

While in the hospital, he was started with 4 units glargine insulin at bedtime and low-dose short-acting aspart for correction. Mealtime insulin was not required. Upon discharge, FBG was 142 mg/dL (7.8 mmol/L).

The patient received intensive diabetic education. He was discharged with 4 units of glargine insulin at bedtime. Genetic testing and consideration of a later trial of sulfonylureas were recommended.

This case demonstrates a common dilemma encountered by many clinicians. The diagnosis of MODY or other genetic variants often is missed because of the lack of awareness by providers as well as the difficulty of obtaining genetic testing. It is important to make the correct diagnosis because of implications for treatment, chronic complications, and need for genetic counseling.

REFERENCES

1. Diagnosis and classification of diabetes mellitus. *Diabetes Care* 2014; 37(Suppl. 1):81–90

2. Stanescu DE, Hughes N, Kaplan B, Stanley CA, De León DD. Novel presentations of congenital hyperinsulinism due to mutations in the MODY genes: HNF1A and HNF4A. *J Clin Endocrin Metab* 2013;97(10):E2026–E2030

3. Shields BM, Hicks S, Shepherd MH, et al. Maturity-onset diabetes of the young (MODY): how many cases are we missing? *Diabetologia* 2010;53:2504–2508

4. Hattersley A, Bruining J, Shield J, Njolstad P, Donaghue KC. The diagnosis and management of monogenic diabetes in children and adolescents. *Pediatr Diabetes* 2009;10(Suppl. 12):33–42

5. Tattersall RB, Fajans SS. A difference between the inheritance of classical juvenile-onset and maturity-onset type diabetes of young people. *Diabetes* 1975;24:44–53

Case 2

Diagnosis of Coexistent Maturity-Onset Diabetes of the Young in a Patient with Type 1 Diabetes

Shazli Azmi, MBChB,[1,2] and Rayaz A. Malik, MBChB, PhD[1,2]

A 23-year-old Caucasian woman was seen in the diabetes clinic. She was diagnosed with type 1 diabetes (T1D) at the age of 11 years following a history of polyuria, polydipsia, lethargy, and dramatic weight loss. She was started on a multidose insulin injection (MDI) regime. Her glycemic control was generally poor and required hospitalization due to diabetic ketoacidosis at the age of 19 years.

When she initially attended our hospital clinic, her BMI was 23 kg/m^2, her blood pressure was 122/83 mmHg, and she had an HbA$_{1c}$ of 107 mmol (11.9%). She had no evidence of background retinopathy or microalbuminuria and minimal neuropathy.

There was a strong family history of diabetes, with her father, paternal grandmother, and great-grandmother all having diabetes. Her father was diagnosed as having T1D at the age of 43 years after checking his random blood glucose using his daughter's glucose meter. He initially was treated with metformin, but within 2 months, treatment failure with metformin lead to the diagnosis of T1D by his primary care doctor, and he was started on an MDI regime (total dose ~18 units daily) with which he maintained excellent glycemic control (HbA$_{1c}$ ~40–44 mmol/mol [5.8–6.2%]). At 50 years of age, however, he was referred to secondary care where he underwent genetic testing and was diagnosed with maturity-onset diabetes of the young (MODY) resulting from a hepatocyte nuclear factor-4-α (HNF4-α) mutation.

MODY is an autosomal-dominant inherited monogenic form of diabetes. In a recent study of 586 participants diagnosed with diabetes at the age of <20 years who were autoantibody negative and had a fasting C-peptide levels of 0.8 ng/mL, 47 (8%) had MODY.[1] Most patients with monogenic diabetes initially are diagnosed as having type 1 or 2 diabetes. It usually presents in patients <25 years old and is due to a single gene defect that affects insulin secretion. There are at least 12 identified monogenic defects.

Optimizing glycemic control in this patient was a challenge. In view of the family history of MODY and mode of inheritance, she underwent genetic testing.

[1]Institute of Human Development, Center for Endocrinology and Diabetes, University of Manchester. [2]Department of Medicine and Manchester Diabetes Center, University of Manchester and Central Manchester NHS Foundation Trust.

DOI: 10.2337/9781580405713.02

The International Society for Pediatric and Adolescent Diabetes (ISPAD) produced consensus guidelines for the diagnosis and management of monogenic diabetes in children.[2] The primary features to consider are as follows:

1. Diagnosis of diabetes before 6 months old.
2. Family history of diabetes with an affected parent.
3. Evidence of insulin production persisting after 3 years from the diagnosis of diabetes, with a detectable C-peptide (>2 nmol/L or 6 ng/mL) when glucose >8 mmol/L (144 mg/dL).
4. Absence of pancreatic islet autoantibodies.

She was found to be heterozygous for a missense mutation, R127W, in exon 4 of the HNF4-α gene due to a substitution of tryptophan for arginine at codon 127.

HNF4-α is also known as MODY1, being one of the first mutations to be identified, and accounts for 10% of MODY cases.[3] Diabetes is diagnosed in the late teens to early twenties when insulin production becomes insufficient and often is misdiagnosed as T1D. MODY1 responds well to sulphonylureas, which act by stimulating the pancreas to secrete insulin. There is a progressive decrease in insulin production, however, eventually necessitating insulin. In patients who are already on insulin, it may be possible to reduce or even stop insulin once sulphonylureas have been initiated. HNF4-α patients may develop vascular complications and may be associated with high serum lipids and metabolic syndrome, and therefore optimal glycemic control is very important.

She was found to be anti-GAD+ve (5.1 U) with weakly positive insulin autoantibody at 1/10 iU/mL antibodies and a C-peptide of 9.1 ng/mL. Therefore, she was diagnosed as having both T1D and MODY1. She was started on gliclazide 80 mg twice daily. She remained on the same daily dose of insulin (66 units per day) and developed episodes of hypoglycemia. Gliclazide was reduced to 80 mg daily, and her glycemic control improved but remained erratic.

In an attempt to promote insulin release in a more regulated manner, the sulphonylurea was switched to a dipeptidyl peptidase-4 (DPP-4) inhibitor (DPP4i), sitagliptin 100 mg daily, as it has a lower risk of hypoglycemia. With the introduction of sitagliptin, there was a reduction in the fluctuations in blood glucose level and fewer hypoglycemic episodes. She was able to decrease the total daily insulin dose to 45 units and her HbA$_{1c}$ improved to 76 mmol/L (9.1%).

The cautionary note of this case is that one should always exclude T1D when diagnosing MODY, as the withdrawal of insulin could have had catastrophic effects in the form of diabetic ketoacidosis.

Making the diagnosis of MODY in a patient with apparent T1D is potentially life changing as one can withdraw insulin therapy safely. It has an impact on relatives as once a mutation in a family is identified, it will allow correct diagnosis in other family members (50% chance that first-degree relatives also will have MODY). There has been one previous report of a patient with coexistent T1D (with positive islet cell autoantibodies) and MODY3 (mutation of HNF1-α).[4] The absence of autoantibodies is a reason to test for MODY as the presence of anti-GAD and insulinoma-associated protein 2 autoantibodies is <1% in MODY.[5] Genetic testing for MODY is expensive, and careful selection of patients to be tested is paramount. Equally important, however, a strong clinical suspicion of MODY and appropriate genetic testing can be life changing.

This case highlights two clinically important issues:

- The necessity of testing patients who are known to have a mutation in the family.
- The importance of excluding T1D, particularly as this patient had a history of ketoacidosis, which does not occur in patients with MODY.

Coexistence of MODY and T1D may be a reason why this patient presented with diabetes early and, despite high doses of insulin, she had erratic and overall poor glycemic control. Given that she has had T1D for 12 years, it is unusual that she has residual β-cell function. Nevertheless, the introduction of DPP4i has reduced her overall requirement of insulin and markedly has improved her glycemic control.

REFERENCES

1. Pihoker C, et al. Prevalence, characteristics and clinical diagnosis of maturity onset diabetes of the young due to mutations in HNF1A, HNF4A, and glucokinase: results from the SEARCH for Diabetes in Youth. J *Clin Endocrinol Metab* 2013;98(10):4055–4062

2. Hattersley A, et al. ISPAD Clinical Practice Consensus Guidelines 2006–2007: the diagnosis and management of monogenic diabetes in children. Pediatr *Diabetes* 2006;7(6): 352–360

3. Shields B, et al. Maturity-onset diabetes of the young (MODY): how many cases are we missing? *Diabetologia* 2010;53(12):2504–2508

4. Bowden SA, Hoffman RP. Triple diabetes: coexistence of type 1 diabetes mellitus and a novel mutation in the gene responsible for MODY3 in an overweight adolescent. *Pediatr Diabetes* 2008;9(2):162–164

5. McDonald TJ, et al. Islet autoantibodies can discriminate maturity-onset diabetes of the young (MODY) from type 1 diabetes. *Diabetic Med* 2011; 28(9):1028–1033

Case 3

An Unusual Clinical Presentation of Diabetes Eventually Diagnosed as a Monogenic Form

VINCE N. MONTES, MD;[1] ALAN CHAIT, MD;[1] AND CRAIG E. TAPLIN, MD[2]

A 31-year-old man of Eastern European decent was evaluated in the endocrinology clinic for suspected type 2 diabetes. He initially presented to an outside clinic 2 years previously with dizziness and was found to have a blood glucose concentration of nearly 400 mg/dL. He apparently did not appear very ill at the time and was sent home with a prescription for pioglitazone with plans for outpatient follow-up. He took the pioglitazone for approximately 6 months and had little success with attaining satisfactory glycemic control. His primary care physician subsequently discontinued the pioglitazone and placed the patient on metformin 1,000 mg twice daily and glipizide 2.5 mg daily. Glycemic control improved with normalized fasting blood glucose levels and HbA$_{1c}$ levels in the 6.2–6.5% range. During the course of his improvement, the patient presented with changes in his vision and was diagnosed with proliferative diabetic retinopathy and vitreous hemorrhage. The patient also had neurologic symptoms that were consistent with peripheral neuropathy, which subsequently improved with the addition of gabapentin.

Interestingly, his family history was significant for diabetes in his mother, who died at 37 years of age secondary to renal failure. He also had a maternal aunt with diabetes, but his four sisters were not known to have diabetes. He has two children, one of which recently was noted to have symptoms of increased thirst and intermittent headaches.

The patient is a lean male who was losing weight prior to the original diagnosis, gained weight on pioglitazone, and stabilized once it was discontinued and he started the glipizide and metformin. On examination in our clinic, he did not have acanthosis nigricans. Laboratory investigation showed negative GAD65 antibodies.

Here we describe a patient with diabetes who does not fit with a classical presentation of either type 1 or type 2 diabetes. He is a thin and young male with diabetic complications, which may be consistent with type 1 diabetes. He has achieved good glycemic control without insulin, however, and did not present with ketoacidosis. He responded well to a combination regimen of

[1]University of Washington, Division of Metabolism, Endocrinology, and Nutrition, Seattle, WA. [2]Department of Pediatrics, University of Washington, Seattle Children's Hospital, Division of Endocrinology and Diabetes, Seattle, WA.

DOI: 10.2337/9781580405713.03

oral sulfonylurea with metformin, but he did not have physical signs of insulin resistance to suggest type 2 diabetes, such as obesity or acanthosis nigricans. He also had negative GAD65 antibodies, which usually are associated with type 1 diabetes and latent autoimmune diabetes of adults (LADA). All of these factors led us to believe that he may have an unusual, monogenic form of diabetes. His family history suggests this as well, given that his mother had significant disease with renal complications.

Around the same time as the patient was being diagnosed and treated, the patient's 8-year-old daughter was referred to the pediatric endocrinology clinic with occasional intermittent headaches and occasional increased thirst, but no persistent polyuria or polydipsia. There was no nocturnal enuresis or unintentional weight loss, abdominal pain, or fruity breath; however, because of the family history of diabetes, further investigation was initiated. Her laboratory testing showed the following:

Random glucose	85 mg/dL
HbA$_{1c}$	6.3% (reference range 4–6%)
Insulin	negative
GAD65	negative
ICA512	negative
ZnT8	negative
Random C-peptide	0.9 ng/mL (reference range 1.0–5.5)

A urinalysis showed glycosuria but no ketonuria. On examination, she was lean with no acanthosis nigricans. A repeat HbA$_{1c}$ in clinic was 5.9%. The family history, evidence of mild hyperglycemia (inferred from A1C), and negative diabetes autoantibodies prompted genetic testing to search for a monogenic cause of diabetes. She was found to be heterozygous for a novel frameshift mutation, c.768delC in the *Hnf1a* gene, an alteration not previously reported in the literature.

Monogenic diabetes can include the originally proclaimed maturity-onset diabetes of the young (MODY) and a maternally inherited diabetes and deafness syndrome. The latter usually includes a personal and family history of deafness, which was not the case here. The former group of diseases include genetic abnormalities in key genes that can cause diabetes associated with non-insulin-dependent diabetes diagnosed at a young age with autosomal-dominant transmission and lack of diabetes autoantibodies.[1] The responsible genetic abnormality identifies the type of disease and results in the different subtypes of MODY (Table 3.1). A defect in hepatocyte nuclear factor-1-α (HNF1-α), formerly called MODY3, is the most common type of MODY, occurring in 52% of MODY patients.[2] It is more common in European patients. The defect results in abnormal insulin secretion, which is improved with oral sulfonylurea treatment.[3] These patients are at great risk for the development of microvascular and macrovascular complications of diabetes.[4] The disease also is characterized by a low renal threshold for glucose, and detection of glycosuria can be used to screen for carriers that do not yet have hyperglycemia, as in the case of the daughter in this report.

Table 3.1 — Different Subtypes of MODY

MODY type	Genetic defect
1	Hepatocyte nuclear factor-4-α
2	Glucokinase gene
3	Hepatocyte nuclear factor-1-α
4	Insulin promoter factor 1
5	Hepatocyte nuclear factor-1-β
6	Neurogenic differentiation factor-1

Because of the clinical presentations of both the father and the daughter, they were highly suspected of having a mutation in HNF1-α. Interestingly, the daughter had her genetic testing first and was found to have a frame-shift mutation in HNF1-α not previously reported. The father subsequently underwent genetic testing and was found to have the same mutation, confirming the diagnosis of HNF1-α diabetes. We are providing the first report of this specific mutation leading to monogenic diabetes of the HNF1-α type.

The treatment regimen for the father includes continuation of the oral sulfonylurea. The metformin has been discontinued. The patient continues to have excellent glycemic control on the oral sulfonylurea alone. The daughter and family were taught to check her blood glucose levels before meals and at bedtime. Fasting glucose levels have remained <100 mg/dL, and postprandial glucose levels are 140–160 mg/dL 7 months after the genetic diagnosis was confirmed. She is not currently on any therapy, but she continues to follow up in the pediatric endocrinology clinic.

The natural progression of HNF1-α diabetes is increasingly worsened glycemic control with progression to insulin dependence.[5] Tight glycemic control and aggressive control of other risk factors are warranted.

REFERENCES

1. Tattersall RB, Fajans SS. A difference between the inheritance of classical juvenile-onset and maturity-onset type diabetes of young people. *Diabetes* 1975;24:44–53

2. Shields BM, Hicks S, Shepherd MH, Colclough K, Hattersley AT, Ellard S. Maturity-onset diabetes of the young (MODY): how many cases are we missing? *Diabetologia* 2010;53:2504–2508

3. Pearson ER, Starkey BJ, Powell RJ, Gribble FM, Clark PM, Hattersley AT. Genetic cause of hyperglycaemia and response to treatment in diabetes. *Lancet* 2003;362:1275–1281

4. Murphy R, Ellard S, Hattersley AT. Clinical implications of a molecular genetic classification of monogenic beta-cell diabetes. *Nat Clin Pract Endocrinol Metab* 2008;4:200–213

5. Fajans SS, Bell GI, Polonsky KS. Molecular mechanisms and clinical pathophysiology of maturity-onset diabetes of the young. *N Engl J Med* 2001;345:971–980

Case 4

A Case of Monogenic Diabetes

Robert H. Slover, MD[1]

This patient presented as a 13-year 10-month-old boy with episodes of hyperglycemia. Several weeks before the visit, he developed symptoms of fatigue, light-headedness, and headaches. His primary care provider (PCP) noted that he had had mononucleosis a year previously and suspected that he might have a recurrence of this disorder. Because his father has a history of diabetes, the PCP checked urine for glucose and found it to be markedly elevated (>1,000 mg/dL). He asked the parents to perform self-monitoring of blood glucose using the father's meter. The family reported fasting glucose levels as high as 170 mg/dL (9.4 mmol/L) with an average of about 137 mg/dL (7.6 mmol/L). The patient had an initial hemoglobin A1C of 8.4%.

He returned to his PCP a week later and had nonfasting blood glucose of 108 mg/dL (6 mmol/L) and no glycosuria. He was then referred to the Barbara Davis Center for Childhood Diabetes for further evaluation.

Significantly, this patient had decided 2 years previously to increase his exercise and change to healthier eating patterns, and he had lost weight. BMI at our visit was 22.5 kg/m². His past history was significant for bilateral myringotomies and motor delay treated with physical therapy and exercise. He also had occupational therapy earlier in childhood to improve fine motor skills. He is in seventh grade and is a good student. A physically active boy, he is involved in football, swimming, running, biking, and trampoline.

The patient's family history is strongly positive for diabetes. The patient's father developed diabetes in his early 20s, but he never required insulin and controls his glucose levels with diet and exercise. The paternal grandfather also had diabetes and did not require insulin. Likewise, a paternal great-grandfather, great uncle, and great aunt also had non-insulin-requiring diabetes. The patient's grandfather died at the age of 44 years, apparently of non-diabetes-related causes, and the other affected family members lived into their 80s. There is no history of diabetes in the mother's family.

On physical examination, he was at the 91st percentile in height and the 93rd percentile in weight with BMI at the 86th percentile (22.72 kg/m²). Vital signs were normal, and physical examination was unremarkable. Patient is Tanner Stage V.

[1]Professor of Pediatrics, University of Colorado School of Medicine, Denver, CO; Director of Pediatrics, Barbara Davis Center for Childhood Diabetes; Wagner Family Chair in Childhood Diabetes.

     DOI: 10.2337/9781580405713.04

Initial laboratory evaluation revealed the following:

Micro-insulin autoantibody (mIAA)	–0.003
GAD	0
Insulinoma-associated protein 2 (IA2)	0
ZnT8RW	–0.001

(All four markers for type 1 diabetes are negative)

IGA transglutaminase	–0.003 (negative)
21 Hydroxylase antibody	0.031 (negative)
C-peptide	5.4 ng/dL (upper normal range)

The patient has a remarkably strong family history and appears to represent the fourth generation of noninsulin diabetes in his family. His father has always been told that he has type 2 diabetes, but he developed his diabetes early in his adult life despite being slim and fit and did not require oral therapy. None of the family members have been tested for monogenic diabetes, although the family history is strongly suggestive of this diagnosis, rather than type 1 or type 2 diabetes. The patient himself presented serendipitously and has no immune markers for type 1 diabetes. He also has a high C-peptide, suggesting robust insulin production.

We have enrolled him in an ongoing monogenic diabetes study.[1] Through participation in that study, he will receive genetic testing for all forms of maturity-onset diabetes of the young (MODY). The father and other family members also will be enrolled.

MODY3 (hepatocyte nuclear factor [HNF-1-α]) is the most common of the forms of MODY, accounting for some 50–55% of MODY cases, with glucokinase deficiency (MODY2) accounting for another 20–25%. MODY 3 often can be treated successfully with diet alone, and MODY2 can be treated with sulfonylureas.[2]

We recommended a sensible diet and exercise with no other medical therapy pending the results of genetic testing. Other family members have not needed sulfonylureas, so MODY3 seems the most likely diagnosis.[3]
The patient has sent glucose readings and a diet history. In the past 3 weeks, his mean fasting glucose has been 139.5 mg/dL (7.7 mmol/L), and mean postprandial glucose has been 157 mg/dL (8.7 mmol/L), with only one value >200 mg/dL (11.1 mmol/L). Diet history documents a healthy diet, but not elimination of all simple sugars, and certainly not a low carbohydrate diet.

This monogenic diabetes is likely to be more common than has been believed, accounting for as much as 1% of young people with diabetes. Unfortunately genetic testing is costly and poorly covered by insurance. In this family, however, we may be able to provide a diagnosis not only for this young teen but also for his father and other affected family members.

REFERENCES

1. Steck AK, Winter WE. Review on monogenic diabetes. *Curr Op Endocrinol, Diabetes, Ob* 2011;18(4):252–258

2. Hattersley A, Bruining J, Njolstad P, Donaghue KC. The diagnosis and management of monogenic diabetes in children and adolescents. *Pediatr Diabetes* 2009:10 (Suppl. 12):33–42

3. Fajans SS, Bell GI. MODY: history, genetics, pathophysiology, and clinical decision making. *Diabetes Care* 2011;34:1878–1884

Case 5

Recurrent Ketoacidosis: Lessons from Multiple Clinical Presentations

Eli Ipp, MD,[1] and Kristina Djekic, MS[1]

PHASE 1

A 33-year-old Mexican American man presents to the emergency department (ED) with a history of nausea, abdominal pain, and weakness. Four months prior he was diagnosed with diabetes after complaints of polyuria, polydipsia, and anorexia. He was treated with glyburide but continued to experience symptoms. He reported a cumulative weight loss of 40 lb in the intervening months and arrived in the ED weighing 69.8 kg, with a BMI of 25 kg/m². He is admitted to the hospital with a diagnosis of ketoacidosis. Laboratory evaluation revealed the following:

Presenting glucose	444 mg/dL (24.7 mmol/L)
β-hydroxybutyrate	10.1 mmol/L
Anion gap	21 mEq/L
Serum bicarbonate	7 mEq/L (see Table 5.1)
HbA$_{1c}$	17.9%

This patient presents with typical features of the onset of type 1 diabetes in a young, lean male. Oral agents fail, he is in poor glycemic control, and after significant weight loss, he presents to the hospital with ketoacidosis. Marked ketosis and severe acidosis signal severe β-cell failure, confirmed by almost unmeasurable plasma C-peptide concentrations (0.03 pmol/mL is the lower limit of measurement in this assay). The patient was discharged with a diagnosis of type 1 diabetes.

Most ketoacidosis seen today in the United States is of a mild to moderate severity, whether it occurs in type 1 or type 2 diabetes.[1] With improvements in health care and access, it is unusual to see severe ketoacidosis unless diabetes is unrecognized or the patient has a functional barrier to health care access, such as inability to communicate or altered mental status that may be unrelated to diabetes. So in a young, lean patient with evidence of a significant catabolic state (>20% unexplained weight loss), marked ketonemia, acidosis, and severe β-cell failure, all of this adds up to typical metabolic decompensation in

---

[1]Division of Endocrinology, Los Angeles Biomedical Research Institute at Harbor–UCLA Medical Center, Los Angeles, CA.

DOI: 10.2337/9781580405713.05

15

Table 5.1—First Admission

Data on presentation to hospital	Value	After recovery from ketoacidosis	Value
Glucose (mg/dL)	444	Weight (kg)	69.8
BOH (mmol/L)	10.1	BMI (kg/m²)	25.0
Anion Gap (mEq/L)	21	Glucose day 2 (mg/dL)	116
Na⁺ (mEq/L)	126	C-peptide day 2 (pmol/mL)	0.04
K⁺ (mEq/L)	4.0	Glucose day 5 (mg/dL)	188
CO_2 (mEq/L)	7	C-peptide day 5 (pmol/mL)	0.07
Cl⁻ (mEq/L)	98	Total cholesterol (mg/dL)	150
BUN (mg/dL)	13	Triglycerides (mg/dL)	307
Creatinine (mg/dL)	1.3	HDL (mg/dL)	25
HbA$_{1c}$ (%)	17.9	LDL (mg/dL)	64

a patient with type 1 diabetes. Because he was diagnosed after the age of 30 and had been off insulin for close to 6 months, a diagnosis of latent autoimmune diabetes of adults (LADA) also could be considered.[2,3]

PHASE 2

Now 34 years old, he presents again to the ED about 1 year after the original diagnosis of diabetes, with polyuria, polydipsia, blurred vision, and dizziness on standing. He reports taking insulin after discharge from the hospital until it ran out 3 months ago when he was on a visit to Mexico. Again he lost weight. On arrival, he now weighs 84 kg and has a BMI of 29.9 kg/m². In the ED, he is once again found to be in ketoacidosis and he is admitted. Metabolic decompensation on this occasion is milder than on the first admission. The serum glucose, β-hydroxybutyrate, and anion gap were not as high, and bicarbonate not as low as before (see Table 5.2).

This patient now presents with a clinical picture quite similar to his previous presentation, precipitated by failure to use insulin. Management was similar to the first admission, and again he was discharged on insulin. But the similarity ends there. Diabetes management should be individualized and that first requires accurate characterization of diabetes.

Yes, this could be a young, nonadherent patient with type 1 diabetes who presented with yet another bout of ketoacidosis. A closer look, however, tells a different story in this patient. First, he presented heavier, with a BMI of almost 30 kg/m². That is surely not unusual in patients with type 1 diabetes, where insulin treatment often is associated with weight gain. But it's more than his weight that is different about this presentation. He also was found to have other unusual features for a patient with type 1 diabetes.

Table 5.2—Second Admission

Data on presentation to hospital	Value
Weight (kg)	84.0
BMI (kg/m²)	29.9
Presenting glucose (mg/dL)	399
BOH (mmol/L)	5.0
Anion Gap (mEq/L)	16
Na⁺ (mEq/L)	129
K⁺ (mEq/L)	5.1
CO_2 (mEq/L)	14
Cl⁻ (mEq/L)	99
BUN (mg/dL)	15
Creatinine (mg/dL)	1.2
After recovery from ketoacidosis	**Value**
Fasting glucose (mg/dL)	120
Fasting C-peptide (pmol/mL)	0.1

He had been off insulin for 3 months. It is unlikely that this is attributed to a honeymoon phase of type 1 diabetes. Insulin independence or decreased requirements are not seen this late in the course of the disease (late year 1/early year 2, after diagnosis). Indeed, this prolonged insulin-free period suggests that the patient must have regained β-cell reserves to keep him out of ketoacidosis for 3 months. C-peptide concentrations during the second admission confirm more β-cell reserve, 2.5-fold higher than on the first admission (although still relatively low), and, though low, are within a range seen in patients with type 2 diabetes who develop ketoacidosis (ketosis-prone type 2 diabetes).[4] Another look at C-peptide in the first admission, where a second sample was obtained (though still suppressed), revealed a doubling of concentrations within a few days, unusual in type 1 diabetes.

Another feature, observable in the first admission, was low high-density lipoprotein (HDL) cholesterol, a finding that is unusual in patients with type 1 diabetes, who on average have higher than normal HDL cholesterol concentrations. On the other hand, low HDL is common in patients with type 2 diabetes, consistent with the metabolic syndrome phenotype seen in the latter.

Thus, after the second admission, this patient is looking less like a patient with type 1 diabetes or LADA, although the latter could explain the later age of onset and insulin independence.[3] In our experience, the clinical phenotype of LADA resembles that of type 1 diabetes in a member of a minority population. The BMI, HDL, and C-peptide in this patient would not be consistent with a diagnosis of autoimmune diabetes.[4]

PHASE 3

Now 46 years old, the patient presents to the ED about 13 years after original diagnosis of diabetes with a nonhealing foot wound after a traumatic work accident 3 weeks prior. The patient is still using insulin for treatment of his diabetes. He has a blood pressure of 165/106 mmHg.

Although limited follow-up data are available, combining findings between three visits for which we have records, we see that the patient satisfies requirements for metabolic syndrome: he is overweight, has hypertension, consistently low HDL cholesterol, hypertriglyceridemia, and hyperglycemia. This is consistent with an underlying etiology of type 2 diabetes, in this case more specifically ketosis-prone diabetes (KPD-2). KPD-2 explains his original presentation. In many younger patients ketoacidosis is characteristic of the first presentation and is not a manifestation of long-standing burned out diabetes.[4,5]

Finally, if possible, we would test for anti-GAD antibodies to confirm our clinical suspicion that this is not autoimmune diabetes, and we would measure C-peptide again. A diagnosis of type 2 diabetes, if accompanied by adequate β-cell reserve might earn him a trial of oral anti-hyperglycemic agents. A diagnosis of type 2 diabetes also merits all of the attention that these patients need for concomitant disorders.

REFERENCES

1. Ipp E, Huang C. Diabetes mellitus and the critically ill patient. In *Current Diagnosis and Treatment in Critical Care, 3rd edition*. Bongard F, Sue D, Vintch J, Eds. New York, Appleton and Lange, 2008

2. Djekic K, Mouzeyan A, Ipp E. Latent autoimmune diabetes of adults is phenotypically similar to type 1 diabetes in a minority population. *J Clin Endocrin Metab* 2012;97(3):E409–413

3. Hawa M, et al. Adult-onset autoimmune diabetes in Europe is prevalent with a broad clinical phenotype: action LADA 7. *Diabetes Care* 2013;36:908–913

4. Linfoot P, Bergstrom C, Ipp E. Pathophysiology of ketoacidosis in type 2 diabetes mellitus. *Diabetic Med* 2005;22:1414–1419

5. Maldonado MR, Otiniano ME, Lee R, Rodriguez L, Balasubramanyam A. Characteristics of ketosis-prone diabetes in a multiethnic indigent community. *Ethn Dis* 2004;14:243–249

Case 6

Ketoacidosis in a Patient with Type 1 Diabetes on a Low-Calorie Meal Replacement Diet

KATY BROWN, DO,[1] AND DANIEL BESSESEN, MD[2]

A 30-year-old woman with type 1 diabetes (T1D) and a BMI of 31 kg/m² was told by her obstetrician that she was having trouble becoming pregnant because of her weight. To improve fertility, she enrolled in a medically supervised low-calorie diet (LCD) weight loss program. She managed her diabetes with an insulin pump and her HbA$_{1c}$ was 6.7%.

Obesity is one of the most common health problems encountered in medical practice, and although individuals with T1D typically have normal weight, given the high prevalence of obesity in the general population, it is becoming more common to encounter patients with T1D who are obese. Although lifestyle changes remain the treatment of choice for all obese patients, some obese individuals with T1D have been treated with LCDs[1] or even bariatric surgery.[2] Currently, it is not clear how best to manage insulin during a diet that is severely restricted in calories and carbohydrate.

The LCD delivered 1,000 kcals/day from five meal replacements (HMR, IHM San Diego CA) with each meal replacement containing 15 grams of protein (38% of calories), 24 grams of carbohydrate (60%), 1 gram of fat (2%), and 160 kcals. Because of the reduction in energy and carbohydrate intake, her insulin pump settings were prophylactically decreased. Basal rates were decreased by 30%, her carbohydrate-to-insulin (I:C) ratio was changed from 1:12 to 1:16, and her correction factor (CF) was changed from 1:10 to 1:60 with a target blood glucose (BG) of 120 mg/dL. For the first 11 days of the LCD, her BG levels were well controlled and she lost ~5 lb. By the 12th day, she began to experience postprandial low BG <70 mg/dL, so she stopped bolusing for most of her meals, especially before exercise.

Much of the rapid weight loss seen immediately following the introduction of a low-calorie or low-carbohydrate diet likely is due to depletion of body glycogen stores and loss of associated water. Although one might think that meal insulin simply would be reduced in proportion to the reduction in dietary carbohydrate, this patient's hypoglycemia on low doses of insulin demonstrate how a reduction in hepatic glycogen stores, which act as a buffer against

---

[1]Fellow in Endocrinology, University of Colorado, School of Medicine, Denver, CO.
[2]University of Colorado, School of Medicine, Chief of Endocrinology, Denver Health Medical Center, Denver, CO.

DOI: 10.2337/9781580405713.06

meal-to-meal changes in glucose levels, can alter meal insulin responses and overall insulin sensitivity.

The frequency of hypoglycemia diminished with these changes. However, during the third week of the diet, her BG rose to 200–300 mg/dL (11.1–16.6 mmol/L) with urinary ketones measuring small to moderate. Total weight loss at this time was 4.4% of her starting body weight. She increased her basal rates, kept her I:C ratio at 1:16, but tightened the CF to 1:40 with frequent corrections every 2–4 h. Despite these changes, she continued to have elevated BG >200 mg/dL (11.1 mmol/L) and mild-moderate urinary ketones.

Ketogenesis occurs when there is a relative or absolute deficiency of insulin, excessive counter-regulatory hormones, especially glucagon; and a source of substrate for ketogenesis, most often free fatty acids (FFA). Ketoacidosis (DKA) differs from ketogenesis in that the production of ketones overwhelms clearance. In type 1 diabetes, DKA most commonly occurs in newly diagnosed individuals, with states of illness (infection, myocardial infarction, trauma) or with nonadherence with insulin therapy.

Starvation ketosis occurs following dramatic reductions in dietary carbohydrate resulting in a marked fall in the insulin-to-glucagon ratio and increased rates of lipolysis. Starvation typically does not cause DKA because glucose levels are normal, and by the time ketogenesis occurs, peripheral utilization of ketones has increased through a process called ketoadaptation.[3] Ketosis also can be produced by ketogenic diets.[4] Moderate to severe starvation DKA has been reported in people consuming very low energy diets (<800 kcal) and very low carbohydrate diets with <50 g/day carbohydrate. Our patient was ingesting 120 g/day of carbohydrate and 1,000 kcals/day raising suspicion for starvation and very low carbohydrate DKA. Although DKA has been reported in a patient with type 1 diabetes and anorexia nervosa who was not eating,[5] to our knowledge, there have not been any reported cases of DKA in individuals with T1D on a LCD.

During the fourth week of the LCD, she awakened with a BG >300 mg/dL, nausea, weakness, and moderate urinary ketones. She changed her infusion site and filled the reservoir using a new vial of insulin. She then bolused >30 units of insulin over the course of 5 h without food intake and BG continued to rise into the 400s. She presented to the emergency department in DKA. Initial laboratory findings are shown in Table 6.1.

A key difference between physiological insulin secretion and insulin delivery in the treatment of T1D is the location of delivery. Normally insulin and glucagon are delivered directly into the portal vein, providing precise control of hepatic glucose metabolism. In the treatment of T1D, insulin is delivered to the periphery, resulting in overinsulinization of the periphery relative to the liver when compared with normal physiology. In addition, the suppression of glucagon that occurs following a meal appears to be insulin dependent. The close anatomic relationship between β and α-cells in the pancreatic islet fosters precise control of glucagon secretion. If insulin is delivered peripherally, this important insulin action is also disrupted. The result is a decrease in the

Table 6.1—Initial Laboratory Findings

Lab	Value	Reference range
Sodium	134	138–146 mmol/L
Potassium	5.2	3.5–4.9 mmol/L
Chloride	104	98–109 mmol/L
Bicarb	22	24–29 mmol/L
Blood urea nitrogen	17	8–26 mg/dL
Creatinine	1.0	0.6–1.3 mg/dL
Blood glucose	425 **High**	70–105 mg/dL
Anion gap	8	
Urinary albumin	>500 glucose, 80 ketones, mod. blood (–) nitrite, (–) leukocytes, WBC 0–5, RBC 0–5	
Venous blood gas	pH 7.295, pCO_2 46, pO_2 21, HCO_3 22.4	
White blood cells	10.4	4.0–11.1 10^9/L
% Neutrophils	76.4%	
Absolute neutrophils	8.8 **High**	1.8–6.6 10^9/L

insulin-to-glucagon ratio in the portal vein, which could favor both increased hepatic glucose production as well as ketogenesis when insulin doses fall during hypocaloric feeding. It may be that in this patient as insulin doses were reduced because of dietary carbohydrate-energy restriction, glucagon levels rose.

Intravenous (i.v.) fluids and 20 units of subcutaneous insulin were administered in the emergency department. Diagnostic studies did not reveal a precipitating cause for her DKA other than the LCD. She was discharged home and resumed her usual diet and insulin program. DKA did not recur.

The temporal association, lack of another precipitating cause, and resolution of her DKA following the resumption of her usual diet all argue for a causative role for the LCD in her DKA. If a person with T1D starts on a diet that is markedly restricted in calories and or carbohydrates, they should consider monitoring ketones. If ketones become positive, consideration should be given to increasing energy and carbohydrate intake modestly and accepting a more gradual weight loss.

REFERENCES

1. Musil F, Smahelová A, Bláha V, Hyšpler R, Tichá A, Lesná J, Zadák Z, Sobotka L. Effect of low calorie diet and controlled fasting on insulin sensitivity and

glucose metabolism in obese patients with type 1 diabetes mellitus. *Physiol Res* 2013;62(3):267–276

2. Chuang J, Zeller MH, Inge T, Crimmins N. Bariatric surgery for severe obesity in two adolescents with type 1 diabetes. *Pediatrics* 2013;132(4): e1031–e1034

3. Cahill GF Jr, Aoki TT. Alternate fuel utilization by brain. In *Cerebral Metabolism and Neural Function*. Passonneau et al., Eds. Williams & Wilkins, Baltimore, MD, 1980

4. Paoli A, Fubini A, Voleck JS, Grimaldi KA. Beyond weight loss: a review of the therapeutic uses of a very-low-carbohydrate (ketogenic) diets. *European J Clin Nutr* 2013;67:789–796

5. Espes, Engstrom, et al. Severe diabetic ketoacidosis in combination with starvation and anorexia nervosa at onset of type 1 diabetes: A case report. *Upsala J Med Sci* 2013;118:130–133

Case 7

Reevaluation after Ketoacidosis
Presentation

Paulina Cruz-Bravo, MD,[1] and Janet B. McGill, MD[1]

A 51-year-old man presented to the emergency department with plasma glucose of 1,170 mg/dl (65 mmol/L) and in ketoacidosis. He was treated with intravenous (i.v.) insulin and transferred to the intensive care unit. Review of systems revealed he had lost 45 lb within the month before his hospitalization because of a prolonged bout of gastroenteritis. Past medical history included hypertension and hyperlipidemia but no history of diabetes. He was discharged 5 days later on 90 units of insulin glargine daily and 25 units of insulin glulisine three times a day with meals.

Diabetic ketoacidosis (DKA) is one of the two most serious acute metabolic complications of diabetes. It is characterized by uncontrolled hyperglycemia, metabolic acidosis, and ketosis. Mortality in adults is <1% but can increase up to 5% in the elderly and patients with coexistent severe illnesses. DKA results from the combination of hyperglycemia, reduced effective insulin concentrations, and a concomitant increase in counter-regulatory hormones.

These processes lead to increased lipolysis and release of free fatty acids into the circulation with the subsequent unrestrained fatty acid oxidation in the liver to ketone bodies, resulting in ketonemia and acidosis.[1]

DKA traditionally has been considered a key clinical feature of type 1 diabetes. Even though onset of type 1 diabetes commonly occurs in childhood and adolescence, it can occur at any age.

Six months later, he presented to the Washington University Diabetes Center for follow-up. He had stopped using insulin glulisine because of hypoglycemia and sometimes skipped insulin glargine. Family history was negative for diabetes and was otherwise noncontributory. Physical exam was normal, with no evidence of acanthosis nigricans. BMI was 30 kg/m². His HbA$_{1c}$ was 4.9% and his meter showed an average glucose of 94 ± 22 mg/dL (5.2 ± 1.2 mmol/L).

Discontinuation of insulin in patients with a history of DKA has been increasingly observed, especially in adult African American and Hispanic individuals that present with unprovoked DKA. Even though their initial clinical

[1]Fellowship in Endocrinology, Diabetes and Metabolism, Division of Endocrinology, Metabolism and Lipid Research, Washington University School of Medicine, St. Louis, MO.

DOI: 10.2337/9781580405713.07

23

presentation was that of type 1 diabetes, these patients often require a short period of insulin therapy with eventual maintenance of glycemic control with only diet or oral antihyperglycemic agents. This variant has been referred in the literature as Flatbush diabetes, diabetes 1.5, idiopathic type 1 diabetes, atypical diabetes, and more recently ketosis-prone diabetes.[1,2]

Balasubramanyam et al. attempted to predict long-term β-cell function in this subset of patients in a cohort of 294 patients presenting with DKA. Preserved β-cell function was defined as a fasting C peptide >1 ng/mL or a peak C-peptide response >1.5 ng/mL after glucagon stimulation test. Those with preserved β-cell function and negative autoimmunity represented 74% of their cohort. These patients exhibited clinical characteristics of type 2 diabetes, were obese, had strong family history, and were newly diagnosed diabetes. β-Cell function was substantially further improved 6–12 months after the index DKA.[3]

Observational studies have reported that these patients can achieve near normoglycemia remission within 10 weeks and ~40% are free of insulin injections at 10 years.[2] The findings of a normal range HbA_{1c} level and significantly less insulin requirements are likely to represent a remarkable improvement in β-cell function. At this point, we are considering that our patient likely has ketosis-prone diabetes.

Further laboratory investigation showed a fasting C-peptide of 3.4 ng/mL. Anti-GAD65 antibody test was undetectable. Insulin glulisine was discontinued, and insulin glargine was reduced initially by 25%. It was further tapered and eventually discontinued within 2 months. Normoglycemia persisted.

Six weeks after discontinuation of insulin, our patient had a 75-g oral glucose tolerance test. The results were as follows:

Fasting glucose	**90 mg/dL (5 mmol/L)**
2 h glucose	**123 mg/dL (6.8 mmol/L)**

These values suggest his diabetes had resolved.[4] On further questioning, he remembered being diagnosed with an episode of acute viral bronchitis and prescribed a short course of high-dose steroids a few weeks before his hospitalization.

Steroid-induced hyperglycemia occurs virtually in all patients with known diabetes. Case-control studies, however, have shown the odds ratio of new-onset diabetes to be around 1.36 to 2.23. The total glucocorticoid dose and duration of therapy were strong predictors of diabetes induction. The predominant mechanism responsible for hyperglycemia is reduced insulin sensitivity both in the liver and skeletal muscle. Many patients exhibit 2 h postprandial glucose concentrations >200 mg/dL (11.1 mmol/L) in the setting of normal fasting glucose; therefore the diagnosis of glucocorticoid induced diabetes should not focus only on fasting glucose values.[5]

The presentation of DKA is rare in patients without a previous history of diabetes. It has been reported previously during pregnancy, when high-dose steroids are used in preterm labor. It also has been reported in the pediatric literature when high-dose steroids have been used for hematological malignancies and for acute rheumatic fever. The combination of a viral gastroenteritis and steroid use contributed to this patient's presentation in ketoacidosis. Often, there is not a precipitating event. Patients with type 2 diabetes who present in DKA should be reevaluated after recovery from the episode so that therapy can be tailored to their needs. The presence of C-peptide and absent antibodies suggested that insulin, or at least multiple daily injections, was not needed in this patient. Surprisingly, he did not have diabetes, and more surprising, he did not have severe hypoglycemia on a relatively high dose of insulin.

REFERENCES

1. Kitabchi AE, et al. Hyperglycemic crises in adult patients with diabetes. *Diabetes Care* 2009;32(7):1335–1343

2. Umpierrez GE. Ketosis-prone type 2 diabetes: time to revise the classification of diabetes. *Diabetes Care* 2006;29(12):2755–2757

3. Balasubramanyam A, et al. Accuracy and predictive value of classification schemes for ketosis-prone diabetes. *Diabetes Care* 2006;29(12):2575–2579

4. American Diabetes Association. Standards of medical care in diabetes—2014. *Diabetes Care* 2014;37(Suppl. 1):S14–80

5. Clore JN, Thurby-Hay L. Glucocorticoid-induced hyperglycemia. *Endocr Pract* 2009;15(5):469–474

Case 8

Metabolic Syndrome-Related Comorbidities Typical of Older Adulthood Complicate Diabetic Ketoacidosis in a Youth with Type 2 Diabetes

Kristen Nadeau, MD, MS[1]

A 13-year-old, obese boy initially presented with DKA and severe dehydration. He developed a sore throat 3 weeks prior to admission (PTA), which resolved without therapy. Concurrently, the family noted symptoms of polyuria and polydipsia, which did not remit. One week PTA, vomiting began, worsening 2 days PTA. On the day of admission, he was confused, sleepy, and complained of headache.

Past medical history was positive for sickle cell trait and obesity. At age 6 years, he weighed 39 kg and blood pressure (BP) was recorded as 150/80 mmHg and at 138/83 mmHg on repeat. He was seen by his primary care provider 4 months PTA at which time blood glucose (BG) was normal. Family history included type 2 diabetes in multiple relatives.

Upon arrival to an outside hospital, vital signs were as follows:

BP	122/84 mmHg
Pulse	140 bpm
Respiratory Rate	46 respirations per minute
Temperature	97°F
O$_2$ sat	100% on RA
Weight	113 kg
Height	6'1"
Body mass index	33 kg/m^2
Glasgow coma scale (GCS)	10

Exam was notable for signs of severe dehydration requiring multiple intravenous (i.v.) attempts. Neurologic exam was nonfocal, but he was extremely agitated, requiring four-point restraints for safety. Initial labs showed the following:

BG	>700 mg/dL
pH	unreadable
Na (sodium)	127 mEq/L
K (potassium)	6.3 mEq/L
Cl (chloride)	112 mEq/L
Blood urea nitrogen (BUN)	41 mg/dL

[1]University of Colorado Denver/Children's Hospital Colorado, Aurora, CO.

 DOI: 10.2337/9781580405713.08

White blood cells (WBC)	$14.1 \times 10^3/\mu L$
	(78% neutrophils,
	20% lymphocytes)
Hematocrit (Hct)	44.3%
Platelets	$275 \times 10^3/\mu L$
Urine	
Specific gravity (SG)	1.015
pH	5.0
Ketones	large
Glucose	large
Protein	30+
Blood	moderate

He received a liter of normal saline (NS) bolus and an insulin drip (0.03 units/kg/h). Repeat BG was unchanged and hypotension developed. He was given a 5-unit bolus, an increased insulin drip (0.09 units/kg/h), and a second NS liter bolus. Vitals improved, and he was transported to the Children's Hospital Colorado (CHC). En route, severe hypotension developed; therefore dopamine was begun, normalizing the BP.

Three and a half hours after presentation, he arrived at CHC emergency room pale, cold, and dry appearing, with capillary refill of 3 sec, minimal response to pain and GCS of 8. He was intubated and labs showed the following:

Arterial blood gas values:	
pH	6.98
pCO_2	25 mmHg
pO_2	49 mmHg
HCO_3	6 mEq/L
Base excess	24.7 mEq/L
BG	1,110 mg/dL
Na	136 mEq/L (152 mEq/L
	corrected for glucose)
K	5.5 mEq/L
Cl	96 mEq/L
CO_2	5 mEq/L
BUN	38 mg/dL
Creatinine (Cr)	3.5 mg/dL
Serum osmolarity	366 mEq/L
Urine	
SG	1.010
Glucose	>1,000 mg/dL
Ketones	15 (mg/dL)
Blood	moderate

Urine and blood cultures were drawn and a third NS liter bolus was given. A computed tomography (CT) scan of the head and a chest X-ray were read as normal.

An hour later, he was transferred to the pediatric ICU with the following labs:

pH	7.05
Na	146 mEq/L (162 mEq/L corrected for glucose)
K	6.3 mEq/L
BUN	41 mg/dL
Cr	3.5 mg/dL
BG	1,084 mg/dL
Ionized Ca	1.2 mmol/L
Magnesium	2.7 mg/dL
Phosphorous	7 mg/dL
Serum osmolarity	367 mOsm/kg H_2O

Additions to his treatment included fentanyl, midazolam, NS (210 cc/h), kayexalate, 500 cc 5% albumin, and cefotaxime. GCS gradually improved; he was extubated and dopamine was discontinued. At 10 h after presentation, he continued to appear combative and dehydrated, and hypernatremia persisted. Intravenous fluids were changed to 1/2 NS plus 20 mEq KCl and 20 mEq Kphos per liter (140 cc/h). At 15 h after presentation, the pH corrected to 7.4, but hyperosmolarity persisted.

Eighteen hours after presentation, hypotension reoccurred, accompanied by hyperthermia, desaturation, unresponsiveness, and a decline in pH to 7.22. He was reintubated and given fentanyl, midazolam, rocuronium, ranitidine, ibuprofen, acetaminophen, 500 cc NS, 500 cc 5% albumin, dopamine, epinephrine, and vancomycin. BP and perfusion improved. Labs were significant for a corrected Na of 167 mEq/L, K of 2.7 mEq/L, CO_2 of 10 mEq/L, BG of 381 mg/dL, and phosphorus of 0.5 mg/dL. Twenty-two hours after presentation, 250 cc of 25% mannitol was given for continued poor mental status. Shortly afterward, a 15-beat run of ventricular tachycardia was noted. Lidocaine was started and an echocardiogram showed a shortening fraction of 26% with reasonable volume. Central venous pressure was 12 mmHg. Because of persistent acidosis, 1 ampule of sodium bicarbonate was given. By 23 hours after presentation, intermittent slow ventricular tachycardia and recurrent hypotension were noted; therefore amiodarone was begun. Little improvement was noted, and final labs showed the following:

Na	158 mEq/L (169 mEq/L corrected for glucose)
K	2.7 mEq/L
Cl	128 mEq/L
CO_2	9 mEq/L
BUN	50 mg/dL
Cr	5.6 mg/dL
BG	769 mg/dL
Ca	4.4 mg/dL
pH	7.15
Serum osmolarity	376 mOsm/kg H_2O

Table 8.1 — Overall Fluid Calculations

	Outside ER	In Flight	TCH ER	PICU#1	PICU#2	Total
TIME	2 h	1.5 h	1 h	15 h	3.5 h	23 h
IN	2,000 cc	300 cc	1,000 cc	5,000 cc	1,050 cc	9,350 cc
OUT	750 cc	200 cc	200 cc	3,600 cc	250 cc	5,000 cc

Pulses were lost and ventricular defibrillation was attempted four times; he was given lasix along with high-dose epinephrine, sodium bicarbonate, and calcium chloride. Twenty-five hours after presentation, the patient was pronounced dead.

Additional labs included creatine kinase (CK) - MB subunit CK-MB 29.7 ng/mL (0–4.9), CK 1,300 units/L (55–1,790), and troponin 20.6 ng/mL (0–0.8).

An autopsy was notable for central obesity, hepatomegaly and marked steatosis, pulmonary edema, diffuse cerebral anoxia without evidence of cerebral edema or tonsillar herniation, cardiomegaly, myocardial hypertrophy, and marked myocardial reperfusion injury with extensive contraction bands. There was no evidence of islet cell inflammation or antibodies.

Table 8.2 — Summary of Vital Signs

Time after admission	BP (mmHg)	HR (bpm)	RR (respirations/min)	Temp (°F)
0	122/84	140	46	97
0:15	200/86	142		
0:45	171/58	122		
1:15	100/60	136		
2:15	137/97	125		
2:45	90/72			
3:13	56/29	142	48	
3:15	No BP	137		
3:26	77/44			
3:30	135/94			
4:10	72/palp			
5:00	125/85	130		
17:45	60/palp		None	40.1
23:15		V tach		
24:30	83/49			
24:40		V fib		

Table 8.3—Summary of Laboratory Values

Time after admit	BG (mg/dL)	Osm (mOsm/ kg H₂O)	pH	Na (mEq/L)	K (mEq/L)	CO₂ (mEq/L)	BUN (mg/dL)	Cr (mg/dL)	Ca (mg/dL)	Mg (mg/dL)	Phos (mg/dL)
0	>700			127	6.3		41				
1:45	>700										
3:45	1,110	366	6.98	136	5.5	5	38	3.5			
4:25	1,084	367	7.05	146	6.3		41	3.5		2.7	7
7:15	827			148	5.1	5	39	3.0		2.1	4.3
9:15	594	348		152	4.2	28			4.9	2.8	2.8
14:15			7.4								
16:15	349	358		161	3.4	9			4.9		
17:45			7.22								
18:30	381			162	2.7	10			4.3	2.3	0.5
19:25	511	367		163	3.1	9				2.6	0.8
24:10	708	366	7.21	155	2.7	7	47	4.9		2.4	0.4
25:24	769	376	7.15	158	2.7	9	50	5.6	4.4		

Diabetic ketoacidosis (DKA) and associated cerebral edema was historically the main source of morbidity and mortality in pediatric type 1 diabetes (T1D).[1] The face of pediatric diabetes, however, has changed with the increase in obesity and type 2 diabetes (T2D).[2] Because of the metabolic syndrome–related comorbidities typical of T2D, the presentation of T2D differs from T1D.

This patient presented with symptoms of DKA, severe dehydration and hypotension. His abrupt clinical onset and severe acidosis might suggest T1D, whereas his obesity, ethnicity, hypertension, liver steatosis, family history of T2D, and lack of islet cell abnormalities point to T2D. Despite evidence of diffuse hypoxia, this was likely secondary to hypotension-induced ischemia. Therefore, cerebral edema or tonsillar herniation does not appear to be causative of death. Instead, the elevated troponin-1 and CK-MB strongly suggest that cardiac abnormalities and myocardial ischemia were the cause of death. On pathology, multiple sections of the heart contained contraction bands, likely formed by exaggerated contraction of myofibrils when perfusion is reestablished after severe hypotension.[3-5] Typically, hypotension results from hypovolemia or septic shock. In contrast, this patient had hypotension and arrhythmias on the background of a markedly enlarged and hypertrophic heart, possibly secondary to hypertension. Hypertrophic myocardium is more susceptible to arrhythmias and has a higher oxygen requirement, making it more vulnerable to poor perfusion.[5] The left ventricular hypertrophy seen with hypertension also is associated with abnormal vasodilatation, impaired endothelial function, and hypercoagulability.[5] These increase the risk for ischemic damage, especially in the setting of dehydration and hyperosmolarity.

The patient presented is not representative of typical pediatric DKA. He had many features of the previously "adult" metabolic syndrome, including obesity, hypertension, hypertrophic myocardium, and fatty liver. He also may have had renal dysfunction, more common at presentation in T2D. Therefore, such a patient cannot be treated with a typical T1D DKA protocol. The approach to DKA in the setting of potential cardiovascular, hepatic, renal, and hematologic dysfunction requires pediatricians to address issues previously delegated to internal medicine.

REFERENCES

1. Rosenbloom AL, Hanas R. Diabetic ketoacidosis (DKA): treatment guidelines. *Clin Pediatr* 1996;35(5):261–266

2. Kaufman FR. Type 2 diabetes mellitus in children and youth: a new epidemic. J *Ped Endocrin Metab* 2002;15(Suppl. 2):737–744

3. Michael LH, Entman ML, Hartley CJ, et al. Myocardial ischemia and reperfusion: a murine model. *Am J Physiol* 1995;269(6 Pt 2):H2147–2154

4. Torok B, Trombitas K, Roth E. Ultrastructural consequences of reperfusion of the ischaemic myocardium. *Acta Morphol Hung* 1983;31(4):315–326

5. Tin LL, Beevers DG, Lip GY. Hypertension, left ventricular hypertrophy, and sudden death. *Curr Cardiol Rep* 2002;4(6):449–457

Case 9

Not Your Usual Diabetic Ketoacidosis

Ruchi Gaba, MD;[1] Susan L. Samson, MD, PhD;[2] and Alan J. Garber, MD, PhD, FACE [3]

A 51-year-old Hispanic woman with no history of diabetes presented to the emergency department with several days of nausea, vomiting, abdominal pain, and shortness of breath. She also reported blurry vision, polyuria, polydipsia, and a 30 lb weight loss over the past 3 months.

She had a past medical history of hypertension. Her mother and maternal grandmother had type 2 diabetes (T2D). She did not smoke or drink alcohol and did not exercise regularly.

Her weight was 73.93 kg (BMI 32.5 kg/m^2). Physical examination revealed signs of volume depletion. She had acanthosis nigricans at the neck. She had no clinical evidence of retinopathy, neuropathy, or nephropathy.

Testing revealed the following:

Metabolic acidosis	arterial pH 6.95, anion gap 20
Serum bicarbonate	5 mmol/l
Serum glucose	>500 mg/dL
Hemoglobin A1c (HbA$_{1c}$)	14.3%

She was diagnosed with diabetic ketoacidosis (DKA) and treated with hydration and intravenous (i.v.) insulin. There was no evidence of a precipitating event. Anti-islet cell and glutamic acid decarboxylase antibodies were absent.

She was discharged from the hospital on day 3 on subcutaneous basal and mealtime insulin (total insulin 30 units/day).

DKA is life-threatening hyperglycemic emergency. Historically, it was most closely associated with type 1 diabetes. In recent years, however, another distinct phenotype has emerged. Ketosis-prone diabetes (KPD) is a heterogeneous syndrome characterized by patients who present with DKA but who do not have type 1 diabetes (T1D), with many having characteristics of T2D, such as high BMI and a family history. Often there is no evidence of a precipitating illness. Initially called Flatbush diabetes, this condition was first described in

[1]Division of Endocrinology Diabetes and Metabolism, Baylor College of Medicine, Houston, TX. [2]Department of Medicine, Baylor College of Medicine, Houston, TX. [3]Departments of Medicine, Molecular and Cellular Biology, Biochemistry and Molecular Biology, Baylor College of Medicine, Houston, TX.

        DOI: 10.2337/9781580405713.09

patients of African ancestry. Now it has been described in a wide variety of geographic and ethnic backgrounds.[1]

The inpatient treatment of DKA is the same regardless of the apparent KPD phenotype. KPD patients should be discharged from the hospital on a regimen that provides basal and mealtime insulin coverage.

Within a few weeks of starting insulin, the patient's insulin requirements gradually declined. She was assessed in the endocrine clinic 4 weeks after hospitalization and her glucose levels were at goal as per ADA guidelines (fasting/preprandial 70–130 mg/dL and bedtime/peak postprandial <180 mg/dL). β-Cell function was assessed by fasting serum C-peptide levels after i.v. glucagon stimulation. Fasting C-peptide was 1.1 ng/mL at baseline and peaked to 3.01 ng/mL after stimulation.

One method of classifying KPD patients takes into account the presence or absence of autoimmunity (A) and β-cell function (β) (see Fig. 9.1).[2] The former is assessed by autoantibody testing, whereas the latter is assessed by the fasting serum C-peptide response to glucagon stimulation. β-Cell testing should be performed a few weeks after resolution of DKA to minimize any acute effects of glucotoxicity.

Patients are classified as β+ if the fasting serum C-peptide concentration is ≥1 ng/mL or if the peak serum C-peptide response to glucagon is at least 1.5 ng/mL; otherwise, they are classified as β–. These cutoffs accurately predict β-cell function and glycemic control after 1 year.[3,4] After the episode of DKA, our patient had partially preserved β-cell function. Hence, she had the phenotype of A–β+.[2,3]

A–β+ patients account for the largest subgroup of KPD. Approximately half of these patients have new-onset diabetes and develop DKA without

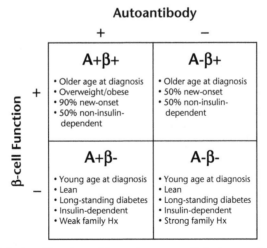

Figure 9.1—Aβ classification of ketosis-prone diabetes and common characteristics.[3]

a clinically evident precipitating factor (unprovoked A–β+ KPD), whereas the remainder have long-standing diabetes before presentation with DKA, which develops in association with acute illness or treatment noncompliance (provoked A–β+ KPD). Most are obese and have strong family history of T2D.[1]

With evidence of improved glycemic control and β-cell function, the patient's insulin doses were decreased by 50%. Two weeks later, blood glucose levels remained at goal. Her insulin was further reduced by 50% (<10 units total/day). She was seen in the endocrine clinic 2 weeks later. HbA$_{1c}$ was 5.6%, and glucose levels were at target. Insulin was discontinued and metformin 500 mg twice daily was introduced. The metformin was doubled to 1,000 mg twice daily within 2 weeks.

Attempts to administer noninsulin diabetes therapies should be made on basis of knowledge of the KPD subgroup and assessment of predictive factors. A–β+ KPD patients have impaired insulin secretion and action at initial presentation, but aggressive diabetes management results in significant improvement in β-cell function and insulin sensitivity, which can allow discontinuation of insulin therapy within a few months.

If blood glucose values over a 2-week period attain ADA goals, then the insulin can be reduced by 50%. If blood glucose values are at goal for another 2 weeks, oral agents can replace insulin injections. If blood glucose remains controlled, then patients can be monitored without pharmacological therapy and can continue lifestyle modification.

Patients should be advised to check for significant ketosis if blood glucose levels rise to >200 mg/dL. If there is no ketosis, then patients are placed on additional oral antidiabetes agents. Conversely, if ketosis develops after decreasing the insulin dose, then insulin should be intensified. The process of insulin withdrawal may require ≥10–14 weeks.

A–β+ patients have the highest frequency of metabolic syndrome among KPD groups, and insulin-sensitizing agents (metformin, thiazolidinedione) should be used.[5] If blood glucose levels are uncontrolled at 8 weeks, then one could consider adding low doses of a sulfonylurea, meglitinide, or α-glucosidase inhibitor. There is limited experience with newer agents, such as incretin-based therapies in this population.

Subsequent visits at 3-month intervals demonstrated good glycemic control with HbA$_{1c}$ between 5.7 and 6.9 %. Fasting C-peptide levels and peak responses to glucagon increased over time. Repeat assessment of β-cell function at 1 year showed a baseline C-peptide 3.17 ng/dL with peak postglucagon level 7.08 ng/dL. At year 2 from DKA, the C-peptide was 4.18 ng/dL with peak postglucagon level 9.98 ng/dL. She is still controlled adequately on metformin 1,000 mg twice daily with no DKA recurrence.

Once patients have been classified for KPD type, assessed for predictive factors, and treated appropriately, it is important that ADA standards of diabetes management are followed. Routine reevaluation of β-cell function every 6 months can be done to track its evolution.

REFERENCES

1. Balasubramanyam A, Nalini R, Hampe CS, Maldonado M. Syndromes of ketosis-prone diabetes. *Endocr Rev* 2008;29(3):292–302

2. Maldonado M, Hampe CS, Gaur LK, D'Amico S, Iyer D, Hammerle LP, Bolgiano D, Rodriguez L, Rajan A, Lernmark A, Balasubramanyam A. Ketosis-prone diabetes: dissection of a heterogeneous syndrome using an immunogenetic and β-cell functional classification, prospective analysis, and clinical outcomes. *J Clin Endocrinol Metab* 2003;88:5090–5098

3. Balasubramanyam A, Garza G, Rodriguez L, Hampe CS, Gaur L, Lernmark A, Maldonado MR. Accuracy and predictive value of classification schemes for ketosis-prone diabetes. *Diabetes Care* 2006;29:2575–2579

4. Maldonado M, D'Amico S, Otiniano M, Balasubramanyam A, Rodriguez L, Cuevas E. Predictors of glycaemic control in indigent patients presenting with diabetic ketoacidosis. *Diabetes Obes Metab* 2005;7:282–289

5. Otiniano ME, Balasubramanyam A, Maldonado M. Presence of the metabolic syndrome distinguishes patients with ketosis-prone diabetes who have a type 2 diabetic phenotype. *J Diabetes Complications* 2005;19:313–318

Case 10

Ketosis-Prone Diabetes

DAVID SAXON, MD,[1] AND NEDA RASOULI, MD[1,2]

A 64-year-old African American man presented to the endocrinology clinic for management of diabetes. His past medical history included CAD s/p STEMI (two stents), CHF (EF 50%, diastolic dysfunction), hypertension, osteoporosis, and hyperparathyroidism. Family history was significant for type 2 diabetes in both his mother and brother. He never smoked, reported drinking two beers per week, and denied use of illicit drugs. At initial outpatient consultation, his weight was 100.6 kg (BMI 31 kg/m^2), blood pressure 145/84 mmHg, and pulse 72. Physical exam was unremarkable. Most recent hemoglobin A1c (HbA$_{1c}$) was 6.8% while taking insulin glargine 45 units at bedtime and approximately 10 units of aspart per meal. He was experiencing rare hypoglycemia.

In type 2 diabetes, β-cell dysfunction is a gradual and progressive process starting with loss of first-phase glucose-induced insulin secretion and leading to impaired second-phase insulin secretion, development of hyperproinsulinemia, and then impaired basal insulin secretion. Amyloid deposition into islet cells results in loss of β-cell mass and chronic exposure to high levels of glucose (glucotoxicity) and free fatty acids (lipotoxicity) causes β-cell apoptosis. Insulin resistance, generally related to obesity, and insulin secretion defects are the major risk factors for the development of type 2 diabetes.[1]

Upon chart review, we found the course of this patient's diabetes to be unique and atypical. He had been diagnosed with diabetes 18 years earlier at the age of 46 years when he presented to an emergency department with diabetic ketoacidosis (blood glucose of 1,200 mg/dL [66.7 mmol/L], positive serum ketones, and HbA$_{1c}$ of 10%). At that time he was discharged on insulin, which he took for 4 months before being switched to oral medications. His blood glucose was well controlled on oral antidiabetes agents (HbA$_{1c}$ <7%); however, 2 years later, he was again hospitalized with a hyperglycemic emergency without a precipitating event. Insulin therapy was restarted, but he was again able to transition to oral medications and was even able to come off of diabetes medications altogether after several months. He remained off all diabetes medications for approximately 11 years until 3 years ago when he was again found to be in a hyperglycemic crisis with an HbA$_{1c}$ of 9.9%

[1]Division of Endocrinology, Diabetes and Metabolism, University of Colorado, Aurora CO. [2]Denver Veterans Affairs Medical Center, Denver CO.

 DOI: 10.2337/9781580405713.10

and no obvious precipitating event. Urine and serum ketones were positive. GAD antibodies were found to be negative. Nine months before that presentation, his HbA_{1c} had been 5.8% off all diabetes medications. He was restarted on insulin at that time and currently is taking insulin glargine 40 units at bedtime and insulin aspart 6 units with meals in addition to a correction factor of 1u:50 mg/dL for blood glucose higher than 150 mg/dL (8.3 mmol/L). His most recent HbA_{1c} on intensive insulin therapy was 6.8% with minimal hypoglycemia. Review of his chart indicated that during periods of near-normoglycemic remission, he did not have any significant change in weight or lifestyle that could explain periods of remission.

β-Cell recovery is not a rare phenomenon in African Americans with type 2 diabetes. A subset of adult African American patients lacking islet antibodies present with severe diabetic ketoacidosis but may soon transition off insulin after just a few months of intensive therapy. This variant of type 2 diabetes has been referred to as Flatbush diabetes, idiopathic type 1 diabetes, diabetes type 1.5, atypical diabetes, and ketosis-prone diabetes (KPD). In one small study, 11 of 26 (42.3%) consecutive African American patients with initial presentation of severe hyperglycemia developed remission with intensive pharmacologic therapy after a mean of 83 days and all but one patient had stayed in remission after an average follow-up period of 349 days.[2] Such cases make it difficult to label patients as having either type 1 or type 2 diabetes, and they bring attention to the heterogeneous nature of diabetes in clinical practice.

In 2006, Balasubramanyam et al. proposed a classification scheme ("Aβ classification") for patients with KPD consisting of four subgroups based on immunologic criteria—that is, the presence or absence of β-cell antibodies (A+ or A-) and recovery or lack of recovery of β-cell function after the initial episode of DKA (β+ or β-). The purpose of such a scheme is to predict which patients presenting with DKA will have preserved β-cell function and thus long-term insulin independence.[3]

Our patient's characteristics of obesity, unprovoked ketoacidosis, absence of β-cell antibodies, and reversible β-cell dysfunction after ketoacidosis with near-normoglycemic remission categorize him as having A- β+ KPD. The pathophysiology of this syndrome is not completely understood, but recently has been investigated using a metabolomics-kinetics approach, which determined that defective oxidation of ketones and accelerated leucine metabolism are key defects of fasting energy metabolism in A- β+ KPD.[4] Studies addressing whether treatment of KPD patients during near-normoglycemic remission period will prolong the period of remission are needed. A study by Banerji et al. of 20 African American patients in near-normoglycemic remission treated with either sulfonylurea (glipizide 2.5 mg daily) or placebo demonstrated that the former led to a significant delay in onset of hyperglycemia over a 3-year period.[5] Other antidiabetes medications without increased risk of hypoglycemia might present a better option to prolong remission.

In brief, KPD is a unique form of diabetes presenting with hyperglycemic crisis followed by the remission of β-cell function. The pathophysiology of this fluctuating β-cell failure is not well understood, and the best management of diabetes during the periods of remission has yet to be thoroughly studied.

REFERENCES

1. Kahn SE. The relative contributions of insulin resistance and β-cell dysfunction to the pathophysiology of type 2 diabetes. *Diabetologia* 2003;46:3–19

2. McFarlane SI. Near-normoglycaemic remission in African-Americans with type 2 diabetes mellitus is associated with recovery of beta cell function. *Diabet Med* 2001;18(1):10–16

3. Balasubramanyam A, Garza G, Rodriquez LVN, Hampe CS, Gaur L, Lernmark Å, Maldonado MR. Accuracy and predictive value of classification schemes for ketosis-prone diabetes. *Diabetes Care* 2006;29:2575–2579

4. Patel SG, Hsu JW, Jahoor F, Coraza I, Bain JR, Stevens RD, Iyer D, Nalini R, Ozer K, Hampe CS, Newgard CB, Balasubramanyam A. Pathogenesis of A⁻β⁺ ketosis-prone diabetes. *Diabetes* 2013;62(3):912–922

5. Banerji MA, Chaiken RL, Lebovitz HE. Prolongation of near-normoglycemic remission in black NIDDM subjects with chronic low-dose sulfonylurea treatment. *Diabetes* 1995;44(4):466–470

Case 11

From a Total Daily Dose of Insulin of 415 Units to No Insulin: A Case of Ketosis-Prone Diabetes

Caroline T. Nguyen, MD,[1] and Jorge H. Mestman, MD[1]

A 29-year-old Mexican American man with no past medical history presented with an 8-day history of sore throat, intermittent subjective fevers, nausea, decreased PO intake, and a 1-day history of altered mental status. Review of systems revealed 3 weeks of polyuria, polydipsia, vision changes, fatigue, and weight loss. He denied recent trauma, surgery, alcohol, or drug use. He has no family history of diabetes.

Physical exam was remarkable for the following:

Temperature	38.4°C
Blood pressure	97/58 mmHg
Heart rate	124 bpm
Respiratory rate (RR)	30–36 respirations/min
O$_2$ saturation	96% on room air
BMI	35 kg/m^2

He presented with somnolence, dry mucous membranes, and mild acanthosis nigricans in the posterior neck and axilla. He was diagnosed with DKA with the following:

pH	7.17
HCO3	14 mmol/L on venous blood gas
Blood glucose	>1,650 mg/dL (91.7 mmol/L)
K+	5 mmol/L
Cr	1.73 mg/dL
Lactate	5.2 mmol/L
Anion gap	22
KUrine ketones	positive
HbA$_{1c}$	14.1%

In the medical intensive care unit, he was treated with a total daily insulin dose of 415 units of insulin with improvement in his glucose, metabolic acidosis, and altered mental status. No precipitating factor could be elucidated. The patient was transitioned and eventually discharged on SQ glargine

[1]Keck School of Medicine, Division of Endocrinology, Diabetes, and Metabolism, University of Southern California, Los Angeles, CA.

DOI: 10.2337/9781580405713.11

70 units qAM/60 units qPM and Humalog 30 units with each meal, and fair control (fingerstick blood glucose) 98–235 mg/dL (5.4–13.1 mmol/L). Our differential diagnosis included type 1 diabetes or latent autoimmune diabetes of adulthood versus ketosis-prone diabetes (KPD).

He returned to the diabetes clinic 2 weeks after discharge and was feeling well with blood glucose 60–198 mg/dL (3.3–11 mmol/L) and a median of 94 mg/dL (5.2 mmol/L). Sixteen percent of his fingerstick blood glucose levels were in the 60s. His HbA_{1c} was 11%, and his anti-GAD65, insulin, and islet-cell antibodies were negative.

Our patient was diagnosed with KPD, sometimes referred to as Flatbush diabetes, as it initially was described in young adult Afro-Caribbean patients from the Flatbush neighborhood in New York City. KPD has since been described in patients of non-African decent, including Chinese, Latinos, and Native Americans. Patients typically present with DKA, but then proceed to have insulin independence of variable duration, with some never requiring insulin.[1]

Table 11.1 shows the four different classification schemes of KPD: *1)* Classically, the ADA has divided these individuals into type 1a and type 1b diabetes. Type 1a diabetes is characterized by autoimmune destruction of the pancreatic β-cells leading to the virtual absence of circulating insulin. Type 1b diabetes may present with DKA but may lack autoantibodies. *2)* A modified ADA system has been proposed in which type 1b diabetes is further divided into two subgroups: *a)* long-term insulin dependence characterized by thin individuals with poor β-cell function, and *b)* noninsulin dependence characterized by obese individuals with preserved β-cell function for a prolonged duration. *3)* In the BMI-based classification system, KPD patients are distinguished by lean (BMI <28 kg/m²) versus obese (BMI ≥28 kg/m²). *4)* The Aβ classification distinguishes four KPD subgroups based on the presence or absence of *a)* autoantibodies

Table 11.1—Classification Systems of Ketosis-Prone Diabetes

Classification system		
ADA	Type 1a:	+ autoantibodies
	Type 1b:	– autoantibodies
Modified ADA classification	Type 1a:	+ autoantibodies
	Type 1b:	– autoantibodies
	•	Insulin-dependent (KPD-ID)
	•	Non-insulin-dependent (KPD-NID)
BMI	Lean:	BMI <28kg/m²
	Obese:	BMI ≥28kg/m²
Aβ	A+β–	autoantibodies +, β-cell function –
	A+β+	autoantibodies +, β-cell function +
	A–β–	autoantibodies –, β-cell function –
	A–β+	autoantibodies –, β-cell function +

and *b)* β-cell functional reserve, measured by fasting or glucagon-stimulated C-peptide. The Aβ classification has been shown to be the most accurate of the four systems in predicting long-term insulin dependence with 99% sensitivity and 96% specificity.[2]

A–β+ (autoantibody negative with β-cell functional reserve) KPD is the most common of the four KPD subgroups.[3] This subgroup, however, is heterogeneous with roughly half developing DKA without an evident precipitating factor and the remainder being associated with a precipitating event. Consequently, A–β+ can be further classified into *1)* "unprovoked DKA" defined as new-onset diabetes and development of DKA without a clinically evident precipitation factor, and *2)* "provoked DKA" defined by long-standing diabetes and development of ketoacidosis in association with acute illness or nonconsistency with antidiabetic treatment (Table 11.2).

Although "provoked DKA" and "unprovoked DKA" both lack autoantibodies, they have been found to have different underlying genetic susceptibilities. Provoked DKA is characterized by a progressive loss of β-cell reserve and increased frequency of HLA susceptibility alleles for autoimmune type 1 diabetes. "Unprovoked DKA" is characterized by reversible β-cell dysfunction with a male predominance and increased frequency of a protective HLA allele for autoimmune diabetes. Unprovoked DKA is predictive of long-term β-cell functional reserve and insulin independence.[4]

Although the cause of A–β+ KPD remains unclear, a distinctive pathogenic sequence involving impaired ketone oxidation, fatty acid utilization for energy, and accelerated leucine catabolism has been shown in this subgroup.[5]

As our patient's clinical and laboratory presentation appeared consistent with KPD, we anticipated that his insulin requirement would continue to decrease over the coming weeks. His daily insulin dose was decreased by 20%. We had an extensive discussion regarding hypoglycemia and further titration of his insulin at home. At follow-up 1 month later, he was off

Table 11.2—KPD A–β+ Group: Autoantibody Negative with β-Cell Functional Reserve

Unprovoked	• New-onset diabetes • DKA without clinically evident precipitation factor • Reversible β-cell dysfunction • Male predominance • Increased frequency of DQB1*0602 (protective HLA allele for autoimmune diabetes)
Provoked	• Long-standing diabetes • DKA in association with acute illness or nonconsistency with antidiabetic treatment • Progressive loss of β-cell reserve • Increased frequency for DQB1*0302 and DRB1*04, HLA susceptibility alleles for autoimmune type 1 diabetes

insulin for 3 weeks with a median glucose of 112 mg/dL (6.2 mmol/L) and one value >200mg/dL (11.1 mmol/L). Fasting C-peptide was 7.07 ng/dL (0.8–3.10) and HbA$_{1c}$ 6.8%. His C-peptide allowed us to further classify him as A–β+ unprovoked KPD.

This case illustrates the current limitations of our historical classification system. Given the differences in underlying pathophysiology and management of KPD, consideration of newer classification systems would be judicious for the future. Key points from this case include: *1)* Antibodies against β-cell proteins and assessment of β-cell functional reserve with fasting or glucagon-stimulated C-peptide often are not done in patients who present with routine DKA with the typical type 1 diabetes phenotype (thin, young). In a subset of patients with atypical presentation (overweight, older, non-Caucasian ethnicity), however, these can be helpful in predicting clinical course and possible discontinuation of insulin. *2)* All patients presenting with DKA initially should be managed with insulin. *3)* Close follow-up is necessary in KPD because initially high insulin requirements may decrease rapidly and patients may be successfully managed with no hypoglycemic agents. Continued follow-up is strongly advised because hyperglycemia returns in the majority of cases.

REFERENCES

1. Balasubramanyam A, Nalini R, Hampe CS et al. Syndromes of ketosis-prone diabetes mellitus. *Endocr Rev* 2008;29:292–302

2. Banergi MA, Dham S. A comparison of classification schemes for ketosis-prone diabetes. *Nat Clin Pract Endocrinol Metab* 2007;3:506–507

3. Nalini R, Gaur LK, Maldonado M, et al. HLA class II alleles specify phenotypes of ketosis-prone diabetes. *Diabetes Care* 2008;31:1195–1200

4. Nalini R, Ozer K, Maldonado M, et al. Presence or absence of a known diabetic ketoacidosis precipitant defines distinct syndromes of "A–β+" ketosis-prone diabetes based on long-term β-cell function, human leukocyte antigen class II alleles, and sex predilection. *Metabolism* 2010;59:1448–1455

5. Patel SG, Hsu JW, Jahoor F, et al. Pathogenesis of A-β+ ketosis-prone diabetes. *Diabetes* 2013;62:912–922

Case 12

The Worst Case Scenario: Severe HHS in a Relatively Young Man

Elizabeth Herman, MD,[1] and Marie E. McDonnell, MD[1]

A 48-year-old man was brought to the emergency department (ED) after being found in his bed unresponsive. The patient's medical history was notable for remote alcohol abuse, hypertension, and hyperlipidemia. He weighed 103 kg. In the ED, the patient was febrile at 101.1°F, BP 151/79 mmHg, HR 80 bpm, and O_2 saturation 99%. Because of the altered mental status, he was intubated for airway protection. On arrival, the fingerstick glucose read "HI" (≥600 mg/dL). The patient had no history of diabetes and a hemoglobin A1c (HbA$_{1c}$) was 5.1% 1 year prior.

A full metabolic workup revealed several abnormalities (Table 12.1). Significant labs included the following:

Sodium	122 mmol/L
Potassium	4.3 mmol/L
Bicarbonate	22 mmol/L
Anion gap (AG)	26
BUN	94 mg/dL
Creatinine	8.3 mg/dL
Glucose	2,108 mg/dL (117.1 mmol/L)
Calculated effective serum osmolality	361 mOsm/kg
Measured total osmolality	410 mOsm/kg
Arterial blood pH	7.2
pCO$_2$	45.6 mmHg
Lactate	3.4 mmol/L (normal 0.5–2.0 mmol/L)
Urinalysis (UA)	negative for ketones
Toxicology screens	negative

A lumbar puncture was consistent with meningitis:

White blood cell	106
Polys	85%
Protein	118 mg/dL (normal 15–45 mg/dL)
Glucose	718 mg/dL (normal 40–70 mg/dL)

[1]Boston University School of Medicine, Section of Endocrinology, Diabetes, Nutrition and Weight Management, Boston MA.

DOI: 10.2337/9781580405713.12

Table 12.1—Admission Laboratory Tests

Complete blood count		Coagulation	
WBC	10.3 k/µL	INR	1.0 sec
Hemoglobin	7.0 g/dL	PTT	30 sec
Hematocrit	21.10%		
Platelets	139 k/µL	**Cardiac enzymes**	
		CK	1,307 units/L
Chemistries		CKMB	2.1 ng/mL
Sodium	122 mmol/L	Troponin	0.086 ng/mL (normal <0.033)
Potassium	4.3 mmol/L		
Chloride	74 mmol/L	**Urinalysis**	
Bicarbonate	22 mmol/L	WBC	0–5
Anion Gap	26	RBC	0.3
Glucose	718 mg/dL (39.9 mmol/L)	Glucose	3+
BUN	94 mg/dL	Protein	1+
Creatinine	8.3 mg/dL	Specific gravity	1.027
Calcium	9.3 mg/dL	Ketones	Negative
Magnesium	3.8 mg/dL	Blood	3+
Phosphorous	3.4 mg/dL	Nitrites	Negative
Albumin	4.7 g/dL	Leukocyte esterase	Negative
AST	28 units/L	**Serum β-hydroxybutyrate**	Not performed
ALT	33 units/L		
Alkaline phosphatase	123 units/L	**Lumbar puncture**	
Lipase	301 units/L	WBC	106
Effective osmolality	361 mOsm/kg	polys	85%
Serum osmolality	401 mOsm/kg	RBC	36
Lactate	3.4 mmol/L (normal 0.5–2.0)	Protein	118 mg/dL (normal 15–45)
		Glucose	718 mg/dL (normal 40–70)
Arterial blood gas			
pH	7.19	**Hemoglobin A1c**	
CO_2	45.6 mmHg	Admission	14.2%
		1 year prior	5.1%

continued

Table 12.1—Admission Laboratory Tests *(continued)*

Urine toxicology		Blood toxicology	
Amphetamines	Negative	Acetaminophen	Negative
Barbiturates	Negative	Ethanol	Negative
Benzodiazepines	Negative	Methanol	Negative
Cocaine	Negative	Salicylates	Negative
Opiates	Negative	Tricyclics	Negative

The patient was administered broad spectrum antibiotics and admitted to the intensive care unit (ICU).

The diagnosis of diabetic ketoacidosis (DKA) and hyperglycemic hyperosmolar syndrome (HHS) has been reviewed in recent literature.[1] Criteria for DKA includes a blood glucose of >250 mg/dL, metabolic acidosis with ph <7.3 or serum bicarbonate <15 mM, and ketonemia. Criteria for HHS include a blood glucose >600 mg/dl and effective serum osmolality >320 mOsm/kg. A patient may present in DKA, HHS, or a combination of the two, often called hyperosmolar ketoacidosis (HKA). In HKA a patient must present with hyperglycemia, metabolic acidosis, ketosis, and hyperosmolarity.

Although the patient was acidemic (arterial pH 7.2) and there was an AG of 26, his UA was negative for ketones. Given the negative ketones, his presentation was not consistent with DKA. Plasma ketone level (β-hydroxybutyrate level or acetone) was not measured. In rare cases, urine ketones can be negative in a patient with severe acidemia because of a shift of ketone body production away from acetoacetate (detected on UA) and toward β-hydroxybutyrate. Plasma ketones should be checked to rule out DKA or HKA, but given the patient had only mild acidemia, it would be unlikely his urine ketones would be falsely negative. In this patient, other causes of acidosis should be considered, including lactic acidosis and septic shock.

To evaluate for HHS, one must calculate the effective osmolality. An effective osmolality (Osm_E) >320 mOsm/kg has been shown to reliably cause altered mental status.[1] If the calculated effective osmolality is <320 mOsm/kg, other sources of altered mental status must be considered. The Osm_E differs from total osmolality as the BUN is not included because BUN flows freely across cell membranes and does not independently cause fluid shifts. In our patient, the effective osmolality was calculated: $[2 \times Na] + [glucose \div 18] = 361$ mOsm/kg.

The presentation was consistent with HHS, with several poor prognostic indicators. HHS mortality far exceeds that of DKA with reported mortality rates of 5–20% compared with <5% for DKA in adults.[2]

In the ED, the patient received 3 L of 0.9% saline and insulin infusion therapy. Given the severely elevated osmolarity, the ICU team was concerned that lowering the glucose too rapidly could cause intracerebral fluid shifts and cerebral edema. Complicating factors included acute kidney injury with decreased urine output and shock requiring vasopressor therapy. In the first 36 h, his fluid management was focused on volume resuscitation. He received normal saline (NS) at 250 cc/h in addition to multiple boluses totaling ~13 L over the first 36 h. Insulin infusion was continued to treat his hyperglycemia. The plasma sodium rose to 160 mmol/L. NS was changed to lactated ringers (LR) to lower hypernatremia and osmolarity, while expanding plasma volume during initial resuscitation. Glucose improved to <250 mg/dL (13.9 mmol/L). After initial volume resuscitation, the central venous pressure (CVP) normalized indicating the patient was now intravascularly replete. Despite this, he remained oliguric and required vasopressors. The free water deficit was calculated as ~4–5 L. Gentle replacement of free water ~1–2 L/day was recommended with a goal decrease in sodium of 4–6 mEq/day. Intravenous (i.v.) fluids were changed to 1/2 normal saline (1/2 NS) to provide free water in addition to enteral free water boluses. Insulin infusion was continued to maintain glucose between 120 and 180 mg/dL (6.7 and 10 mmol/L). Sodium only modestly improved with free water and oliguria and renal failure persisted. Continuous veno-venous hemofiltration (CVVH) eventually was initiated with improvement in electrolytes.

> It is unclear how best to treat the metabolic disarray typical of HHS to improve prognosis. A gradual reduction in osmolarity as a marker of effective and safe HHS therapy may be less important in adults than in children, although this dogma is not supported by recent studies. Data from recent pediatric studies no longer support the previous thought that changes in osmolarity cause cerebral edema, but rather suggest it may be linked to low overall brain perfusion and insufficient volume resuscitation, and the failure to correct these quickly enough.[3] In our experience, with usual treatment aimed at reestablishing perfusion (measured by urine output, hemodynamics, and cognitive function) and insulin and electrolyte repletion, osmolarity usually declines within the recommended guidelines. NS is the fluid of choice until reperfusion is established. After reperfusion, NS can be continued if the corrected sodium is low, ½ NS or LR can be used if the corrected sodium is normal or elevated. The recommendation is for the (Osm_E) to fall no more than 5 mOsm/kg/h until the effective osmolarity reaches 320 mOsm/kg.[1] In our patient, the effective osmolarity declined at a rate of 0.8 mOsm/kg/h in the initial 24 h, in keeping with this guideline. On the basis of this patient's weight of 103 kg, however, it is possible that 13 L over 36 h was inadequate, and fluid replacement may have been overly cautious in the initial 12–24 h. Our patient's hypernatremia was another poor prognostic indicator. One retrospective analysis showed in ICU patients sodium >149 mEq is an independent risk factor for mortality.[4]

Despite aggressive management with pressors, CVVH, and broad spectrum antibiotics, the patient remained persistently febrile and critically ill. Meningitis cultures and serologies were negative. The course was further complicated by rhabdomyolysis with CK peaking at 113,234 units/L and

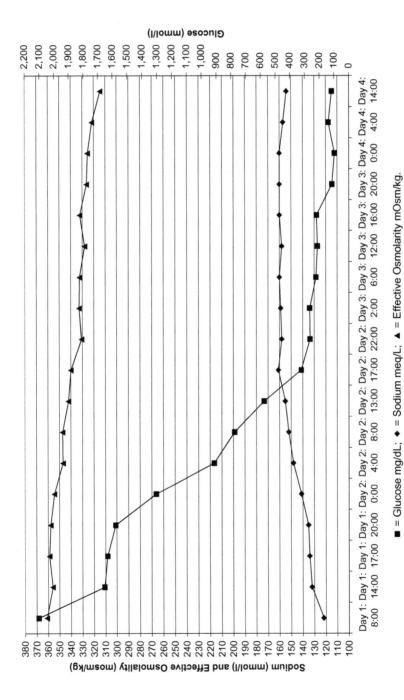

Figure 12.1—Change in sodium, effective osmolality, and glucose over time.

hypophosphatemia to 0.7 mg/dL. He continued to be oliguric, vasopressor-dependent with significant cardiovascular instability, and on mechanical ventilation. He died after 11 days in the ICU.

Recent case reports have described a unique idiopathic syndrome of patients presenting with HHS complicated by hyperthermia, rhabdomyolysis, and severe hypophosphatemia. The patients reported have all been under the age of 22 years and have a higher mortality then is seen in typical HHS. Patients with similar presentations should be evaluated for other causes of hyperthermia, including intoxications (such as MDMA or cocaine). Our patient had a negative urine and serum toxicology ruling this out. The etiology and full nature of this severe form of HHS remains unclear.[5]

REFERENCES

1. Steenkamp DW, Alexanian SM, McDonnell ME. Adult hyperglycemic crisis: a review and perspective. *Curr Diab Rep* 2013;13(1):130–137

2. Umpierrez G. Diabetic ketoacidosis and hyperglycemic hyperosmolar syndrome. In *Clinical Diabetes*. V Fonseca, Ed. Elsevier, 2006

3. Glaser N, Kuppermann N. DKA-related cerebral edema and intravenous fluid therapy: potential pitfalls of uncontrolled retrospective studies. *J Pediatr* 2008;152(1):145; author reply 7–9

4. Linder G, et al. Hypernatremia in the critically ill is and independent risk factor for mortality. *Am J Kidney Dis* 2007;50(6):952–957

5. Hollander AS, Olney RC, Blackett PR, Marshall BA. Fatal malignant hyperthermia-like syndrome with rhabdomyolysis complication the presentation of diabetes mellitus in adolescent males. *Pediatrics* 2003;111:1447–1452

Case 13

Unusual Cause of New-Onset Diabetes

Kᴇʟsᴇʏ M. Sʜɪᴋᴜᴍᴀ, MD,[1] ᴀɴᴅ Jᴏʀɢᴇ H. Mᴇsᴛᴍᴀɴ, MD[1]

 21-year-old woman presented with complaints of severe nausea, vomiting, and abdominal pain. She was diagnosed with a perivaginal infection and found to be in diabetic ketoacidosis (DKA) with the following:

Serum glucose	488 mg/dL
pH	6.97
HCO$_3$	6 mmol/L
HbA$_{1c}$	12.3%

She was treated with intravenous (i.v.) fluids and insulin. Despite resolution of her DKA and underlying infection, she continued to require at least 375 units of subcutaneous insulin a day. Upon further questioning, the patient reported being admitted to three different hospitals with similar episodes of DKA over the past 3.5 months. Following each hospitalization, she had been discharged on more than 200 units of insulin per day. Despite compliance with her diabetes regimen, she continued to have significant hyperglycemia. Before this time, she had never experienced hyperglycemia or prior hospitalizations.

Severe insulin resistance from secondary causes includes an expansive range of pathophysiological states and endocrine disorders. Those that require a total daily insulin dose of >2 units/kg/day (or >200 units/day) generally are considered to involve severe insulin resistance.[1] In addition to the metabolic syndrome, a variety of rare endocrine disorders and receptor defects may contribute to severe insulin resistance. The insulin receptor is a heterotetrameric transmembrane receptor composed of two (α) and two (β) subunits. The intracellular β subunits activate a tyrosine kinase upon binding of insulin to its receptor. This tyrosine phosphorylation starts a cascade of intracellular signaling, which eventually leads to the stimulation of cellular glucose and amino acid uptake, lipogenesis, and glycogen synthesis.[2] Disruption in the insulin receptor itself or at another point in the postreceptor cascade plays a role in various forms of severe insulin resistance.

The differential diagnosis for high insulin requirements is broad, but in an adult, it includes syndromes of severe insulin resistance types A, B, and C,

[1]Keck School of Medicine, Division of Endocrinology, Diabetes and Metabolism, University of Southern California, Los Angeles, CA.

DOI: 10.2337/9781580405713.13

endocrine disorders (acromegaly, pseudoacromegaly, thyrotoxicosis, Cushing's syndrome, pheochromocytoma), lipodystrophy, drugs, subcutaneous insulin resistance, HIV infection, gustatory, increased insulin clearance, and impaired absorption.

Physical exam revealed a young overweight female (BMI 27 kg/m²) with a small amount of acanthosis nigricans at the posterior neck, but otherwise unremarkable exam. She had no evidence of acrochordia, hirsutism, virulization, or coarse facial features. Inpatient glucose control was achieved on a regimen of glargine 75 units b.i.d., and Humalog 32 units before each meal (QAC), and she was discharged with close follow-up.

Following hospital discharge, she was seen in the diabetes clinic, and her insulin regimen was adjusted to glargine 100 units b.i.d., along with U500 16 units QAC. Her glycemic control had improved significantly. Because of her persistent severe insulin resistance, she underwent further evaluation for secondary causes. Her medical history included secondary amenorrhea for the past 3 months but no headaches, vision or voice changes, or change in the size of her hands. She did admit to a sensation of "puffy feet," but denied an increased shoe size. She denied recent weight gain or stretch marks. There were no recent changes in oral intake, over-the-counter medication use, or any history of sexually transmitted diseases or HIV infection. She was not currently sexually active. There was no family history of diabetes or other endocrinopathies.

Given her age and the general paucity of physical findings, the differential diagnosis was focused on severe insulin resistance syndromes and possible endocrine disorders.

Severe insulin resistance syndrome A is characterized by acanthosis nigricans, hyperandrogenism in lean patients, the absence of auto-antibodies to the insulin receptor, and oligoamenorrhea with an onset in reproductive age females. Patients generally have low or normal triglyceride levels. The syndrome is caused by mutations in the insulin receptor gene. Severe insulin resistance syndrome type B is characterized by nonspecific autoimmune features in association with acanthosis nigricans in the periocular, perioral, and labial regions, and generally is seen in middle-aged women. Laboratory evaluation shows low triglycerides but high fatty acids, elevated erythrocyte sedimentation rate, leukopenia, hypergammaglobulinemia, and positive antinuclear antibodies. The syndrome is caused by autoantibodies to the insulin receptor. Severe insulin resistance syndrome C (also known as HAIRAN [hyperandrogenism, insulin resistance, acanthosis nigricans]) is similar in phenotype to type A, but most patients are obese. The underlying defect of this disorder is unknown.[1,2]

Subsequent endocrine workup revealed the following:

IGF-1	**1,699 ng/mL**
Follicle-stimulating hormone (FSH)	**2.6 mIU/mL**
Luteinizing hormone (LH)	**<0.1 mIU/mL**
Estradiol	**<5 pg/mL**

Lipid panel showed the following:

Total cholesterol	225 mg/dL
Triglyceride	596 mg/dL
High-density lipoprotein (HDL)	86 mg/dL

Thyroid function, cortisol, and prolactin were within normal limits. Pregnancy and HIV screens were negative. C-peptide levels were normal at 3.16 ng/mL with a glucose of 287 mg/dL, and anti-GAD and islet cell antibodies were negative.

Given the degree of elevation in IGF-1, acromegaly was suspected. Growth hormone levels were obtained and found to be elevated at >200 ng/mL. The patient underwent pituitary MRI, which showed a large 2.3 cm sellar mass. She was referred to neurosurgery for evaluation for surgical resection of her mass. Preoperatively, she was started on octreotide therapy as a temporizing measure because of her severe insulin resistance and marked elevation in growth hormone.

The mechanisms by which growth hormone excess in acromegaly leads to insulin resistance are complex and not fully elucidated. Growth hormone elicits a lipolytic effect, inducing hydrolysis of triglycerides to free fatty acids and glycerol.[3] It also worsens insulin resistance at the cellular level, not by a direct effect on the insulin receptor but by the uncoupling of downstream insulin-stimulated protein kinases, such as phosphatidylinositol-3-kinase and protein kinase B (Akt), thereby altering gene transcription and leading to decreased glucose transport into adipocytes.[4,5]

Concomitant to starting the patient on octreotide therapy, her insulin dosages were reduced in anticipation of decreasing insulin requirements because of a decrease in her growth hormone excess. Her regimen was changed to Lantus 50 units b.i.d. and Humalog 40 units QAC. Over the next few months, her IGF-1 levels decreased, and her HbA$_{1c}$ improved to 6.7%. She currently is awaiting surgical resection of her pituitary lesion.

Her case illustrates the importance of clinical suspicion and further evaluation for underlying causes in the face of severe insulin resistance, even though acromegaly usually does not present with insulin resistance of such severity.

REFERENCES

1. Ovalle F. Clinical approach to the patient with diabetes mellitus and very high insulin requirements. *Diabetes Res Clin Pract* 2010;90(3):231–242

2. Tritos NA, Mantzoros CS. Syndromes of severe insulin resistance. *J Clin Endocrinol Metab* 1998;83(9):3025–3030

3. Colao A, et al. Systemic complications of acromegaly: epidemiology, pathogenesis, and management. *Endocrine Rev* 2004;25(1):102–152

4. Takano A, et al. Growth hormone induces cellular insulin resistance by uncoupling phosphatidylinositol 3-kinase and its downstream signals in 3T3-L1 adipocytes. *Diabetes* 2001;50(8):1891–1900

5. Saltiel AR, Kahn CR. Insulin signalling and the regulation of glucose and lipid metabolism. *Nature* 2001;414(6865):799–806

Case 14

What Type of Diabetes?

Anthony L. McCall, PhD, FACP[1]

This patient is a 65-year-old woman who was referred to the clinic for continued treatment of her diabetes. Patient was diagnosed 5 years before her first visit (now 2 years later) with diabetes. Fasting glucose levels were elevated on routine blood work. Because her GAD-65 was positive and her C-peptide levels were low, she was uncertain about whether she had type 1 or type 2 diabetes. Her first HbA$_{1c}$ was 7%. Although BMI was normal, she lost 10 lb and watched her diet. Her HbA$_{1c}$ decreased to the 6.2–6.6% range. She was given a sliding-scale lispro and instructed to take 2 units if her blood glucose levels were >200 (11.1 mmol/L). When the patient attempted to follow this recommendation, she became hypoglycemic to ≤50 mg/dL (2.8 mmol/L) within 1–1.5 h after insulin injection. She never took oral antihyperglycemics. She had a history of gestational diabetes during her second pregnancy, which was diet controlled. Post delivery she had normal blood glucose levels.

Recently, fasting blood glucose levels were 80–90 (4.4–5 mmol/L), while 2 h postprandial blood glucose levels were 116–204 mg/dL (6.4–11.3 mmol/L). She had one symptomatic hypoglycemia to 60 mg/dL (3.3 mmol/L) without the use of insulin. She had a normal retinal exam and denied neuropathy symptoms. She had hyperlipidemia in the past, although her high-density lipoprotein (HDL) has always been high. She has been on simvastatin since 2009. Her 40 mg dose was decreased to 20 mg daily because of cramps. She also took aspirin 81 mg daily, calcium carbonate 600 mg daily, and levothyroxine 125 mcg 30–60 min before breakfast.

Her exam revealed the following:

Blood pressure	140/82 mmHg
Pulse	68 bpm
Height	1.638 m (5' 4.5")
Weight	55.339 kg (122 lb)
BMI	20.62 kg/m²

[1]University of Virginia School of Medicine and Health System, Charlottesville, VA.

DOI: 10.2337/9781580405713.14

Lab Results (date 1/12)

Component (reference range)	Value
HbA_{1c}	6.5%
Sodium (136–145 mmol/L)	138
Potassium (3.4–4.8 mmol/L)	3.7
Chloride (98–107 mmol/L)	101
CO_2 (23–31 mmol/L)	26
BUN (9.8–20.1 mg/dL)	24 (H)
Creatinine (0.6–1.1 mg/dL)	0.7
Glucose (74–99 mg/dL)	127 (H)
ALT (<55 units/L)	27
CALC GFR (mL/min/1.73 m^2)	>60
Cholesterol (<200 mg/dL)	221 (H)
Triglycerides (60–240 mg/dL)	54 (L)
HDL Cholesterol (35–85 mg/dL)	108 (H)
LDL Cholesterol (<130 mg/dL)	104
LDL-to-HDL Ratio (<2.8 ratio)	1.0
Cholesterol-to-HDL Ratio (<4.4 ratio)	2.0
Albumin, Ur (µg/mL)	16.0
Creatinine, Ur (mg/dL)	81.3
Microalbumin-to-Creatinine Ratio (<30 mg alb/g cre)	19.7
C-Peptide (0.50–2.00 ng/mL)	1.16
TSH (0.45–4.50 µIU/mL)	1.60
Free T4 (0.7–1.5 ng/dL)	1.31

When considering what type of diabetes this woman may have, her history of GAD Ab positivity, hyperthyroidism, lean body habitus, and elevated HDL are more indicative of an autoimmune etiology, such as late autoimmune diabetes in adults (LADA), resulting in the gradual β-cell loss over time as in type 1 diabetes.[1,2] This patient has kept her HbA$_{1c}$ within target range with diet and exercise for >8 years. When she will lose insulin secretory function is not clear. Her glycemic pattern indicates glucose intolerance after meals, but her fasting levels are normal. Her pancreatic insulin is sufficient to control her fasting glycemia.

Three treatment strategies seem plausible.[3] One would be to continue to monitor her A1C levels and act upon them once they increase over a threshold (e.g., 7%). Another would be to start small doses of basal insulin at 3–4 units in the morning to decrease her daytime hyperglycemia but avoid overnight hypoglycemia. A third option would be to start a dipeptidyl peptidase (DPP)-4 inhibitors that might aid insulin secretion and suppress meal glucagon if she has hyperglycemia but not risk hypoglycemia. The patient was advised to think about these options. We indicated that her HbA$_{1c}$ value was stable at ≤7%, but it was not necessary to make a change now. We mentioned there was evidence supporting the use of insulin relatively early in type 1 diabetes to preserve insulin secretion and that we may suggest a low-dose morning administration of nonpeaking insulin, such as glargine or detemir, that likely would wear off before the next morning and might be helpful and safer. Although a GLP-1 or DPP-4 inhibitor has theoretical appeal, no current evidence supports such use and probably would be a less desirable choice.

Based on frequent sampling of her blood glucose levels, her glycemic pattern is as follows (mg/dL):

FPG	2h PPG	pre-lunch	2h PPG	pre-supper	2h PPG
85	145	127	171	102	141

Her trend of HbA$_{1c}$ over 3 years very gradually increased and then recently came down as she was more vigorous in her lifestyle activity and dietary reduction in high-glycemic foods (Fig. 14.1):

This patient might be treated as a person with type 2 diabetes but has numerous features that are atypical and a strong family history of autoimmune disease: type 1 diabetes and autoimmune thyroid disease. She has a markedly elevated HDL, very low triglycerides, and is of lean body habitus and was never overweight—all not characteristic of type 2 diabetes.

When she was given insulin therapy with rapid analog using a sliding scale for postprandial hyperglycemia, she had repeated hypoglycemia to 50 mg/dL (2.8 mmol/L) or lower and was frightened by these and stopped insulin. Use of basal insulin now seems inappropriate at this point as her HbA$_{1c}$ is at goal and her fasting glucose is well controlled. A DPP-4 inhibitor or GLP-1 agonist might cause little or no hypoglycemia and works in a glucose-dependent fashion primarily affecting postprandial glucose. With no trials of such treatment in LADA, we

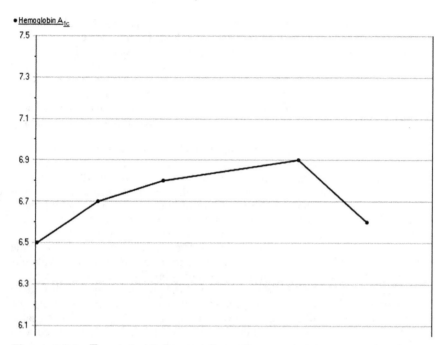

● Hemoglobin A$_{1c}$

Figure 14.1 — Trends in HbA$_{1c}$ over 3 years.

were reluctant to try them. Secretagogues like sulfonylureas would risk hypoglycemia and may accelerate insulin secretory loss. Her good glycemic control is important to sustaining her endogenous insulin production. She already has good control, however, and precisely when to intervene is unclear. This patient has a fairly stable course with >8 years of glycemic control that has kept her doing well. It is attractive to consider that if her HbA$_{1c}$ continues to rise gradually, that a small dose of levemir might be given in the morning and should avoid overnight lows. The most recent data on her HbA$_{1c}$ indicated that she still showed considerable benefit from increased activity and being careful with high-glycemic-load meals.

Most LADA patients are moderately stable but typically benefit from earlier insulin intervention.[4,5] A gradual progression from small doses of basal insulin to basal plus one or two rapid analog injections and eventually to full basal bolus therapy is used with gradual progression over months to years. This patient has a slower onset than average (possibly related to details of her immune abnormalities) and at some point probably will need a progressive insulin regimen. The potential for trials of immune intervention should be raised, but so far there has been some disappointment in the balance of efficacy and safety for immune interventions in type 1 diabetes, although good glycemic control and possibly vitamin D have shown some promise.

REFERENCES

1. Chaillous L, Bouhanick B, Kerlan V, Mathieu E, Lecomte P, Ducluzeau PH, Delamaire M, Sonnet E, Maugendre D, Maréchaud R, Rohmer V, Saï P, Charbonnel B. Clinical and metabolic characteristics of patients with latent auto-immune diabetes in adults (LADA): absence of rapid beta-cell loss in patients with tight metabolic control. *Diabetes Metab* 2010;36(1):64–70

2. Hillman M, Törn C, Landin-Olsson M; DISS study group. The glutamic acid decarboxylase 65 immunoglobulin G subclass profile differs between adult-onset type 1 diabetes and latent autoimmune diabetes in adults (LADA) up to 3 years after clinical onset. *Clin Exp Immunol* 2009;157(2):255–260

3. Guglielmi, C. Palermo, A. Pozzilli, P. Latent autoimmune diabetes in the adults (LADA) in Asia: from pathogenesis and epidemiology to therapy. *Diabetes Metab Res Rev* 2012;28(Suppl. 2):40–46

4. Brophy, S, Davies, H, Mannan, S, Brunt, H., Williams, R. Interventions for latent autoimmune diabetes (LADA) in adults. *Cochrane Database Syst Rev* 2011(9):CD006165

5. Montes, VN, Hirsch, IB. Treatment of LADA with etanercept. *Diabetes Care* 2012;35(5):e36

Case 15

Type 1 Diabetes versus LADA in a Patient Misdiagnosed with Type 2 Diabetes

Cecilia C. Low Wang, MD[1]

A. is a 42-year-old African American man referred for poorly controlled diabetes. He takes metformin 1 g b.i.d. and glargine insulin; his glargine dose recently was lowered from 45 units to 40 units daily. Review of his glucose monitoring device download revealed episodes of severe hyperglycemia up to the low 300s mg/dL (16.6 mmol/L) in the mornings, with hypoglycemic episodes as low as 40 mg/dL (2.2 mmol/L) fasting and midday. He has a physically demanding job and reports never skipping a meal; he feels hypoglycemic when he delays a meal. These episodes occur approximately twice a week, but hypoglycemia was detected four times per week on his blood glucose meter download. He denied peripheral neuropathy, blurry vision, polyuria, or weight changes. His family history included a parent with hypertension and a grandparent with diabetes. His medications included glargine 40 units SC QD, metformin 1 g bi.d., aspirin 81 mg q.i.d., and lisinopril 10 mg q.i.d.. He had no other medical problems and did not smoke or drink alcohol. His exam revealed the following:

BP	124/74 mmHg
Pulse	58 bpm
Height	1.829 m (6')
Weight	82 kg (180 lb)
BMI	24.4 kg/m^2

He was a well-appearing African American man in no acute distress. Thyroid was mildly enlarged without discrete nodules. Feet were in excellent condition with intact sensation to 10 g monofilament. Labs included the following:

A1C	9.1%
Total cholesterol	119 mg/dL
HDL cholesterol	62 mg/dL
Triglycerides	48 mg/dL
LDL cholesterol	47 mg/dL
Creatinine	1.3 mg/dL (0.4–1.2)
Urine microalbumin-to-creatinine ratio	16 (0–30 mg/G)

[1]Department of Medicine Division of Endocrinology, Metabolism and Diabetes; University of Colorado Anschutz Medical Campus School of Medicine, Aurora, CO.

DOI: 10.2337/9781580405713.15

This patient's diabetes history is significant for frequent hypoglycemia. Contributing factors include a physically strenuous occupation and too much basal insulin as evidenced by hypoglycemia when he delays a meal. He is relatively lean with low LDL cholesterol and high HDL cholesterol. Additional diabetes history is needed to design an approach to glycemic management.

His initial diagnosis of type 2 diabetes was made at age 23 years after hospitalization for flu-like symptoms. Whether he had diabetic ketoacidosis was unclear. He was started on insulin, but this was stopped after a few months because of hypoglycemia, and he was placed on "pills for diabetes." He remained on these for 5 years and then started on insulin for the next 14 years before presentation. He had no known chronic complications of diabetes, but he had not undergone a recent dilated retinal exam.

The patient describes a history concerning for late autoimmune diabetes of adulthood (LADA) versus type 1 diabetes. He had marked highs fluctuating with severe lows and a lean metabolic phenotype, suggestive of absolute insulin deficiency. LADA was first described as a form of diabetes diagnosed during adulthood with an indolent course, associated with diabetes autoantibodies and a slowly evolving autoimmune insulitis.[1] Part of the definition of LADA included not requiring insulin treatment for at least the first 6 months after diagnosis. Action LADA, a European study group, recently found that of 6,810 patients with adult-onset diabetes, 9.7% had diabetes autoimmunity mainly in the form of anti–glutamic acid decarboxylase (GAD) antibodies.[2] The distinction between LADA and adult-onset type 1 diabetes is not defined clearly using such criteria as age at diagnosis, history of DKA, or timing of insulin requirement after initial diagnosis. Furthermore, little information is available for ethnic minority populations. Recently, a retrospective study of GAD-antibody-positive patients with diabetes in the Los Angeles area found few phenotypic differences between patients with "typical" type 1 diabetes and LADA in an ethnic minority population,[3] suggesting that the distinction may not be clinically meaningful. The term "diabetes" is an umbrella term encompassing a heterogeneous group of metabolic disorders characterized by hyperglycemia. Only 5–10% of patients with adult-onset diabetes have diabetes-related autoimmunity, but even this single distinguishing feature encompasses different clinical phenotypes.[4] Younger age of onset (<50 years of age) and higher titer long after diagnosis (GAD antibody titer >4 units/mL) may be associated with higher likelihood of "requiring insulin" for control and survival.[5]

AL felt clammy and lightheaded during his clinic visit; a point of care glucose was <30 mg/dL (1.7 mmol/L). He was given three packets of glucose gel (total 45 g) with a resulting increase in blood glucose (BG) to 120 mg/dL (6.7 mmol/L). He was sent home with multiple packets of glucose gel and apple juice. He had heard of glucagon injections but had never received a prescription for it.

He almost certainly has hypoglycemia unawareness; his blood glucose meter download indicated the presence of undetected hypoglycemia, and he was able to speak and function normally without apparent cognitive dysfunction with a point-of-care (POC) glucose of <30 mg/dL (1.7 mmol/L). His documented fasting hyperglycemia was concerning for the Somogyi effect in response to overnight episodes of hypoglycemia. His basal insulin dose likely was providing prandial coverage and causing hypoglycemia with inadvertently delayed meals. His A1C likely reflected multiple episodes of undetected hypoglycemia averaged with severe hyperglycemia.

His glargine dose was decreased to 20 units daily and lispro insulin was started at a fixed dose of 6 units before breakfast and dinner because he was physically active during the day. He was reluctant to take insulin during the day because of a dusty and dirty work environment. The metformin was continued initially, and he was instructed to check his fingerstick BG at least twice a day, alternating among four possible time points (fasting/before breakfast, pre-lunch, pre-dinner, and bedtime) to provide enough data over the course of a week to make further adjustments to his insulin regimen.

His C-peptide was <0.1 (0.8–3.5 ng/mL) with simultaneous glucose of 119 mg/dL and glutamic acid decarboxylase antibody level of >250 (0–5 IU/ mL). At his follow-up visit, his overall average BG was 221 ± 115 mg/dL, range 61–546 mg/dL (3.4–30.3 mmol/L). He was having hypoglycemia with BG levels <70 mg/dL (3.9 mmol/L) only once a week, mostly occurring in the afternoon or evening after significant exertion. Repeat POC A1C was 9.2%.

He was considered to be an excellent candidate for continuous glucose monitoring and an insulin pump. The metformin was discontinued as it should be done in most cases of poorly controlled LADA. Making the diagnosis of LADA changed the overall approach to glycemic management in this patient. Diabetes-related autoimmunity should be considered in many patients with adult-onset diabetes.

REFERENCES

1. Tuomi T, Groop LC, Zimmet PZ, Rowley MJ, Knowles W, Mackay IR. Antibodies to glutamic acid decarboxylase reveal latent autoimmune diabetes mellitus in adults with a non-insulin-dependent onset of disease. *Diabetes* 1993;42(2):359–362

2. Hawa MI, Kolb H, Schloot N, Beyan H, Paschou SA, Buzzetti R, Mauricio D, De Leiva A, Yderstraede K, Beck-Nielsen H, Tuomilehto J, Sarti C, Thivolet C, Hadden D, Hunter S, Schernthaner G, Scherbaum WA, Williams R, Brophy S, Pozzilli P, Leslie RD; Action LADA Consortium. Adult-onset autoimmune diabetes in Europe is prevalent with a broad clinical phenotype: Action LADA 7. *Diabetes Care* 2013;36(4):908–913

3. Djekic K, Mouzeyan A, Ipp E. Latent autoimmune diabetes of adults is phenotypically similar to type 1 diabetes in a minority population. *J Clin Endocrinol Metab* 2012;97(3):E409–E413

4. Merger SR, Leslie RD, Boehm BO. The broad clinical phenotype of type 1 diabetes at presentation. *Diabet Med* 2013;30(2):170–178

5. Katahira MI, Hanakita M, Ito T, Suzuki M, Segawa S. The age of onset of diabetes and glutamic acid decarboxylase titer measured long after diagnosis are associated with the clinical stage of slow-onset type 1 diabetes. *Diabetes Res Clin Pract* 2013;99(2):93–97

Case 16

Type 1 Diabetes Can Present at Any Age

David S.H. Bell, MB[1]

CASE 1

A 49-year-old white man was diagnosed as having diabetes at age 34 years when he presented with polyuria, polydypsia, weight loss, and a blood glucose level of 367 mg/dL (20.4 mmol/L). He was placed on a diabetic diet for 2 years, and when his glucose levels were not controlled by diet alone, he was started on metformin and a sulfonylurea for 9 years until basal insulin was added at the age of 43 years. Even after three hospital admissions for diabetic ketoacidosis, short-acting insulin had not been added to his regimen.

When he finally saw an endocrinologist, his perception was that he had type 2 diabetes since that was what he always had been told. Reluctantly, he accepted the endocrinologist's opinion that he had type 1 diabetes. Finally, he was convinced by an undetectable C-peptide level and a GAD antibody level of greater than 30 IU/mL (normal <1 IU/mL). With this diagnosis, basal bolus therapy was intensified and there were no further hospital admissions for ketoacidosis. However, because of 15 years of undertreated diabetes, he had developed symptomatic distal symmetrical polyneuropathy, which was confirmed clinically by absent ankle jerks and decreased vibration sense in the feet and a loss of pinprick sensation to the knee bilaterally.

> Even after three hospital admissions for DKA, this patient's primary care physician still believed that this patient had type 2 diabetes. With a symptomatic late onset of diabetes in a patient who was never obese or had any of the manifestations of insulin resistance and who had developed ketoacidosis on three occasions, the presence of type 1 diabetes should have been recognized at a much earlier stage. In most patients with late autoimmune diabetes in adults (LADA) insulin should be started earlier, particularly if glycemia is poorly controlled when LADA diagnosis is made.

CASE 2

A 46-year-old white woman presented with candida vaginitis and was found to have a blood glucose level of 319 mg/dL (17.7 mmol/L). On further

[1]Clinical Professor, University of Alabama. Birmingham, AL.

DOI: 10.2337/9781580405713.16

questioning, she reported thirst, nocturia, and a 15-lb weight loss. Her BMI was 20 kg/m^2. She was started on metformin and a sulfonylurea because she was diagnosed as having type 2 diabetes. Although her blood glucose levels became well controlled (HbA$_{1c}$ 6.8%) on the metformin-sulfonylurea combination, she continued to lose weight. Upon consulting an endocrinologist, she was found to have a C-peptide of 1.8 ng/mL and a GAD antibody level of 274 IU/mL. She was placed on a basal bolus insulin regimen, and after 3 months, her HbA$_{1c}$ was 6.5%, and she had regained weight to her usual BMI of 23 kg/m^2. Some of the details of this case history have been previously published.[1]

Studies of European populations have shown that between 10 and 20% of diabetes developing after age 40 years is type 1 diabetes as evidenced by the presence of GAD antibodies. In the United Kingdom Prospective Diabetes Study (UKPDS), a study of patients with an onset of diabetes after age 40 years, the presence of GAD antibodies predicted that within 6 years insulin therapy would be needed. Similarly, in studies performed in subjects of European origin presumed to have type 2 diabetes, if GAD antibodies were present, insulin therapy was required within 1 year.[2,3]

The autoimmune attack on the pancreatic β-cells in type 1 diabetes is directed only at cells that are producing insulin. If the function of these cells can be taken over with exogenous insulin, and the production of endogenous insulin declines or ceases, the β-cells may be protected from the body's autoimmune attack. Alternatively, when secretagogues such as a sulfonylurea are utilized, the β-cell will be stimulated and potentially subject to a more intense autoimmune attack so that the progression toward total β-cell destruction will accelerate. Therefore, earlier utilization of insulin and avoidance of sulfonylurea might result in preservation of or a slower deterioration of β-cell function.[4] This preservation will result in reduced hypoglycemia and lower postprandial glucose levels and thus a lower HbA$_{1c}$.

CASE 3

A 50-year-old white man was admitted to the hospital for placement of a coronary artery stent and was found to have symptomatic hyperglycemia. His BMI was 28 kg/m^2, his waist circumference 38", and his waist-to-height ratio was 0.49. His HDL was 52 mg/dL and his fasting triglycerides 148 mg/dL (triglyceride-to-HDL ratio 2.85) and he was not hypertensive. Therefore, he had none of the manifestations of the insulin resistance syndrome. He was, however, based on his age, assumed to have type 2 diabetes and started on metformin.

On consulting with an endocrinologist, based on the clinical findings, a C-peptide level of 1.8 ng/mL, and a GAD antibody of 8.0 IU/mL (normal <5 ng/mL), he was diagnosed as having type 1 diabetes. He was immediately started on basal bolus insulin therapy.

In this case, the lack of features of the metabolic syndrome should have alerted the clinicians to suspect type 1 diabetes. Type 1 diabetes can occur even in obese subjects who have the features of the insulin resistance syndrome, however, so ideally with new-onset diabetes a GAD antibody level should be ordered, and if it is positive, insulin therapy should be initiated.[1]

GAD antibody testing is expensive, however, and a cheaper screening test would be preferable. C-Peptide is the fragment of the proinsulin molecule that remains when the α- and β-chains of the insulin molecule separate. C-Peptide, because of its longer half-life, is a better measure of endogenous insulin production than serum insulin levels and is more economic. In GAD-antibody-positive subjects, C-peptide levels at the time of diagnosis are in the low or low-normal range, whereas in type 2 diabetes, C-peptide levels are either high normal, high, or very high. Therefore, if the C-peptide level is low or low normal, a GAD antibody titer should be ordered to establish whether the patient has type 1 or type 2 diabetes.[1,5]

REFERENCES

1. Bell DSH. Should anti-glutamic acid decarboxylase antibody levels be determined in new-onset diabetes? *Endocr Pract* 2000;6(2):214–216

2. Turner R, Stratton I, Horton V, Manley S, Zimmet P, Mackay IR, Shattock M, Bottazzo GF, Holman R. UKPDS 25: autoantibodies to islet-cell cytoplasm and glutamic acid decarboxylase for prediction of insulin requirement in type 2 diabetes. UK Prospective Diabetes Study Group. *Lancet* 1997;350(9087):1288–1293

3. Pozzilli P, Di Mario U. Autoimmune diabetes not requiring insulin at diagnosis (latent autoimmune diabetes of the adult): definition, characterization, and potential prevention. *Diabetes Care* 2001;24(8):1460–1467

4. Kobayashi T, Nakanishi K, Murase T, Kosaka K. Small doses of subcutaneous insulin as a strategy for preventing slowly progressive beta-cell failure in islet cell antibody-positive patients with clinical features of NIDDM. *Diabetes* 1996;45(5):622–626

5. Bell DSH, Ovalle F. The role of C-peptide levels in screening for latent autoimmune diabetes in adults. *Am J Ther* 2004;11(4):308–311

Case 17

Is This Type 2 Diabetes, Type 1 Diabetes, or Late Autoimmune Diabetes in Adults?

DEVJIT TRIPATHY, MD, PhD;[1] SHEILA PINKSON, MPAS, PA-C;[1]
MAUREEN KOOPS, MD;[1] AND RALPH A. DEFRONZO, MD[1]

A 55-year-old African American woman was referred for management of uncontrolled diabetes. She was diagnosed with type 2 diabetes (T2D) when she was 44 years old during a routine physical exam and initially was started on metformin. After 2 years, glyburide was added, and 4 years later, glargine insulin was initiated following hospitalization for hyperglycemia with ketosis. She was discharged home on insulin, metformin, and glyburide. She reported that her glycemic control was still poor and she experienced wide swings in her glucose values, ranging from 60 to 400 mg/dL (3.3–22.2 mmol/L). At presentation, she was on glipizide, metformin, glargine, and premeal aspart insulin. On further questioning, she revealed that she had a history of hypothyroidism and pernicious anemia. Her vitamin B_{12} deficiency was so severe that it led to myelopathy and permanent weakness in her lower extremities. She has been on B-12 and levothyroxine. She denied skin pigmentation or history of adrenal insufficiency. Her other medications included simvastatin and lisinopril. She had a family history of T2D in both parents, but she denied any family history of other autoimmune diseases.

On examination, she was a moderately built woman in a wheelchair and was alert and oriented. There was no vitiligo. She had mild bilateral pitting edema and pedal pulses were intact. Her HbA_{1c} was 12.6% and blood glucose values throughout the day ranged from 100 to 400 mg/dL (5.5–22.2 mmol/L). Her clinical characteristics at the time of diagnosis are shown in Table 17.1.

The question arises as to what type of diabetes this patient has: type 1 diabetes (T1D) or T2D? On the basis of the clinical features, she did not fit into a clinical picture of a classical case of T2D. Although her diabetes was diagnosed when she was 44 years old, her BMI was 25 kg/m², she required insulin after approximately 4 years, and she has history of ketoacidosis and demonstrated wide swings in blood glucose levels. Also, her lipid profile was not consistent with that usually seen in T2D. She possibly does not have T1D, as she was diagnosed at 44 years of age on a routine physical and was on oral agents for approximately 4 years before requiring insulin. Of note, she has

[1]Audie L. Murphy VA Hospital, South Texas Veterans Health Care System, San Antonio, TX.

 DOI: 10.2337/9781580405713.17

Table 17.1 — Clinical Characteristics at the Time of Onset of Diabetes

Age (years)	44
BMI (kg/m²)	25.4
HbA$_{1c}$ (%)	12.6
Triglycerides (mg/dL)	118
HDL (mg/dL)	40
LDL (mg/dL)	128
Total cholesterol (mg/dL)	192

several autoimmune conditions and a history of diabetic ketoacidosis. Because of these features, GAD antibody was ordered and was noted to be very high (225 IU/mL).

Although diabetes is traditionally classified as T1D and T2D, there is significant heterogeneity at the time of presentation.[1] With a large number of youth now presenting with T2D, there is significant overlap with features of both T1D and T2D. Soon after islet cell antibody (ICA) was identified in T1D, Groop, Botazzo, and Doniach described the presence of ICA in approximately 10% of patients with clinical T2D.[2] ICA-positive patients with T2D were leaner, had lower fasting C-peptide, and progressed more rapidly to insulin requirement; thus, the term late autoimmune diabetes in adults (LADA) was coined. Later Tuomi et al. characterized this condition further and proposed the following diagnostic criteria: *1)* onset of diabetes after 35 years old, *2)* should be managed on oral hypoglycemic agents for at least 6 months, *3)* markers of autoimmunity, and *4)* GAD antibody should be present.[3] The prevalence of LADA varies in different populations with higher prevalence in the Scandinavian countries ~9%, about ~5% in the U.S., and <5% in Asian countries.[1,4] The genetic and metabolic characteristics of LADA patients are intermediate between T1D and the T2D. Although patients with LADA have more severe β-cell dysfunction and fewer features of metabolic syndrome compared with T2D, in the prediabetic state, there was no difference in measures of insulin secretion or insulin sensitivity between subjects with or without GAD antibody.

Clinically, individuals with an onset of diabetes between 20 and 40 years old are the most challenging for classification into T1D or T2D. Although T2D in youth is now seen relatively commonly, several cases of T1D are presenting at a later age. Thus, age of onset becomes a difficult differentiating factor. Other factors, such as insulin requirement and the presence of autoantibodies, help differentiate between T1D and T2D. Because the insulin requirement also may depend on personal preference or bias, testing for autoantibody appears to be the most helpful criteria. In our case, the patient had onset of diabetes after 35 years, was managed on oral agents for 4 years, and had high titers of GAD antibody.

We probably should not routinely screen all T2D patients for the presence of autoantibodies. The utility of antibody testing in management of T2D has not been tested and should be limited to a select group of patients in whom there is a diagnostic dilemma, such as the following: *1)* those with age of onset of diabetes 10–40 years old, *2)* those with ketosis-prone diabetes regardless of the age of onset, and *3)* patients with clinical T2D who have other autoimmune diseases. In our case, the patient had features of multiple autoimmune conditions (i.e., pernicious anemia and hypothyroidism), which suggests the possibility of polyglandular autoimmune syndrome.

The next important question addresses how to manage LADA. Few randomized trials have compared different agents in the treatment of LADA. A recent meta-analysis showed that sulfonylureas were associated with worse metabolic control and should be avoided in LADA.[5] The decision to start insulin should be based not on the antibody status but rather on the individual's glycemic control. In patients with poor glycemic control, insulin should be initiated as soon as the diagnosis of LADA is made. Novel therapeutic agents, such as dipeptidylpeptidase (DPP)-4 inhibitors, have been shown to maintain fasting and stimulated C-peptide levels, although the effects on glycemic control have been poor. There is no evidence for or against other drugs, such as glucagon-like peptide 1 (GLP-1) analogs or sodium-glucose co-transporter (SGLT)-2 inhibitors, in the treatment of LADA.

Although clinically, LADA may be classified as a distinct subtype of diabetes, it appears to be a continuum of varying degree of immune dysfunction seen in T1D and metabolic abnormalities seen in T2D. Sulfonylureas should be avoided in the treatment of patients with LADA. Newer drugs like GLP-1 analogs and SGLT-2 inhibitors might play an important role in the management of LADA in future.

REFERENCES

1. Tuomi T, Santoro N, Caprio S, Cai M, Weng J, Groop L. The many faces of diabetes: a disease with increasing heterogeneity. *Lancet* 2014;383(9922)1084–1094

2. Groop LC, Bottazzo GF, Doniach D. Islet cell antibodies identify latent type I diabetes in patients aged 35-75 years at diagnosis. *Diabetes* 1986;35:237–241

3. Tuomi T, Carlsson A, Li H, Isomaa B, Miettinen A, Nilsson A, Nissen M, Ehrnstrom BO, Forsen B, Snickars B, Lahti K, Forsblom C, Saloranta C, Taskinen MR, Groop LC. Clinical and genetic characteristics of type 2 diabetes with and without GAD antibodies. *Diabetes* 1999;48:150–157

4. Hawa MI, Kolb H, Schloot N, Beyan H, Paschou SA, Buzzetti R, Mauricio D, De Leiva A, Yderstraede K, Beck-Neilsen H, Tuomilehto J, Sarti C, Thivolet C, Hadden D, Hunter S, Schernthaner G, Scherbaum WA, Williams R, Brophy S, Pozzilli P, Leslie RD; Action LADA Consortium. Adult-onset autoimmune diabetes in Europe is prevalent with a broad clinical phenotype: Action LADA 7. *Diabetes Care* 2013;36:908–913

5. Brophy S, Davies H, Mannan S, Brunt H, Williams R. Interventions for latent autoimmune diabetes (LADA) in adults. *Cochrane Database of Systematic Reviews* 2011:CD006165

Case 18

A Common Misdiagnosis

Irene E. Schauer, MD, PhD[1,2]

M. is a 59-year-old Caucasian man referred to an endocrinology clinic for assistance with levothyroxine dosing for his hypothyroidism post I-131 ablation for Graves' disease about 8 years earlier. He had been noting increasing fatigue and weight loss that he associated with his thyroid medication and requested endocrinology consultation. His primary provider had decreased his LT4 dose by 15% 1 month prior to his endocrine visit in response to a reported thyroid-stimulating hormone (TSH) of 0.25 μIU/mL. The patient had noted no improvement in his symptoms with this change. His past medical history was also notable for an extensive, largely negative evaluation for chronic gastrointestinal pain, and a diagnosis of type 2 diabetes 3.5 years earlier. His medications included metformin (500 mg twice a day), levothyroxine (175 mcg 6 days a week), omeprazole, simvastatin (20 mg once daily), and lisinopril (2.5 mg once daily). He had been tried for a time on a sulfonylurea, but had hypoglycemia during exercise and was returned to metformin. As instructed, he was only checking occasional morning blood glucose levels, and these were all low to mid-100s mg/dL. He reported regular exercise, a generally active lifestyle, and no family history of diabetes.

On exam, he was a tall, thin, physically fit appearing Caucasian male in no acute distress. His thyroid was not palpable, and he appeared clinically euthyroid. Cardiopulmonary and abdominal exams were benign. His BMI, blood pressure, and most recent labs are shown in Table 18.1.

In light of his history of one known autoimmune disease, his healthy blood pressure and lipids, and his active lifestyle and lean body habitus, labs were ordered to reevaluate his diagnosis of type 2 diabetes (Table 18.1, column 2). Anti-GAD antibody was strongly positive and C-peptide, although within normal limits, was arguably low for his glucose level at the time. His diagnosis was revised to adult-onset type 1 diabetes.

Although the majority of adult-onset diabetes is type 2 diabetes, it is important to recognize that a significant portion is not. Recent literature from the Sweden-based ANDIS project places the percentage of adult-onset (age >35 years)

[1]Department of Medicine, University of Colorado Anschutz Medical Campus School of Medicine, Aurora, CO. [2]Research/Endocrine Sections, Denver Veterans Affairs Medical Center, Denver, CO.

DOI: 10.2337/9781580405713.18

Table 18.1—Baseline and Endocrine Visit Labs

	6 months prior	Endocrine visit
BMI (kg/m²)	23.4	23.6
Blood pressure (mmHg)	114/76	116/73
TSH (μIU/ml)	0.41	2.75
Total T4 (μg/dL)	13.7	15
T3RU (%)	32	
Total T3 (ng/dL)	118	
HbA$_{1c}$ (%)	7.5	8.5
HDL (mg/dL)	56	
Triglycerides (mg/dL)	86	
Anti-GAD Ab (units/ml)		>50
C-peptide (ng/mL)		1.6
Glucose (mg/dL)		128

diabetes that is autoantibody positive at about 7–12%, depending on the antibody titer cutoff that is used to define positivity.[1] These individuals are variably categorized as adult-onset type 1 diabetes or late autoimmune diabetes of adulthood (LADA). Although arguably a continuum of the same condition, autoimmune diabetes, recent evidence suggests that these diagnoses differ in the T-cell populations and autoantibodies, and therefore possibly the pathogenesis, involved.[2,3] It is clear, however, that these individuals represent a population that is clinically distinct from type 2 diabetes, and recognition of this condition has important clinical implications.[4]

First, the autoantibody positivity reflects a state of increased β-cell destruction and, as such, mandates closer attention to the level of glucose control and a more rapid transition to insulin therapy. The adult-onset autoantibody positive diabetes typically follows a more indolent course than younger-onset definitive type 1 diabetes, with a relatively long "honeymoon" phase not requiring insulin. These individuals, however, convert to insulin requirements much more rapidly and inevitably than do those who have type 2 diabetes. In addition, a recent Cochrane review[5] of intervention studies in LADA concluded that sulfonylurea treatment is contraindicated in this population, leading to a more rapid transition to insulin requirement (2-year conversion of 30% vs. 5% in the nonsulfonylurea group, $P < 0.001$). The review also cited evidence that earlier insulin therapy may help preserve β-cell function and maintain C-peptide levels for a longer period.

Our case patient was reasonably well controlled on metformin for >3 years. A trial of sulfonylurea treatment was not, perhaps fortunately, tolerated (likely because of his relatively normal insulin sensitivity, along with his highly active lifestyle). At the time of his endocrinology consult, he was rarely checking blood glucose levels and was unaware of the deterioration in his glycemic control. The initiation of once-daily basal insulin was sufficient to restore glycemic control (current A1C 5.8%) without causing any issues with hypoglycemia. He was continued on metformin for minimization of his insulin requirement and demand on his remaining β-cells, as well as for theoretical benefits for cardiovascular health.

Recognition of LADA/adult-onset type 1 diabetes is also important in that it promotes awareness of and clinically appropriate screening for other autoimmune conditions. Our case patient initially presented with vague and chronic complaints of diffuse abdominal pain, fatigue, and difficulty regaining weight that he lost with his original transition to diabetes. Although he attributed these symptoms to his thyroid condition, his normal TSH and lack of response to dose change argued against this. In light of his autoimmunity, celiac disease and adrenal insufficiency were immediately on the differential diagnosis, as recommended by the ADA standards of care. A random cortisol level of 14.8 µg/mL ruled out adrenal insufficiency and a celiac panel was negative. Complete blood count (CBC) and vitamin D levels revealed a mild anemia (hematocrit [Hct 37.1], mean corpuscular volume [MCV 84]) and an arguably progressive vitamin D insufficiency (25OH-vitamin D: 27.5 ng/mL in May 2011; 22.5 ng/mL in November 2011) concerning for antibody-negative celiac disease. A small bowel biopsy did not reveal any evidence of celiac disease. Follow-up labs revealed progression of his anemia (Hct to 29.8, MCV 74). Although his low MCV argued against pernicious anemia alone, vitamin B_{12} levels were also checked and showed a recent progression to mild vitamin B_{12} insufficiency (vitB$_{12}$: 895 to 386 to 249 pg/mL over a 2-year period). At this time, the full etiology of his anemia remains unclear. Extensive gastrointestinal workup failed to reveal any evidence of bleeding, and hematology workup revealed no evidence of hemolysis or a bone marrow defect. He was given a series of parenteral iron administrations and prescribed vitamin B_{12} and his anemia has resolved.

REFERENCES

1. Groop L, Pociot F. Genetics of diabetes—are we missing the genes or the disease? *Molec Cell Endocrinol* 2014;382:726–739

2. Ramachandra GN, Brooks-Worrell BM, Palmer JP. Latent autoimmune diabetes in adults. *J Clin Endocrinol Metab* 2009:94:4635–4644

3. Nambam, B, Aggarwal S, Jain A. Latent autoimmune diabetes in adults: a distinct but heterogeneous clinical entity. *World J Diabetes* 2010;1:111–115

4. Appel, SJ, Wadas TM, Rosenthal RS, Ovalle F. Latent autoimmune diabetes of adulthood (LADA): an often misdiagnosed type of diabetes mellitus. *J Amer Acad Nurse Practitioners* 2009;21:156–159

5. Brophy, S, Davies H, Mannan S, Brunt H, Williams R. Interventions for latent autoimmune diabetes (LADA) in adults (review). *Cochrane Library* 2011;9:1–79

Case 19
Almost All Nonobese Young People with an Acute Onset of Diabetes Have Type 1 Diabetes

David S.H. Bell, MB[1]

CASE 1

A 24-year-old college senior who was a starting linebacker on a Division 1 football team and who had an excellent chance of being drafted by the National Football League (NFL), developed polyuria, polydypsia, and weight loss. In spite of a blood glucose of >300 mg/dL (16.7 mmol/L) the team doctor decided that he had type 2 diabetes and started him on a low-calorie diet without either insulin or oral agents. This resulted in a catastrophic weight loss of >30 lb. He then was started on a sulfonylurea, which controlled his glucose to a range between 100 mg/dL and 150 mg/dL (5.5–8.3 mmol/L), but this did not decelerate his weight loss. The resultant severe weight loss ruined his chances of being drafted by the NFL and resulted in the loss of significant future income.

When he finally saw an endocrinologist, his GAD antibody level was high and C-peptide was undetectable. To obtain glycemic control and regain weight, he needed continuous subcutaneous insulin infusion (CSSI or pump therapy) because of severe and frequent hypoglycemia, which had occurred without adequate glycemic control on basal bolus insulin therapy.

This patient clearly had type 1 diabetes, which at the time of onset could have been diagnosed with a positive GAD antibody. Because insulin is an anabolic hormone, the weight loss could have been reversed and the weight even could have increased with insulin therapy.[1] Indeed, a high-caloric diet matched with insulin therapy would have enhanced his prospects for the NFL. Furthermore, starting a sulfonylurea instead of insulin might improve glycemic control in some patients, but it will accelerate weight loss because of persistently lower insulin levels that despite lowering blood glucose levels somewhat, cannot suppress catabolism and maintain muscle mass.[2]

CASE 2

A 22-year-old white man, who was also a lineman in a Division 1 college football team, during his junior season developed nocturia and lost 10 lb.

[1]Clinical Professor, University of Alabama, Birmingham, AL.

 DOI: 10.2337/9781580405713.19

He finally was diagnosed as having diabetes with a fasting blood glucose of 340 mg/dL (18.9 mmol/L). His C-peptide was measured and was in the lower normal range, and because his insulin antibody level was normal, he was diagnosed by the team physician as having type 2 diabetes and started on metformin. While on metformin, he continued to lose weight, and sitagliptin was added to his regimen. This did not affect the weight loss, which continued. When he was finally assessed by an endocrinologist, his C-peptide level was 2.1 ng/mL (normal fasting 0.8–3.5 ng/mL), and his GAD antibody titer was 11.25 units/mL (normal 0–1.45 units/mL). He was therefore started on insulin. The goal of insulin therapy in conjunction with a high-calorie diet was to restore his weight to its previous level and maintain this weight gain until the end of his college career when his calorie intake and insulin doses would be lowered. When the training staff were informed that he had type 1 diabetes and would need insulin therapy, the coach awarded a "medical redshirt" (i.e., the patient kept his scholarship but did not retain a place on the team for medical reasons).

Once again this patient clearly had type 1 diabetes, which would have been diagnosed if the correct antibody had been ordered.[3] In addition, he could, with the help of insulin therapy, have been able to play his senior year. After the coach's discriminatory decision, the player realized that if he turned down the "medical redshirt" offer, his playing time would have been very limited and not worth the "pain and effort of practice."

CASE 3

The Case 2 patient's future brother-in-law also developed diabetes. He was asymptomatic when he attended a "job fair" on the campus of a state university where he had his glucose checked and with a reading of 270 mg/dL (15 mmol/L) diabetes was diagnosed. He was referred to the campus diabetes center, where he was seen only by a physician extender, and based on a positive C-peptide reading, he was told that he had type 2 diabetes and was started on metformin.

Fifteen months later he saw an endocrinologist. At that time his C-peptide level was 1.1 ng/mL (normal fasting 0.8–3.5 ng/mL) and his GAD antibody level was 6.6 IU/mL (normal 0–5.0 IU/mL). He had lost 12 lb (7% of his body weight) over the previous 15 months with metformin therapy and his BMI was 22 kg/m². With insulin he returned to his usual body weight of 170 lb.

In this case, the clinical history should have been enough to suspect type 1 diabetes. Utilizing a C-peptide level to distinguish between type 1 and type 2 diabetes may not always be appropriate because during the early phase of type 1 diabetes, the C-peptide level is often normal.[4] This is especially true when high glucose levels are reversed irrespective of the method that is utilized to lower the glucose. This occurs because relieving "glucotoxicity" results in increased insulin sensitivity and improved endogenous insulin release.

In addition, ~10% of patients with type 1 diabetes permanently retain endogenous insulin production. These patients are usually of the HLA B_8/DR_3 haplotype and also more frequently have other autoimmune diseases, such as Hashimoto's thyroiditis, leading to hypothyroidism, pernicious anemia, Addison's disease, or hypoparathyroidism.[5]

Diagnosing type 1 diabetes is not difficult with a typical clinical presentation. Appropriate utilization of laboratory tests should confirm and not contradict the clinical impression.

REFERENCES

1. Malone JI. Growth and sexual maturation in children with insulin-dependent diabetes mellitus. *Curr Opin Pediatr* 1993;5(4):494–498

2. Maruyama T, Tanaka S, Shimada A, Funae O, Kasuga A, Kanatsuka A, Takei I, Yamada S, Harii N, Shimura H, Kobayashi T. Insulin intervention in slowly progressive insulin-dependent (type 1) diabetes mellitus. *J Clin Endocrinol Metab* 2008;93(6):2115–2121

3. Bingley PJ, Williams AJ. Islet autoantibody testing: an end to the trials and tribulations? *Diabetes* 2013;62(12):4009–4011

4. Weir GC, Bonner-Weir S. Islet β cell mass in diabetes and how it relates to function, birth, and death. *Ann NY Acad Sci* 2013;1281:92–105

5. Keenan HA, Sun JK, Levine J, Doria A, Aiello LP, Eisenbarth G, Bonner-Weir S, King GL. Residual insulin production and pancreatic ß-cell turnover after 50 years of diabetes: Joslin Medalist Study. *Diabetes* 2010;59(11):2846–2853

Case 20
Symptomatic Postprandial Hyperglycemia

Amita Maturu, MD,[1] and Michael McDermott, MD[1]

A 54-year-old woman was referred to our clinic for evaluation of spells. The patient noted intermittent symptoms of palpitations, difficulty concentrating, and diaphoresis lasting several hours once or twice a week. For days following the spells she had anorexia and lost 15 lb during the course of a year. Her primary care physician completed an extensive spell workup before referral to endocrinology and no clear cause was identified.

A spell can be defined as a "sudden onset of a symptom or symptoms that are recurrent, self-limited, and stereotypic in nature." The common differential diagnosis for episodic symptoms from an endocrinology perspective includes pheochromocytoma, thyrotoxicosis, menopause, medullary thyroid carcinoma, pancreatic islet cell tumors, carcinoid syndrome, and hypoglycemia.[1]

An oral glucose tolerance test (OGTT) was performed during the course of her workup. The reason it was ordered is unclear, but the results were surprising in this patient without a known history of diabetes. Her results revealed the following:

Baseline blood glucose	87 mg/dL (4.8 mmol/L)
30-min glucose	197 mg/dL (10.9 mmol/L)
60-min glucose	320 mg/dL (17.8 mmol/L)
120-min glucose	278 mg/dL (15.4 mmol/L)

She noted spell symptoms during the 5-h OGTT, which resolved after several hours. Given her lean stature, there was a concern for type 1 diabetes. Her hemoglobin A1c (HbA$_{1c}$) was found to be 5.5%. A C-peptide level was 2.8 ng/mL with a serum glucose of 155 mg/dL (8.6 mmol/L). Antiglutamic acid decarboxylase, anti-insulin, and anti-islet cell antibodies were negative.

The diagnosis of diabetes can be made with an HbA$_{1c}$ ≥6.5%, a fasting plasma glucose ≥126 mg/dL (7 mmol/L), or an oral glucose tolerance test with a plasma glucose ≥200 mg/dL (11.1 mmol/L). This patient clearly fits the diagnosis of diabetes based on her OGTT (albeit her HbA$_{1c}$ was 5.5%); however, the type of diabetes she has is less clear. Her lean stature and lack

[1]Division of Endocrinology, Diabetes and Metabolism, University of Colorado, Aurora, CO.
DOI: 10.2337/9781580405713.20

of family history point more toward type 1 diabetes. The C-peptide level is not informative as it was not conclusively high or low. Her antibodies were negative, but this does not exclude type 1B diabetes, which is characterized by negative β-cell autoimmunity markers, lack of HLA association, and fluctuating insulin levels.[2] As she is likely early in the course of her disease, further data and time should allow for proper classification.

At the time of endocrinology consultation, a thorough medical history was obtained. Her past medical history was significant for degenerative disk disease and a hysterectomy and bilateral oophorectomy 10 years ago. Her home medications included estrotest 1.25 mg, vicodin as needed for back pain, and trazodone daily for insomnia. She had no family history of neuroendocrine tumors. She denied any tobacco or illicit drug exposure. She did consume one glass of wine nightly. The patient confirmed postprandial hyperglycemia and reported several self-monitored blood glucose readings >200 mg/dL (11.1 mmol/L) after meals. She noted that her postprandial hyperglycemia occurred only after eating high-carbohydrate foods. She reported symptoms of palpitations, diaphoresis, weakness, and difficulty concentrating associated with the hyperglycemia.

We hypothesized that the patient's symptoms were due to an exaggerated physical response to fluctuating blood glucose. Adrenergic symptoms have been noted in patients with elevated blood glucose that rapidly decline to normal, sometimes termed relative hypoglycemia [3] Furthermore, studies have demonstrated decreased energy and reduced cognitive function during hyperglycemic episodes in patients with type 2 diabetes.[4] Fluctuating blood sugars in the absence of hypoglycemia is not a common consideration in the differential diagnosis of a spell, but given that other causes had been ruled out, this seemed to best explain the patient's subjective complaints and objective findings.

To reduce postprandial blood glucose fluctuations, we prescribed repaglinide 0.5 mg before breakfast and lunch (highest carbohydrate meals). The patient was asked to monitor her blood glucose closely while taking this medication. She had two symptomatic hypoglycemic episodes about 4 h after taking the medication and self-discontinued repaglinide. She continued to have spells during the day, but noted if she skipped breakfast and lunch, she no longer had symptoms. For 1 month, she ate only one meal in the evening, resulting in the resolution of her spells but an additional 10 lb weight loss. She then developed symptomatic fasting hypoglycemia (self-monitoring) with resolution of her symptoms after drinking juice.

This patient meets criteria for suspicion of Whipple's triad (symptoms of hypoglycemia, documented hypoglycemia, resolution of symptoms with oral intake). Our differential diagnosis for hypoglycemia in this patient included adrenal insufficiency, surreptitious insulin use, IGF-2 producing parenchymal tumor, malnutrition, or an insulinoma.[5]

We admitted the patient for a standard 72-h fast for further evaluation. She developed symptomatic hypoglycemia approximately 35 h into the fast.

Table 20.1—Laboratory Testing during 72-h Fast

Lab test	Value	Normal reference range
Serum glucose	53 mg/dL	70–199 mg/dL
Insulin	<1 μIU/mL	2–23 μIU/mL
Proinsulin	<2.5 pmol/L	≤26.8 pmol/L
C-Peptide	0.1 ng/mL	0.8–3.5 ng/mL
β-Hydroxybutyrate	40.7 mg/dL	0.0–3.0 mg/dL
Glucagon stimulated glucose (30 min)	55 mg/dL	N/A
Glucagon stimulated glucose (60 min)	62 mg/dL	N/A

Labs obtained at this point are outlined in Table 20.1. Results were not consistent with endogenous hyperinsulinemia or surreptitious insulin use. An adrenocortotropic hormone (ACTH; cosyntropin) stimulation test was negative, ruling out adrenal insufficiency. A computed tomography scan of the abdomen and pelvis was performed, and no abnormalities were noted (no evidence of a parenchymal tumor). After this extensive negative workup, we concluded that her hypoglycemia was due to malnourishment. This diagnosis was consistent with her elevated β-hydroxybutyrate level during the fast and the limited glucose response to glucagon.

We advised the patient to consume at least three meals daily to improve her nutritional stores. We prescribed acarbose (25 mg) before lunch and dinner to reduce postprandial fluctuations. Since starting this medication, she has been eating three meals regularly without experiencing recurrent spell symptoms. Her self-monitored blood glucose levels remained <200 mg/dL (11.1 mmol/L) following meals, but most recently she stopped monitoring closely given the drastic improvement in her symptoms.

Our patient may have the beginning stages of antibody-negative type 1 diabetes of adulthood. She is extremely sensitive to blood glucose fluctuations, and her spells were due to rapid increase and then decrease of her blood glucose levels following high-carbohydrate meals. Because of the severity of her symptoms, she limited her oral intake and eventually developed hypoglycemia associated with malnutrition. By prescribing acarbose, we were able to reduce her symptomatic postprandial fluctuations and allow her to eat regular meals.

REFERENCES

1. Van Loon, et al. The evaluation of spells. *Netherlands J Med* 2011;69:7–8

2. Aguilera E, et al. Adult-onset atypical (type 1) diabetes: additional insights and differences with type 1A diabetes in a European Mediterranean population. *Diabetes Care* 2004;27(5):1108–1114

3. Sandler B. *Diet prevents polio*, 1st ed. Lee Foundation for Nutritional Research, 1951.

4. Sommerfield, et al. Acute hyperglycemia alters mood state and impairs cognitive performance in people with type 2 diabetes. *Diabetes Care* 2004;27(10): 2335–2340

5. Ng CL. Hypoglycemia in nondiabetic patients–an evidence. *Aust Fam Physician* 2010;39(6):399–404

Case 21

A Patient with Newly Diagnosed, Asymptomatic Hyperglycemia

Aidan McElduff, MD[1]

A 31-year-old man was found to have a fasting plasma glucose of 8.3 mmol/L (150 mg/dL) at a routine medical examination. He was asymptomatic. His past medical history was unremarkable. There was no family history of diabetes. He worked as an air traffic controller, which was the reason for his routine medical examination. His laboratory results revealed the following:

Weight	80.30 kg
Height	177.0 cm
BMI	25.6 kg/m²
Pulse	regular
Blood pressure	140/80 mmHg

The feet were in good condition with no evidence of sensory neuropathy. The ankle jerks were preserved. The pedal pulses were palpable. There were no carotid bruits. Urinalysis, including albuminuria, was negative. Physical examination was otherwise unhelpful.

In an asymptomatic patient with elevated venous plasma glucose the diagnosis of diabetes should be confirmed by a repeat measurement. The repeat measurement need not be a glucose measurement. In this case, a hemoglobin A1c (HbA$_{1c}$) of 8.4% confirmed the diagnosis of diabetes.[1]

A screen for islet cell antibodies revealed a high titer of IA-2 antibodies with negative GAD and insulin antibodies, confirming this as type 1 diabetes. This has been called late autoimmune diabetes in adults (LADA), although in reality, it is simply slowly evolving type 1 diabetes that, therefore, usually presents in adults.

When a patient is first seen with newly diagnosed diabetes, it is worth considering the underlying etiology, as this may help determine the most appropriate therapeutic approach, particularly if the patient does not have the typical features of type 2 diabetes (older, fatter, inactive with a positive family history).

Type 1 diabetes presents classically with weight loss, polyuria, polydipsia, and ketosis in a younger patient; however, it can be detected at any stage in its evolution.[2] The presence of a variety of islet cell autoantibodies confirms the

[1]Discipline of Medicine, Sydney University, Sydney, NSW, Australia.

DOI: 10.2337/9781580405713.21

diagnosis of type 1 diabetes, but their absence does not exclude this diagnosis. Without a specific identification as type 1 diabetes, many practitioners and patients are slow to start insulin even when treatment does not achieve the target HbA_{1c}.[3]

In a young patient with a strong, particularly an autosomal dominant, family history, genetic mutations have been found that cause dysfunction of pancreatic β cells,[4] and autoantibodies are almost always absent. This is known as maturity-onset diabetes of the young (MODY), although this name likely will be replaced by the name of the specific mutations: MODY accounts for 1 to 2% of cases of diabetes. It is usually diagnosed before the age of 25 years. The six genes listed in Table 21.1 account for most cases of MODY. The most common conditions are MODY 2 and 3. It is important because identifying the mutation may significantly alter treatment.

Mutations in the hepatic nuclear factor genes result in MODY 1 and 3. These mutations are associated with hyperglycemia that leads to microvascular complications so these patients require treatment. They may have been born large, and experienced postnatal hypoglycemia, and they have glycosuria. The mutations produce an insulin deficiency picture that is likely to be mistaken for type 1 diabetes, but the patients do not become totally insulin deficient with time. These patients may be particularly sensitive to therapy with sulfonyl-ureas. Early in the disease, glycemic control may be better with a sulfonylurea than with insulin.

In MODY 2 a mutation causes a defect in glucokinase—a glycolytic enzyme. This results in fasting hyperglycemia, but little postprandial hyperglycemia. During a glucose tolerance test, despite the fasting hyperglycemia, the rise in blood glucose after a glucose load is <3 mmol/L (54 mg/dL).

Recognizing MODY 2 is important, as it is not associated with microvascular complications and thus it does not require intensive treatment to control blood glucose. There are, however, two major cautions: the hyperglycemia is often first detected during pregnancy and may require treatment. The risk

Table 21.1—The Genetics of Maturity-Onset Diabetes of the Young (MODY)

Condition	Gene affected	Chromosome affected
MODY 1	HNF-4-α	Chromosome 20
MODY 2*	glucokinase	Chromosome 7
MODY 3**	HNF-1-α	Chromosome 12
MODY 4	IPF-1	Chromosome 13
MODY 5	HNF-1	Chromosome 17
MODY 6	NeuroD1	Chromosome 2

*13% of MODY cases
**70% of MODY cases

to the fetus depends on whether the fetus also has the mutation. Unaffected fetuses are at risk of being oversized, whereas affected fetuses may be undersized if the mother's hyperglycemia is treated.[5] The second is that a glucokinase mutation does not protect against developing type 2 diabetes. The risk is thought to be the same as in the general population.

A prototype MODY Probability Calculator is available at www.diabetes genes.org/content/mody-probability-calculator. At this time it is also worth considering the possibility of an undiagnosed disease or a medication is contributing to the hyperglycemia.[1] This should be a clinical assessment.

His questions were related to therapy and to the problems hypoglycemia or poorly controlled diabetes would cause with his employment.

Hypoglycemia can result in a sudden impairment of cognitive function placing the patient, and anyone depending on the patient's cognitive skills, in danger. The risk of hypoglycemia as a result of pharmacological treatment restricts or limits many activities that we take for granted. This is best documented with driving (see "Diabetes and Employment" and "Diabetes and Driving" in the ADA Standards of Care).

Initial therapy was a diet and exercise regimen, metformin, and linagliptin targeting a normal BMI and HbA$_{1c}$ in the absence of hypoglycemia. Twenty-one months later, the BMI was 23.7 kg/m^2 and the HbA$_{1c}$ 5.8%. He has not experienced any hypoglycemia. He has passed his 6 monthly employment reviews.

REFERENCES

1. American Diabetes Association. Standards of medical care in diabetes, 2015. *Diabetes Care* 2015;38(Suppl. 1):S1–S93

2. Zinman B, Kahn SE, Haffner SM, O'Neill MC, Heise MA, Freed MI. Phenotypic characteristics of GAD antibody-positive recently diagnosed patients with type 2 diabetes in North America and Europe. *Diabetes* 2004;53:3193–200

3. Peyrot M, Rubin RR, Lauritzen T, Skovlund SE, Snoek FJ, Matthews DR, Landgraf R, Kleinebreil L, and International DAWN Advisory Panel. Resistance to insulin therapy among patients and providers. Results of the cross-national Diabetes Attitudes, Wishes, and Needs (DAWN) study. *Diabetes Care* 2005;28:2673–2679

4. Shields BM, Hicks S, Shepherd MH, Colclough K, Hattersley AT, Ellard S. Maturity-onset diabetes of the young (MODY): how many cases are we missing? *Diabetologia* 2010;53:2504–2508

5. Colom C, Corcoy R. Maturity onset diabetes of the young and pregnancy. *Best Pract Res Clin Endocrinol Metab* 2010;24:605–615

Case 22

Glucokinase Maturity-Onset Diabetes of the Young and Pregnancy

Jill Apel, MD,[1] and Chung-Kay Koh, MD[1]

A 31-year-old woman with maturity-onset diabetes of the young (MODY) with the glucokinase gene mutation (GCK-MODY) presented for preconception counseling She was diagnosed at age 28 years after her mother was diagnosed with GCK-MODY. Her fasting blood glucose levels were mildly elevated and HbA$_{1c}$ ranged 6.5–6.8%. Her only sibling also was diagnosed with GCK-MODY. Her mother had mildly elevated glycemia during her pregnancies but was not treated. The birth weights of the patient and her sister were ~7 lb.

MODY encompasses monogenic disorders of β-cell dysfunction with autosomal dominant transmission. It often is diagnosed before the age of 25 years and is estimated to cause up to 5% of diabetes diagnosed before the age of 45 years.[1] It is characterized by persistent endogenous insulin secretion and an absence of β-cell autoimmunity, obesity, or insulin resistance. The subtypes of MODY are classified by the affected gene, and each has its own disease characteristics.

GCK-MODY, formerly known as MODY2, is the second most common subtype of MODY. It is caused by a mutation of the glucokinase gene on chromosome 7. Glucokinase is a key regulatory enzyme in glucose metabolism and glucose-stimulated insulin secretion. A heterozygous inactivating mutation of the GCK gene increases the set point for glucose-stimulated insulin secretion, but it does not affect the insulin secretion capacity. This manifests as persistent, mild hyperglycemia and a mildly elevated HbA$_{1c}$ (<8%). Outside of pregnancy, it requires no treatment because it does not predispose to microvascular or macrovascular complications.[2]

Genetic testing for GCK-MODY should be considered in patients who are not obese with β-cell autoantibody negative diabetes diagnosed at a young age, an autosomal-dominant pattern of inheritance, insulin independence, and persistent mildly elevated fasting glucose. It can be detected during screening for diabetes in pregnancy. A recent study of a predominantly white European population found the prevalence of GCK-MODY in pregnancy is 0.1% and the prevalence in women with gestational diabetes is 0.9%.[3] Their results suggest that pregnant women with a normal prepregnancy BMI (<25 kg/m^2) and a fasting glucose ≥99 mg/dL (5.5 mmol/L) should be tested for GCK-MODY.

[1]Division of Endocrinology, Rush University Medical Center, Chicago, IL.

                                        DOI: 10.2337/9781580405713.22

It is important to make the diagnosis of GCK-MODY because it is treated differently from diabetes in pregnancy.

Our patient wants to know the effect of her GCK-MODY on future offspring.

Usually, maternal hyperglycemia causes increased fetal insulin secretion resulting in an increased birth weight. In maternal GCK-MODY, the effect on birth weight depends on whether the baby inherits the mutation (Table 22.1).[4] Babies without the mutation are exposed to maternal hyperglycemia, secrete more insulin, and have an average 600-g increase in birth weight. Babies with maternally inherited GCK-MODY have an increased set point for glucose-stimulated insulin secretion and therefore secrete a normal amount of insulin in with maternal hyperglycemia and have a normal birth weight. Babies with paternally inherited GCK-MODY have an increased set point for glucose-stimulated insulin secretion but are exposed to the normal glucose levels of the mother. This causes decreased insulin secretion and an average 500-g decrease in birth weight.

The decision to treat GCK-MODY during pregnancy is based on the genotype of the fetus. The fetal genotype is inferred by fetal growth assessed by abdominal circumference measurement on ultrasound at the beginning of the third trimester (27 weeks). If the fetus is not large (abdominal circumference ≤75th percentile for gestational age), the fetus may have GCK MODY and no treatment is needed for maternal hyperglycemia. If the fetus is large (abdominal circumference >75th percentile for gestational age), the fetus most likely does not have the mutation and the treatment goal is maternal euglycemia to prevent macrosomia and postnatal hypoglycemia. This can be achieved by treatment with insulin or glyburide.

Our patient wants to know the effect of her GCK MODY on the long-term health of future offspring.

A study of 447 subjects from 37 GCK-MODY pedigrees looked at long-term outcomes of maternal GCK-MODY and the inheritance of GCK-MODY. As adults, subjects were grouped by the presence of maternal GCK-MODY, the inheritance of GCK-MODY, both, or neither. Of those without GCK-MODY, there was no difference in the fasting plasma glucose, 2 h glucose during an oral glucose tolerance test, insulin secretion, or insulin sensitivity in

Table 22.1—Birth Weight in Children with GCK-MODY Mutation

Maternal mutation	Fetal mutation	Change in birth weight	Therapy
+	−	+ 600 g	Aim for euglycemia
−	+	− 500 g	None
+	+	No change	None—do not treat hyperglycemia

those born to mothers with or without GCK-MODY. There was also no difference in these variables comparing subjects with GCK-MODY born to mothers with or without GCK-MODY. These results imply that maternal GCK-MODY does not independently increase the risk of metabolic disease.[5]

The diagnosis of GCK-MODY is important because it is treated differently from diabetes in pregnancy. The treatment is based on the genotype of the fetus, which is inferred by fetal growth.

REFERENCES

1. Thanabalasingham G, Pal A, Selwood MP, Dudley C, Fisher K, Bingley PJ, Ellard S, Farmer AJ, McCarthy MI, Owen KR. Systematic assessment of etiology in adults with a clinical diagnosis of young-onset type 2 diabetes is a successful strategy for identifying maturity-onset diabetes of the young. *Diabetes Care* 2012;35:1206–1212

2. Thanabalasingham G, Owen KR. Diagnosis and management of maturity onset diabetes of the young (MODY). *BMJ* 2011;343:d6044

3. Chakera AJ, Spyer G, Vincent N, Ellard S, Hattersley AT, Dunne FP. The 0.1% of the population with glucokinase monogenic diabetes can be recognized by clinical characteristics in pregnancy: the Atlantic Diabetes in Pregnancy cohort. *Diabetes Care* 2014;37:1230–1236

4. Hattersley AT, Beards F, Ballantyne E, Appleton M, Harvey R, Ellard S. Mutations in the glucokinase gene of the fetus result in reduced birth weight. *Nat Genet* 1998;19:268–270

5. Velho G, Hattersley AT, Froguel P. Maternal diabetes alters birth weight in glucokinase-deficient (MODY2) kindred but has no influence on adult weight, height, insulin secretion or insulin sensitivity. *Diabetologia* 2000;43:1060–1063

Case 23

Latent Autoimmune Diabetes of the Adult (LADA) in an Elderly Patient

Monica Shah, MD;[1] Mahtab Sohrevardi, MD;[1] and David Baldwin, MD[1]

An 80-year-old woman presented to endocrine clinic with complaints of weight loss, anorexia, and severe bilateral lower extremity pain and numbness. Two years ago she was diagnosed with type 2 diabetes; her BMI was 17 kg/m², blood pressure (BP) was 100/75 mmHg, and HbA$_{1c}$ was 7.4%. She was treated with metformin 1,000 mg twice daily, but her blood glucose levels remained in the 200s mg/dL (11.1 mmol/L). She had not tried any other medications. She had been told to limit her diet to control her diabetes and her weight decreased from 120 to 80 lb.

The patient has a sister with thyroid disease and a daughter with multiple sclerosis. On physical exam, BP was 110/78 mmHg; heart rate was 68 (standing); and thyroid, cardiac, and abdominal exams were normal. She had considerable muscle wasting and neurologic examination revealed diminished vibratory sensation in the lower extremities. Repeat HbA$_{1c}$ was 8.8%. Additional lab work was notable for positive glutamic acid decarboxylase (GAD), islet cell, and thyroid peroxidase antibodies, thyroid-stimulating hormone (TSH) 15.4 μIU/mL, free T4 0.7 ng/dL, and low vitamin B$_{12}$.

At the time of evaluation, this patient was struggling with severe weight loss and peripheral neuropathy, symptoms characteristic of diabetic neuropathic cachexia. This syndrome was first described by Ellenberg in 1973 and most commonly occurs in middle-age men with fairly well-controlled type 2 diabetes but also may occur in women and in those who have type 1 diabetes.[1] Neuropathic pain and weight loss are both severe and rapidly progressive with patients losing up to 100 lb. Interestingly, most symptoms resolve within a year, although no specific therapy has been found to be effective, including improved glucose control.[2]

This patient has poorly controlled diabetes, which progressed to requiring insulin in a short period of time. She has a very low BMI, and a concurrent diagnosis of Hashimoto's thyroiditis. Her family history of autoimmune disease and the rapid evolution to insulin dependence suggested the diagnosis of late autoimmune diabetes of the adult (LADA). LADA is characterized by anti-islet-cell, anti-GAD, or anti-insulin antibodies, which are serologic markers of chronic β-cell destruction. LADA patients share clinical features with type 2 diabetes patients, such as older age of onset

[1]Division of Endocrinology, Rush University, Chicago, IL.

DOI: 10.2337/9781580405713.23

and a slower progression; however, unlike most type 2 patients, they have low or normal BMI.[3] Most LADA patients initially are treated for type 2 diabetes. The United Kingdom Prospective Diabetes Study detected anti-GAD positivity in 10% of enrolled patients with presumed type 2 diabetes.[4] Of the antibodies associated with LADA, anti-GAD is the most prevalent. It is also the most sensitive marker, as it is present in the early stages of the disease and has a long duration in the serum. Other islet-cell antibody titers may decrease over time.

Proposed diagnostic criteria for LADA include the following: age of diagnosis >30 years, presence of autoantibodies, and the lack of a requirement for insulin for at least 6 months after diagnosis. When seeing patients with type 2 diabetes with a low BMI or a personal and family history of autoimmune disorders, it is important to keep the possible diagnosis of LADA in mind. Our patient fits the criteria for LADA; however, her advanced age of diagnosis is unusual.

In one European study, 6,156 patients with type 2 diabetes were screened for LADA. The 541 patients who tested positive for GAD antibody were younger at diagnosis than GAD-negative patients and were more likely to be female and to be leaner.[5]

Patients with GAD antibodies also may have other endocrine autoimmune disorders; therefore, testing for thyroid disorders is appropriate.

After a diagnosis of LADA was confirmed, metformin was stopped, and the patient was started on insulin glargine 4 units b.i.d. and lispro 2–3 units t.i.d. with meals, as well as levothyroxine and vitamin B$_{12}$.

Patients with LADA will progress to insulin dependence faster than patients with type 2 diabetes; however, our patient progressed within 1 year. One possible explanation is the presence of multiple autoantibodies. Patients with isolated GAD antibodies develop β-cell failure more slowly as compared with patients having multiple autoantibodies. Of those LADA patients with two or three autoantibodies, 74% developed β-cell failure within 5 years.[3] It has been proposed that LADA patients with multiple autoantibodies may benefit from earlier initiation of insulin therapy. Their insulin requirement usually is much lower than with type 2 patients.

One year later, HbA$_{1c}$ was 6.8%, her weight had recovered to her baseline 130 lb, and neuropathic symptoms had resolved. Her doses of glargine and lispro remained stable.

REFERENCES

1. Ellenberg M. Diabetic neuropathic cachexia. *Diabetes* 1973;23:418–423

2. Neal JM. Diabetic neuropathic cachexia: a rare manifestation of diabetic neuropathy. *South Med J* 2009;102:327–329

3. Borg H. A 12-year prospective study of the relationship between islet antibodies and B-cell function at and after the diagnosis of adult-onset diabetes. *Diabetes* 2002;51:1754–1762

4. Pozzilli P, Di Mario U. Autoimmune diabetes not requiring insulin at diagnosis (latent autoimmune diabetes of the adult): definition, characterization, and potential prevention. *Diabetes Care* 2001;24:1460–1467

5. Hawa MI, Kolb H, Schloot N, Beyan H, et al. Adult-onset autoimmune diabetes in Europe is prevalent with a broad clinical phenotype: Action LADA-7. *Diabetes Care* 2013;36:908–913

Case 24

A Diagnostic Dilemma in a Patient with Elevated Glycosylated Hemoglobin

SHALINI PATURI, MD,[1,2] AND JANICE L. GILDEN, MS, MD, FCP, FACE[1,2]

A 19-year-old African American woman was referred to the endocrine clinic for evaluation of elevated hemoglobin A1c (A1C) of 6.5% (repeat value 6.9%) and a fasting plasma glucose (FPG) of 105 mg/dL (5.8 mmol/L). There were symptoms of mild fatigue and increased thirst. Over the past 4 months, she also experienced a 10 lb weight gain, with no changes in diet or exercise. There were no known medical problems, and she did not take any medications, alcohol, or recreational drugs. Family history was significant for diabetes in her maternal grandfather. Physical exam showed a thin female (BMI 21 kg/m²), without acanthosis nigricans, skin tags, striae, or other abnormalities.

According to the American Diabetes Association, diabetes is defined by the following: *1)* A1C ≥6.5%; or *2)* FPG ≥126 mg/dL (7.0 mmol/L); or *3)* 2 h plasma glucose (PG) ≥200 mg/L (11.1 mmol/L) during an oral glucose tolerance test (OGTT); or *4)* in a patient with classic symptoms of hyperglycemia or hyperglycemic crisis, a random PG ≥200 mg/L (11.1 mmol/L). Furthermore, if a patient meets the diabetes criterion for A1C (two results ≥6.5%), but not the FPG (<126 mg/dL or 7.0 mmol/L), or vice versa, that person is considered to have diabetes.[1] It is important to recognize that plasma venous blood often is used for laboratory determination, and glucose values can be different from capillary fingerstick glucose measurements. Furthermore, blood glucose values have a coefficient of variation that is up to 14%.[2]

Recent epidemiological studies have reported that when matched for FPG, African Americans (with and without diabetes) have higher A1C and fructosamine levels than Caucasians, but lower levels of 1,5-anhydroglucitol,[3] suggesting possible postprandial hyperglycemia.

[1]Endocrinology Division, Department of Medicine, Rosalind Franklin University of Medicine and Science/Chicago Medical School, North Chicago, IL. [2]Endocrinology Section, Department of Medicine, Captain James A. Lovell Federal Health Care Center, North Chicago, IL.

This research was supported in part by the Captain James A. Lovell Federal Health Care Center.

DOI: 10.2337/9781580405713.24

Table 24.1—A1C Measurements over Time

Date	A1C	Fasting blood glucose	Fructosamine
11/12	6.5%	—	—
03/13	6.9%	—	—
04/13	7.0%	106 mg/dL	—
05/13	—	94 mg/dL	—
07/13	6.9%	105 mg/dL	271 µmol/L (190–270)
08/13	7.1%	96 mg/dL	—

We then ordered a 3-h 75-g OGTT. Results were as follows:

FPG	112 mg/dL (6.2 mmol/L)
1 h PG	124 mg/dL (6.8 mmol/L)
2 h PG	120 mg/dL (6.6 mmol/L)
3 h PG	102 mg/dL (5.6mmol/L)
Concurrent A1C	7.0%

The patient was thought to have impaired fasting glucose (IFG). Her A1C result, however, met criteria for diabetes, suggesting an average blood glucose (BG) of 154 mg/dL (8.5 mmol/L), contradictory to the FPG and OGTT results (Table 24.1).

Racial minority groups in the U.S. previously have been reported to have IGT with higher A1C levels, after adjustment for factors likely to affect glycemia.[4]

Because of the discrepancy between A1C and BG, a continuous glucose monitoring (CGM) study was performed for 5 days.

In a CGM study, a subcutaneous sensor measures interstitial glucose every 5 minutes and transmits data to a wireless monitor. Capillary fingerstick glucose measurements are used for verification of accuracy. Data are expressed as glucose values at the time-points over 24 h each day for the duration of study. Currently available CGM devices measure interstitial glucose, whereas fingerstick devices measure capillary BG. Because of the physiologic lag in equilibration between these two compartments, an increase or decrease in glucose levels will first be apparent in the blood, followed by the interstitial fluid.

CGM study data revealed an average BG of 124 mg/dL (6.8 mmol/L) (range = 76–164 mg/dL [4.2–9.1 mmol/L]), without hypoglycemia (Fig. 24.1).

This patient's blood glucose did not correlate with the elevation of A1C. This discrepancy also can occur when there is an alteration in the glycation process or red cell survival, such as in hemoglobinopathies, iron deficiency anemia, or chronic kidney disease, or from medications.[5]

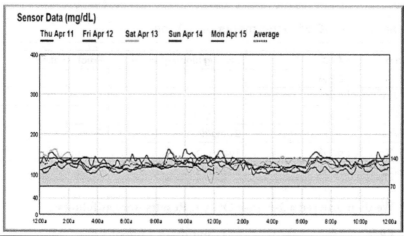

Time	3 am–6 am	Pre-breakfast	Post-breakfast	Prelunch	Postlunch	Predinner	Postdinner	11 pm–3 am
Average in mg/dL	117	132	130	133	110	111	110	130
Min–max mg/dL	93–143	119–146	117–152	119–144	105–120	103–118	105–120	102–162

Figure 24.1 — Continuous glucose monitoring data over 5 days.

The patient's iron levels and binding studies were normal: iron saturation 21% (10–50), iron 73 µg/dL (50–170), ferritin 10 ng/mL (8–252), and TIBC 351 µg/dL (250–450). A hemoglobin electrophoresis showed a pattern of heterozygous positivity for the -α 3.7 (α-plus-thalassemia mutation), and DNA testing indicated that this patient was positive for the -α 3.7 α-globin deletion on one chromosome.

Individuals with this type of thalassemia trait are usually clinically normal. In conditions in which the red cell survival or hemoglobin structures are abnormal, the value of A1C does not accurately reflect the glycemic levels. Useful alternative measurements can be glycated proteins, like fructosamine.

The fructosamine level was 271 µmol/L (190–270), equating to an A1C of 6.2%. On the same day, A1C was 6.9% and FPG was 105 mg/dL (5.8 mmol/L).

When using the criteria for diagnosing diabetes, physicians should be aware that limitations may exist for using A1C because of ethnicity, hemoglobinopathies, and altered red cell turnover. Furthermore, utilizing other evaluation techniques, such as CGM studies and glycated proteins, can add further valuable clinical information.

REFERENCES

1. American Diabetes Association. Standards of medical care in diabetes, 2015. *Diabetes Care* 2015;38(Suppl. 1):S1–S93

2. American Diabetes Association. Tests of glycemia in diabetes. *Diabetes Care* 2004;27(Suppl. 1):S91–S93

3. Selvin E, Steffes MW, Ballantyne CM, Hoogeveen RC, Coresh J, Brancati FL. Racial differences in glycemic markers: a cross-sectional analysis of community-based data. *Ann Intern Med* 2011;154:303–309

4. Herman WH, Ma Y, Uwaifo G, et al. Diabetes Prevention Program Research Group. Differences in hemoglobin A1C by race and ethnicity among patients with impaired glucose tolerance in the Diabetes Prevention Program. *Diabetes Care* 2007;30:2453–2457

5. Gillery P, Hue G, Bordas-Fonfrede M, Chapelle JP, Drouin P, Levy-Marchal C, Perier C, Selam JL, Slama G, Thivolet C, Vialettes B. Hemoglobin A1C determination and hemoglobinopathies: problems and strategies. *Ann Biol Clin* 2000;58:425–429

Case 25

An Unexplained Decline in HbA$_{1c}$ in Spite of Persistent Hyperglycemia

DAVID S.H. BELL, MB[1]

A 35-year-old white woman was diagnosed with type 1 diabetes at age 12 years, and had persistently poor glycemic control with HbA$_{1c}$ ranging from 10 to 13%. Some details of this case have been presented previously.[1] Her historically poor glycemic control had resulted in the development of proliferative diabetic retinopathy (treated with panretinal photocoagulation), cataracts, diabetic nephropathy, recurrent pyelonephritis, distal symmetric polyneuropathy, entrapment, autonomic neuropathies, and trigger fingers. She also had euthyroid Hashimoto's thyroiditis, lumbar and cervical disk disease, depression, and dermatitis herpetiformis.

While her home glucose monitoring readings were in the 250–350 mg/dL range and her serum glucose measured at clinic visits were in the 250–400 mg/dL range, her HbA$_{1c}$ had declined from the usual 10–13% range to the 6–7% range and had remained at that level for >2 years. Subsequently there was a further fall in the HbA$_{1c}$ to the 3–4% range in spite of continued poor glycemic control by glucose readings.

Her home glucose meter readings were compared with clinic serum glucose levels, and her home glucose monitoring equipment was found to be accurate. In addition, her serum fructosamine levels, which estimate average glucose over a 3-week period by measuring the glycosylation of albumin, were elevated at 3.6 mmol/L (upper limit of normal 2.6 mmol/L).

When confronted with a patient with diabetes and poor glycemic control but an artifactually low HbA$_{1c}$, several etiologies should be considered. The first consideration should be etiologies that decrease the life span of the red blood cell, such as hemolytic anemia, spherocytosis, elliptocytosis, hemoglobin F, or any other hemoglobinopathy. In this case, there was no evidence of abnormal red blood cell morphology. In addition, any acute or chronic blood loss, recent blood transfusion, pregnancy, or recent childbirth can all decrease the HbA$_{1c}$ level.[1]

A review of her medication showed that she had been prescribed dapsone by her dermatologist for dermatitis herpetiformis. When her HbA$_{1c}$ had dropped to the 6–7% range, treatment with dapsone 50 mg daily had been initiated. Because of poor clinical response, her dapsone was later

---

[1]Clinical Professor, University of Alabama, Birmingham, AL.

  DOI: 10.2337/9781580405713.25

increased to 100 mg, which coincided with the decrease in her HbA_{1c} to the 3–4% range.

Dapsone ($x_1 4^1$-diaminodiphenylsulfone) is used in the treatment of leprosy and in the prophylaxis of toxoplasmosis, pneumocystis carinii pneumonia, and malaria. Dapsone also can be used in combination with trimethoprim as an alternative therapy for pneumocystis carinii pneumonia. Other uses include the therapy of brown recluse spider bites, inflammatory bowel disease, relapsing polychrondritis, leishmaniasis, pyoderma gangrenosum, necrobiosis lipoidica diabeticorum, and many connective tissue disorders. The efficacy of dapsone in these diseases is mediated through its anti-inflammatory effect, which is why it is preferentially utilized in the therapy of dermatitis herpetiformis.

Although dapsone can cause hemolysis and reduce the life span of the erythrocyte, especially in the presence of glucose-6-phosphate dehydrogenase deficiency, its major effect in reducing the HbA_{1c} is mediated through increased methemoglobin formation, which causes the iron in hemoglobin to be oxidized from the ferrous to the ferric form so that oxygen cannot bind to methemoglobin. In addition, methemoglobin will not spike in the HbA_{1c} location because of a different electrical charge, thus artifactually lowering the HbA_{1c} value. Furthermore, methemoglobin may not be glycosylated in the same manner or at the same rate as hemoglobin.[1,2]

When HbA_{1c} does not reflect the practitioner's estimate of glycemic control, confirmation with a fructosamine or other methods of assessing glycemic control should be performed. When used for necrobiosis diabeticorum or dermatitis herpetiformis in patients with diabetes, dapsone will lower HbA_{1c} because of the excess formation of methemoglobin.

REFERENCES

1. Albright ES, Ovalle F, Bell DSH. Artifactually low hemoglobin A1C caused by use of dapsone. *Endocrine Practice* 2002;8(5):370–372

2. DeGowin RL. A review of therapeutic and hemolytic effects of dapsone. *Arch Intern Med* 1967;120(2):242–248

Case 26

What to Do with Discrepant HbA$_{1c}$ and SMBG Results? The Utility of Fructosamine and Glycated Albumin

TATIANA GANDRABURA, MD,[1] AND DANIEL J. RUBIN, MD, MSc[1]

A 59-year-old white man with a history of orthotopic liver transplant for cryptogenic cirrhosis developed diabetes 1 year post-transplant. His post-transplant immunosuppression regimen consisted of tacrolimus, mycophenolate, and prednisone. The patient presented to the clinic for diabetes management, at which time he was taking glipizide extended release 5 mg daily. The patient checked his blood glucose two times daily (premeal average 170 mg/dL, postmeal average 184 mg/dL; Table 26.1). At this time, the hemoglobin A1c (HbA$_{1c}$) was 5.8% and the hematocrit was 39.9%. Sitagliptin 100 mg daily was added to the glipizide.

HbA$_{1c}$ is the conventional marker for monitoring chronic glycemic control in diabetes. It is the product of nonenzymatic glycation of the hemoglobin β-chain at the valine terminal residue.[1] HbA$_{1c}$ is tightly correlated with average blood glucose levels, making it a useful index of glycemic control. With normal red blood cell (RBC) life span, the HbA$_{1c}$ reflects peripheral blood glucose levels over the preceding 2–3 months. Conditions that affect RBC life span, however, also affect the extent of glycation. A decrease in RBC life span, such as that caused by hemolytic anemia, lowers HbA$_{1c}$, whereas an increase in RBC life span, such as that associated with iron deficiency, raises HbA$_{1c}$.[2]

The estimated average blood glucose predicted by the HbA$_{1c}$ of 5.8% is 120 mg/dL, significantly lower than the self-monitored blood glucose (SMBG) values. We entertained the possibility that anemia of chronic disease was falsely lowering the HbA$_{1c}$ value, despite the low-normal hematocrit. Fructosamine and glycated albumin levels were obtained at the next visit.

In the setting of anemia and discrepant HbA$_{1c}$ and SMBG values, alternative markers of glycemic control may be helpful, namely, fructosamine, glycated albumin, and 1,5-anhydroglucitol (1,5-AG).[2,3] Fructosamine, so named for its similarity to fructose, is produced when blood glucose forms ketoamines by covalently binding to serum proteins. The largest component of fructosamine is glycated albumin, which is formed via glycation of serum albumin, the most abundant serum protein. Based on the half-life of albumin, both fructosamine and glycated albumin reflect glycemic control over the prior 2–3 weeks.[1,2]

---

[1]Temple University School of Medicine, Philadelphia, PA.

DOI: 10.2337/9781580405713.26

Neither of these alternative markers of glycemic control is affected by changes in RBC life span. Fructosamine, however, is influenced by the concentration of serum proteins and low-molecular-weight substances in the plasma, such as bilirubin, hemoglobin, and uric acid.[2] In contrast, because glycated albumin is reported as a ratio of glycated albumin to total serum albumin it is not affected by the concentration of serum albumin. The third alternative marker of glycemic control is 1,5-AG, a serum monosaccharide that is excreted in the urine at an accelerated rate in the presence of glycosuria. Fructosamine and glycated albumin increase in the presence of hyperglycemia, whereas 1,5-AG decreases. Because the level of 1,5-AG depends on reabsorption at the renal tubules, it is not recommended for glucose monitoring in patients with impaired renal function.

The patient returned 3 months later (February 2013) having gained 11 lb, with the following (Table 26.1):

Premeal SMBG values	313 mg/dL (average)
Postmeal values	413 mg/dL (average)
HbA$_{1c}$	8%
Hematocrit	37.1%
Fructosamine	466 µmol/L
Glycated albumin	2.9%

Table 26.1 — Glucose and Laboratory Values

Component reference range	November 2012	February 2013	August 2013	November 2013
SMBG, mean ± SD Overall			213 ± NA	
Premeal	170 ± 23	313 ± 87	NA	141 ± 32
Postmeal	184 ± 35	413 ± 105	NA	181 ± 40
HbA$_{1c}$ <5.7%	5.8 (H)	8.0 (H)	7.8 (H)	6.4 (H)
Estimated average BG by HbA$_{1c}$ (mg/dL)	120	183	177	137
Fructosamine 190–270 µmol/L	NA	466 (H)	329 (H)	321 (H)
Estimated average BG by fructosamine (mg/dL)	NA	285	185	175
Glycated albumin 0.8–1.4%	NA	2.9 (H)	1.5 (H)	1.2
Hematocrit 38.5–50.0%	39.9	37.1 (L)	33.5 (L)	32.5 (L)
Albumin 3.5–5.0 g/dL	4.3	4.1	4.0	4.1

BG, blood glucose; H, high; L, Low; NA, not available; SMBG, self-monitored blood glucose.

The HbA$_{1c}$ corresponds to an average blood glucose of 183 mg/dL, while the fructosamine predicts an average blood glucose of 285 mg/dL.[4] Correlations of glycated albumin with blood glucose have not been determined. Although both the HbA$_{1c}$ and fructosamine underestimated the average blood glucose, the fructosamine was more accurate. The glipizide was increased to 10 mg, and insulin glargine was soon added.

A few months later (August 2013), the blood glucose, fructosamine, and glycated albumin levels had improved, but the HbA$_{1c}$ was little changed. The basal insulin was increased. By November 2013, the blood glucose values were further improved, along with slight decreases in fructosamine and glycated albumin. In contrast, the HbA$_{1c}$ dropped significantly and still underestimated the SMBGs. A decline in the hematocrit over the preceding 9 months is noted.

HbA$_{1c}$ may underestimate average blood glucose levels in the setting of certain anemias. In such cases, fructosamine and glycated albumin can serve as useful alternatives to HbA$_{1c}$ for assessing chronic glycemia.

REFERENCES

1. Klonoff DC. Serum fructosamine as a screening test for type 2 diabetes. *Diabetes Technol Therap* 2000;2(4):537–539

2. Kim KJ, Lee BW. The roles of glycated albumin as intermediate glycation index and pathogenic protein. *Diabetes Metab J* 2012;36(2):98–107

3. Zheng CM, Ma WY, Wu CC, Lu KC. Glycated albumin in diabetic patients with chronic kidney disease. *Clin Chim Acta* 2012;413(19–20):1555–1561

4. Lindsey CC, Carter AW, Mangum S, et al. A prospective, randomized, multi-centered controlled trial to compare the annual glycemic and quality outcomes of patients with diabetes mellitus monitored with weekly fructosamine testing versus usual care. *Diabetes Technol Therap* 2004;6(3):370–377

Case 27

A "Tricky" Low HbA$_{1c}$

Chiara Mazzucchelli, MD;[1] Caterina Bordone, MD;[1] Davide Maggi, MD, PhD;[1] and Renzo Cordera, MD[1]

A 63-year-old Caucasian woman was referred to our diabetes clinic for evaluation of an unexplained drop in HbA$_{1c}$ in the past year without an apparent cause. She was diagnosed with type 2 diabetes (T2D) 5 years earlier upon routine laboratory screening. At the time of diagnosis, she was asymptomatic with a BMI of 29.5 kg/m^2. She had had two uncomplicated pregnancies. Soon after her T2D diagnosis, she was started on therapy with a fixed combination of glyburide and metformin t.i.d. (2.5 mg + 400 mg, respectively; increased later to 5 mg + 400 mg). She also had hypertension treated with enalapril 20 mg/day. Since then, her HbA$_{1c}$ had been measured every 6 months and remained stable at 59 mmol/mol (7.5%) on the higher dose of glyburide. With no apparent reason, her HbA$_{1c}$ dropped to 42 mmol/mol (6%) during the past year. This low value, within the nondiabetic range, was confirmed 6 months later. She did not report any symptomatic hypoglycemia or a change in BMI. Blood glucose self-monitoring carried out twice weekly indicated poor glycemic control inconsistent with her HbA$_{1c}$ values. Her general practitioner recommended decreasing her antidiabetic therapy by half, but her HbA$_{1c}$ was still 42 mmol/mol (6%) 3 months later. At time of presentation, mild anemia was present. Upon obtaining further, it was discovered that she had started therapy with dapsone for pemphigus 15 months earlier.

HbA$_{1c}$ is the product of nonenzymatic covalent ketoaminic linkage of glucose with Val residues in the N-terminus β-chain of hemoglobin. It is the most useful surrogate glucose control marker employed in clinical practice and is used to titrate antidiabetic therapy. HbA$_{1c}$ correlates with the average blood glucose concentration in the preceding 3 months and with risk of both microvascular complications of diabetes and with hypoglycemia. It recently has been proposed as a diagnostic criterion for diabetes. Recent "mega trials" have lent support to the notion that an optimal HbA$_{1c}$ value in subjects with T2D is not equal for all. In some groups of patients, relatively low HbA$_{1c}$ values may even be dangerous. A recent consensus statement emphasizes that the goal HbA$_{1c}$ for each patient should be determined carefully by taking into account several clinical and social parameters.[1] Therefore, it is of paramount importance for clinicians and patients to use reliable and accurate HbA$_{1c}$ measurements for

[1]Department of Internal Medicine, University of Genova, Genova, Italy.

DOI: 10.2337/9781580405713.27

clinical decision making. Falsely elevated or decreased values for HbA$_{1c}$ may have important clinical consequences, such as hypoglycemia or prolonged periods of hyperglycemia.

The HbA$_{1c}$ value depends on two main factors: *1)* the average blood glucose concentration and *2)* red cell aging. Because glucose influx into red cells is not insulin regulated, the amount of intra–red cell glucose is strictly dependent on plasma glucose concentration: the higher the blood glucose, the higher the HbA$_{1c}$ level. In addition, aged red cells accumulate more glycosylated hemoglobin than younger ones. As a consequence, both genetic and acquired conditions associated with pathological hemolysis and shortened red cell life span are linked with lower than predicted HbA$_{1c}$ values.

In this patient the recent drop in HbA$_{1c}$ values could not be ascribed to an improvement in overall glucose control. Hence, an acquired cause of non-glucose-dependent HbA$_{1c}$ decrease had to be pursued.

This patient has been taking dapsone for several months. Dapsone, a synthetic sulfone, commonly is recommended as an anti-inflammatory agent to treat several allergic and autoimmune diseases. Dapsone is responsible for oxidation of the heme moiety and induces red cell death by increasing reactive oxygen species, thus shortening red cell life span. It causes severe hemolysis in G6PD-deficient patients, but even in subjects with normal G6PD, dapsone can induce subclinically increased hemolysis.[2] Older red cells are more damaged by oxidative stress than younger cells, resulting into a significant decrease in hemoglobin A1C values, as published in a few clinical reports.[3] Dapsone therapy was the most likely cause of unexpectedly low HbA$_{1c}$ values in our patient.

When HbA$_{1c}$ measurement is not reliable, alternative methods to measure glucose control may be employed, such as fructosamine determination or continuous glucose monitoring (CGM). Fructosamine, a glycated serum protein, estimates average glucose concentration in the previous 2 weeks. Fructosamine is glycosylated by the same mechanism that produces HbA$_{1c}$. Fructosamine concentration, however, is not routinely measured and its correlation with clinical outcomes has not been investigated extensively.

Recently, CGM has become available. This is a procedure that measures interstitial subcutaneous glucose every 5 min. CGM has been developed to detect glucose variability (especially in T1D) and the occurrence of asymptomatic hypoglycemia. CGM can be utilized to measure average glucose concentration in the previous 6 days. It has been shown that in patients with stable glucose control, the 6-day average glucose concentration correlates very well with HbA$_{1c}$ and can be used to calculate a predicted HbA$_{1c}$ value.[4,5] In this case, we performed CGM for 6 days and found an average blood glucose of 11.5 mmol/L, which predicted an HbA$_{1c}$ of 73 mmol/mol (8.8%), whereas the measured HbA$_{1c}$ was 42 mmol/mol (6%). We made an assumption of a linear relationship between HbA$_{1c}$ and 6-day average blood glucose levels and calculated a correction factor of 1.7, the result of the predicted HbA$_{1c}$ divided by the measured HbA$_{1c}$. We used this correction factor to calculate the actual HbA$_{1c}$ and to titrate her antidiabetic therapy. Further studies are required to validate this method of estimating the HbA$_{1c}$. The patient is still taking dapsone.

We have adjusted her antidiabetic therapy with guidance from the corrected HbA_{1c}, while avoiding acute hypo- or hyperglycemia.

REFERENCES

1. American Diabetes Association. Standards of medical care in diabetes, 2015. *Diabetes Care* 2015;38(Suppl. 1):S1–S93

2. Pallais JC, Mackool BT, Bishop Pitman M. A 52-year-old man with upper respiratory symptoms and low oxygen saturation levels. *N Eng J Med* 2011;364:957–966

3. Bertholon M, Mayer A, Francina A, Thivolet CH. Interference of dapsone in HbA_{1c} monitoring of a T1DM with necrobiosis lipoidica. *Diabetes Care* 1994;17:1364–1368

4. Nathan DM, Kuenen J, Borg R, Zheng H, Schoenfeld D, Heine RJ. Translating the A1C assay into estimated average glucose values. *Diabetes Care* 2008,31:1473–1478 (correction Diabetes Care 2009,32:207)

5. Nielsen JK, Gravholt CH, Djurhuus CB, Brandt D, Becker J. Heinemann L, Christiansen JS. Continous subcutaneous glucose monitoring shows a close correlation between mean glucose and time spent in hyperglycemia and HbA_{1c}. *J Diabetes Sci Technol* 2007;1:857–863

Case 28

Use of Insulin U-500 in a Patient with Severe Insulin Resistance

Hussain Mahmud, MBBS,[1] and Mary T. Korytkowski, MD[2]

A 60-year-old woman with 20-year history of type 2 diabetes presented to the clinic for management of diabetes. She was started on insulin 15 years ago. Her current glycemic regimen included insulin detemir 60 units twice daily, and insulin aspart according to the following scale: blood glucose (BG) <200 mg/dL (11.1 mmol/L) = 0 units, 200–250 = 18 units, 250–300 = 24 units, >300 = 30 units. She was averaging >200 units of insulin per day with all self-monitored blood glucose readings >200 mg/dL (11.1 mmol/L), and occasionally >400 mg/dL (22.2 mmol/L). Her last HbA$_{1c}$ was 10.5%. She reported following a strict 1,500 calorie per day diet, leading to 5 kg weight loss over the preceding 4 months. She endorsed polyuria, nocturia, numbness, and tingling in the lower extremities and hands.

Type 2 diabetes is a chronic disease that is characterized by insulin resistance and progressive β-cell failure. After conventional modalities of treatment (diet, exercise, and noninsulin therapies) fail to maintain desired levels of glycemic control, insulin therapy is required. Average total daily insulin requirements for many patients with type 2 diabetes are 0.5–0.8 units/kg/day. In the presence of more pronounced insulin resistance, however, the insulin requirements can increase to 1–2 units/kg/day or more. Severe insulin resistance is defined as "insulin requirements in excess of 200 units a day for more than 2 days" and can present in a number of different conditions (see Table 28.1).

The patient was a normotensive middle-aged Caucasian woman with a BMI of 37.3 kg/m², without a Cushingoid or lipodystrophic appearance. She had mild acanthosis over the neck and nonpigmented stretch marks over the abdomen. There was no evidence of hirsutism or lipohypertrophy at insulin injection sites. She was started on metformin and insulin U-500.

Insulin U-500 (Humulin R U-500, Eli Lilly and Company, Indianapolis, IN) contains 500 units of insulin in every milliliter (five times more concentrated than Humulin R U-100). It is approved by the Food and Drug Administration (FDA) for use in insulin-resistant patients who require daily insulin doses of >200 units. The advantage of insulin U-500 is the ability to deliver a

[1]Clinical Assistant Professor of Medicine, Division of Endocrinology, University of Pittsburgh Medical Center, Pittsburgh, PA. [2]Professor of Medicine, Division of Endocrinology, University of Pittsburgh Medical Center, Pittsburgh, PA.

     DOI: 10.2337/9781580405713.28

Table 28.1 — Causes of Severe Insulin Resistance

Obesity

Stressful conditions such as severe infection or steroid use

Pregnancy

Polycystic ovary syndrome

HAIR-AN syndrome (hyperandrogenism, insulin resistance, and acanthosis nigricans)

Hemochromatosis

Cushing's syndrome

Werner syndrome

Acanthosis nigricans

Lipodystrophy (congenital and acquired)

Genetic defects of the insulin receptor gene

      Type A insulin resistance syndrome

      Leprechaunism

   Rabson–Mendenhall syndrome

Insulin receptor antibodies

---

large dose of insulin in smaller volumes with a single injection. Although it was approved in 1997, its usage has increased steadily over the past few years because of the continuing obesity and type 2 diabetes epidemics. Clinical experience has shown that it frequently has time action characteristics reflecting both prandial and basal activity. It takes effect within 30 min, but when compared to U-100 regular insulin at high doses, insulin U-500's peak concentration and action profile is blunted with a prolonged duration of activity (Fig. 28.1).[1]

When prescribing insulin U-500, it is important to remember that the dose of insulin U-500 and the corresponding number of units on the insulin syringe are not equivalent. This can lead to medication errors and hypoglycemia. Preferably, a prescription for insulin U-500 should state all three permutations of the insulin order (volume, unit-marks on an insulin U-100 syringe, and actual units) to avoid confusion for the patient, nurse, and pharmacist. For example, an order for 90 units of insulin U-500 may state, "administer 0.18 mL of U-500 regular human insulin, which equals the 18 unit-mark on a U-100 insulin syringe, which is equivalent to 90 actual units of regular human insulin."

The patient was initiated on metformin 500 mg twice daily and insulin U-500 at the 20 unit-mark on an insulin syringe (100 units, 0.20 mL) before breakfast, 16 unit-mark (80 units, 0.16 mL) before lunch, and 16 unit-mark (80 units, 0.16 mL) before dinner. She started this after a diabetic education visit, with special instructions regarding insulin U-500 administration. All prior insulin orders were discontinued. The patient had

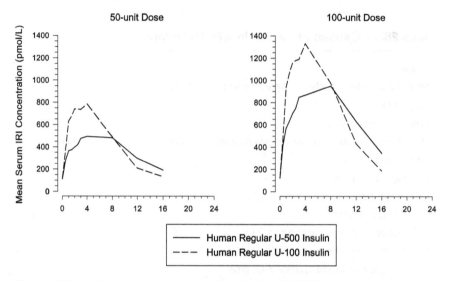

Figure 28.1 — Mean serum immunoreactive insulin (IRI) concentrations over time during a euglycemic clamp after a single dose of 50 units (left) and 100 units (right) of human regular U-500 and U-100 insulin. Adapted from de la Peña A, et al. *Diabetes Care* 2011;34:2496–2501.

immediate improvement in glycemic control with mild hyperglycemia at lunch and occasional hypoglycemia at dinner and during the night. The breakfast insulin U-500 dose was raised while lunch and dinner insulin U-500 doses were lowered gradually.

During insulin U-500 initiation, the patient's U-100 dose may be converted directly into U-500 if glycemic control is adequate. The dose, however, can be increased empirically by 10–20% if the HbA$_{1c}$ is >10%.[2] The longer duration of action of insulin U-500 allows its use for multiple daily injections without the use of basal insulin. Some providers use it in addition to long- or rapid-acting insulin with satisfactory results.[3] If the total daily insulin dose before the initiation of insulin U-500 is between 200 and 300 units and two insulin injections are being used, the insulin U-500 may be divided into two or three daily injections, with 60% of the insulin being given in the morning and 40% of the insulin being given at dinner. In case of three daily injections, 40% of the insulin may be administered at breakfast and 30% at lunch and dinner. If the total daily insulin dose is 300–600 units, about 40–45% of the insulin dose can be administered before breakfast, 30–40% before lunch, and 20–30% before dinner.[4] Because of the pharmacodynamics of U-500 insulin, dose changes are based on trends rather than on glucose levels at each dose.

One year after insulin U-500 initiation, the patient's current glycemic regimen is composed of metformin 1,000 mg twice daily, insulin

U-500 24 unit-marks (120 units, 0.24 mL) before breakfast, 13 unit-marks (65 units, 0.13 mL) before lunch, and 13 unit-marks (65 units, 0.13 mL) before supper. The most recent HbA_{1c} was 7.1%, without significant hypoglycemia. Despite following a strict 45 g carbohydrate per meal diet, she has gained 7 kg since her initial office visit.

Insulin U-500 is an extremely effective method of treatment of type 2 diabetes with severe insulin resistance. Multiple studies have shown improvement in HbA_{1c} (mean HbA_{1c} reduction 1.59%) after insulin U-500 initiation.[5] Patients also report greater satisfaction with its use, likely because of reductions in the number of insulin injections and better glycemic control. Use of insulin U-500 has been associated with significant weight gain (mean weight gain 4.38 kg).[5]

REFERENCES

1. de la Peña A, Riddle M, Morrow LA, Jiang HH, Linnebjerg H, Scott A, et al. Pharmacokinetics and pharmacodynamics of high-dose human regular U-500 insulin versus human regular U-100 insulin in healthy obese subjects. *Diabetes Care* 2011;34:2496–2501

2. Lane WS, Cochran EK, Jackson JA, Scism-Bacon JL, Corey IB, Hirsch IB, Skyler JS. High-dose insulin therapy: is it time for U-500 insulin? *Endocr Pract* 2009;15:71–79

3. Lowery JB, Donihi AC, Korytkowski MT. U-500 insulin as a component of basal bolus insulin therapy in type 2 diabetes. *Diabetes Technol Ther* 2012;14(6):505–507

4. Cochran E, Gorden P. Use of U-500 insulin in the treatment of severe insulin resistance. *Insulin* 2008;3:211–218

5. Reutrakul S, Wroblewski K, Brown RL. Clinical use of U-500 and regular insulin: review and meta-analysis. *J Diabetes Sci Technol* 2012;6(2):412–420

Case 29

Effective Use of U-500 Insulin via Insulin Pump in a Type 2 Diabetes Patient with Severe Insulin Resistance

Vijay babu Balakrishnan, MD,[1] and Elias S. Siraj, MD[1]

A 57-year-old man with a 25-year history of type 2 diabetes (T2D) presented to the endocrine clinic for a second opinion about recent worsening of glycemic control despite the use of increasing doses of insulin. He had been on various oral agents during the early years of his diabetes but for the past 15 years had been on insulin. In the past, he had been on various insulin regimens consisting of glargine, lispro, and premixed insulins, with an average total daily dose (TDD) of 270–300 units. About 2 years ago, his regimen was changed from premixed 70/30 insulin to U-500 regular insulin after his control continued to get worse despite appropriate increases in insulin doses.

He had no family history of diabetes. Comorbidities included hypertension, hyperlipidemia, and coronary artery disease. He also had retinopathy, nephropathy, and neuropathy. He weighed 205 lb (BMI of 30 kg/m^2). Blood pressure was 140/90 mmHg. He had no acanthosis nigricans and features of Cushing's syndrome or acromegaly. No evidence of lipodystrophy or lipohypertrophy.

Worsening of insulin resistance with increasing insulin requirement may occur in patients with T2D for several reasons. Some may require more than 200 units of insulin daily, which is considered as extreme insulin resistance. Most commonly, this resistance could be due to worsening obesity, comorbid conditions, concurrent medications, inadequate dietary restraint, sedentary lifestyle, and infections.

It is important, however, to rule out rare causes of severe or worsening insulin resistance, such as the following:

- Endocrinopathies, including Cushing's syndrome or acromegaly
- Extreme insulin-resistance syndromes,[1] including
  o Type B syndrome with autoantibodies against the insulin receptor
  o Inherited disorders, such as leprechaunism with insulin-receptor mutations
  o Lipodystrophic states

A careful evaluation of our patient did not reveal any features and findings suggestive of those disorders.

---

[1]Section of Endocrinology, Diabetes and Metabolism, Temple University School of Medicine, Philadelphia, PA.

DOI: 10.2337/9781580405713.29

Over the next 18 months, despite an increase in his TDD of U-500 insulin from 450 to 775 units (equivalent of U-100), his HbA$_{1c}$ stayed as high as 12.7% and most of his blood glucose readings ranged from 300 to 400 mg/dL (16.7–22.2 mmol/L). Pioglitazone and metformin were added. Because glycemic control did not improve with huge doses of U-500 insulin, additional investigations were done. An assay for insulin antibodies was negative. An insulin absorption study performed for 8 h following a supervised injection of 55 units of U-500 showed a delayed increase in insulin levels was associated with a delayed drop in blood glucose levels.

Treatment of extreme insulin resistance is best done by a multipronged approach. The role of caloric restriction and exercise cannot be understated. Insulin sensitizers like metformin and thiazolidinediones help improve insulin resistance by decreasing hepatic glucose production and improving insulin responsiveness in peripheral tissues. Increasing the dose of insulin is another approach to overcome the extreme insulin resistance.

Use of high-dose insulin in such patients may be limited by the volume of insulin necessary, when using the standard insulin preparation U-100, containing 100 units/mL. U-500 regular insulin (U-500), which is five times more concentrated (500 units/mL) than U-100 insulin, is a treatment option for such patients. A unique aspect of U-500 is the physical effect of slowed absorption in comparison with U-100 insulin, resulting in a pharmacokinetic profile close to that of NPH insulin.[2] U-500 usually is started twice daily, but it could be given three to four times daily in severe cases.

In a recent meta-analysis, use of U-500 insulin was associated with a significant HbA$_{1c}$ reduction of 1.59%. This was achieved at an expense of weight gain of 4.38 kg and an increase in insulin TDD of 51 units.[3]

In our patient, insulin antibodies, which at high titers can significantly impair insulin action, were negative. The delayed insulin absorption in our patient suggests that there may be unknown factors delaying the U-500 insulin absorption leading to inadequate control and subsequent increase in insulin requirement.

Ultimately, the patient was switched from U-500 insulin injections given in three doses (TDD of 775 units) to an insulin pump using U-500 insulin (starting TDD of 330 units).

U-500 insulin like any other insulin can be delivered using an insulin pump. A growing body of evidence supports its use in patients receiving huge doses of insulin. Most studies have demonstrated the efficacy of using U-500 via insulin pumps in improving HbA$_{1c}$ but have not shown any significant change in daily insulin requirement, body weight, or risk of hypoglycemia.[3,4]

The patient had few days of reasonable blood glucose levels, but then started to experience frequent hypoglycemic episodes necessitating a reduction in his insulin doses. Over 8 weeks, his TDD dropped from 330 to 190 units. His most recent HbA$_{1c}$ was 6.4% and his self-monitored blood glucose readings ranged from 51 to 120 mg/dL (2.8–6.7 mmol/L).

Our patient had a tremendous improvement in glycemic control, with HbA$_{1c}$ dropping from 12.7 to 6.4%, accompanied by a decrease in the insulin TDD of about 75%. This happened within 3 months of converting from a split-dose regimen using U-500.

It is unclear why there was such a dramatic decrease in TDD on starting the insulin pump. The results of the insulin absorption study showed a delayed rise in the insulin levels after injection of U-500. We hypothesize that there may be some local factors affecting the absorption of insulin from the subcutaneous tissue. It is possible that the factors may be more active following bolus injections of large amounts of U-500, as compared with continuous infusion. The presence of insulin degrading enzymes in the subcutaneous tissue, such as insulinase or glutathione-insulin transhydrogenase, cannot be ruled out and has been implicated in few cases of extreme insulin resistance.[5] Local antibodies in the subcutaneous tissue, which may not be detected in the peripheral blood, also may play a role in this mechanism. Saturation of binding sites of local antibodies with continued presence of insulin leading to better bioavailability might explain the progressive reduction of insulin requirements.

The use of U-500 regular insulin for insulin pump is an effective alternative for patients with T2D and severe insulin resistance who are not meeting glycemic goals with the use of subcutaneous insulin regimens or those who have difficulty in using U-100 insulin because of high insulin requirements. The use of U-500 in insulin pumps may result in striking improvements of glycemic control within a relatively short time and, at least in some patients, may result in dramatic reductions in total daily insulin requirements.

REFERENCES

1. Parker V, Semple RK. Genetic forms of severe insulin resistance: what endocrinologists should know. *Eur J Endocrinol* 2013;169(4):71–80

2. Cochran E, Musso C, Gorden P. The use of U-500 in patients with extreme insulin resistance. *Diabetes Care* 2005;28(5):1240–1244

3. Reutrakul S, Wroblewski K, Brown RL. Clinical use of U-500 regular insulin: review and meta-analysis. *J Diabetes Sci Technol* 2012;6(2):412–420

4. Lane WS, Weinrib SL, Rappaport JM, Hale CB, Farmer LK, Lane RS. The effect of long-term use of U-500 insulin via continuous subcutaneous infusion on durability of glycemic control and weight in obese, insulin-resistant patients with type 2 diabetes. *Endocr Pract* 2013;19(2):196–201

5. Duckworth WC, Bennett RG, Hamel FG. Insulin degradation: progress and potential. *Endocr Rev* 1998;19:608–624

Case 30

U-500 Insulin Pump Case

Anthony L. McCall, MD, PhD, FACP[1]

A 49-year-old man presented for follow-up of uncontrolled type 2 diabetes with moderate peripheral neuropathy, hyperlipidemia, obesity, and hypertension. His last endocrine visit was 7 years ago, when he was obese and insulin resistant. This patient was initially on multiple injections of NPH and regular insulin and then converted to injection of U-500 regular insulin twice daily with improved control. He was then placed on an insulin pump, which he still uses with U-500 insulin only.

His current settings are as follows (all values are one-fifth of actual settings except for basal rates that have been corrected for actual doses per hour by multiplying the pump setting by 5):

12:00 A.M.:	3 units (0.6 units/h of U-100 insulin)
7:30 A.M.:	4.25 units
1:00 P.M.:	5 units
6:00 P.M.:	6.45 units
8:30 P.M.:	4.55 units

Insulin-to-carbohydrate (I:C) ratio for pump setting is 1:10 (actual I:C ratio is 1:2 because of the U-500 insulin). Insulin sensitivity factor (ISF) was not estimated by the patient, but based on a self-report of use of about 300 units daily of U-500 insulin, it would be expected to be about 5, which means a five-point drop for every additional unit of premeal bolus of insulin. Because he is using U-500, however, when he takes what his pump thinks is an extra unit, he is actually taking five times that amount, and the pump setting would be 25. The disjunction between his pump settings and his actual dosing can be confusing to pharmacists, educators, and physicians working with him. We prefer to state the apparent and actual doses to clarify the real rates and doses given.[1,2]

The patient states he only checks his blood glucose levels when he is "feeling bad." Thus, he reports a few scattered morning self-monitored blood glucose values, usually <150 mg/dL (8.3 mmol/L). He did not bring his meter and no pump download was available. He also reports a few scattered evening blood glucose values, usually in the low to mid-300 mg/dL

[1]James M. Moss Professor of Medicine, University of Virginia, School of Medicine and Health System, Charlottesville, VA.

DOI: 10.2337/9781580405713.30

(16.7 mmol/L). He endorsed eating out for supper with friends and favors heavy, fatty meals of the takeout variety. He typically boluses *after* supper instead of before he eats, despite being encouraged in the past to use post-meal dosing only for uncertainty about what he was going to eat or because of premeal hypoglycemia.

In recent weeks, he has been getting more exercise after finding a new job at the local auto shop. He claims he is on his feet 6–8 h/day. He does not perform any physical activity outside of work. We have encouraged him to use moderate-duration and intensity exercise as a therapeutic, especially to help with meal control.

His last HbA_{1c} was 7.8% in June 2013. Because of a history of cirrhosis with varices and history of gastrointestinal bleeding, which was thought to be related to non-alcoholic fatty liver disease (NAFLD)/non-alcoholic steatohepatitis (NASH) we are not certain that his values for blood glucose levels would show concordance with the predicted values based on his HbA_{1c}.

We recommended the following changes to this patient:

- Making dietary modifications to avoid high-fat, high-carbohydrate content items
- Changing the timing of his bolus dosing for his supper to 30 min before meal to minimize lows during the night as well as minimizing highs before bedtime
- If continuing 1:10 I:C ratio pump setting (real values 1/2) results in high glucose >200 mg/dL, then going to a 1:9 ratio
- Encouraging walking 20 min or more at least 3 days/week
- Measuring and recording blood glucose levels before breakfast, lunch, and supper and 3–4 h after supper
- Better controlling lipids and blood pressure

This patient illustrates care in very obese insulin-resistant patients. Several issues are brought out by his comorbidities and use of U-500 insulin in his pump, which is not common but increasingly is being used.[3] This patient has suboptimally controlled diabetes and uses an insulin pump to provide him with insulin in sufficient quantities. He is insulin resistant for several reasons, including obesity, frequent consumption of high-fat and high-carbohydrate meals, and liver cirrhosis. He times his insulin boluses improperly and checks his blood glucose levels infrequently. His basal insulin profile is what has been referred to as an "insulin staircase" and "cliff effect." This usually indicates that basal rates are at least partly being raised to compensate for inadequate meal control resulting from insufficient planned meal insulin (see Fig. 30.1).

First, this patient must improve his diet. Second, the patient needs to use correction doses of insulin to achieve better glucose control, especially at the evening meal based on his monitoring. On the basis of a total daily dose (estimated by the patient) of about 60 "apparent" units, he is actually taking 300 units of regular insulin daily or more. His HbA_{1c} of 7.8% is higher than previously and yet is likely falsely low because of his anemia (Hgb 8.2, Hct 25.8), liver disease, and potential shortened red cell survival.

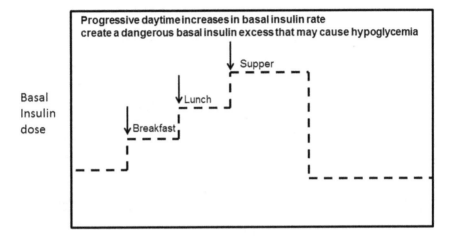

Figure 30.1— Insulin staircase and cliff effect in pump users: The pattern suggests use of basal insulin infusion rates to treat meals. Some insulin pump users inadvertently overuse basal insulin to aid in meal hyperglycemia control. This is observed quite commonly in those needing extended bolus configurations with insulin pump (square wave or dual wave). The marked drop in basal rate overnight may indicate the daytime overdose of basal insulin as well. To improve this situation, one may reduce the basal rates so that adequate mealtime boluses can be safely given. Thus, the total daily dose may not be incorrect, but a high risk of hypoglycemia is associated with an imbalance between meal and basal insulin.

The usual relationship of HbA$_{1c}$ to blood glucose values is shown in Table 30.1. The usual relationship often is altered and reticulocytosis (with less glycation of immature red cells) may explain a component of the altered relationship.

The timing of U-500 insulin probably is altered in comparison to U-100 insulin, probably because of the very high amounts being given and perhaps because of his insulin resistance.[4] With somewhat delayed peaks of action, the use of a postmeal dose probably represents a substantial temporal mismatch between caloric intake and insulin needs. Because he eats high-fat, high-glycemic-load meals often for lunch or late in the day, there may be less mismatch than there would be for a low-fat meal and the persistence of regular insulin for ≥6–8 h. The confusion about how much insulin he is actually taking

Table 30.1—Correlation of A1C with Average Glucose

A1C (%)	Mean plasma glucose	
	mg/dL	mmol/L
6	126	7.0
7	154	8.6
8	183	10.2
9	212	11.8
10	240	13.4
11	269	14.9
12	298	16.5

These estimates are based on ADAG data of ~2,700 glucose measurements over 3 months per A1C measurement in 507 adults with type 1, type 2, and no diabetes. The correlation between A1C and average glucose was 0.92. A calculator for converting A1C results into eAG, in either mg/dL or mmol/L, is available at http://professional.diabetes.org/eAG. *Source*: American Diabetes Association. Standards of medical care in diabetes, 2015. *Diabetes Care* 2015;38 (Suppl. 1):S35

can be serious because his pump settings represent a fivefold difference than his actual doses. Great care should be taken to document his actual doses and their relationship to the insulin pump settings.

REFERENCES

1. McCall AL. Insulin therapy and hypoglycemia. *Endocrinol Metab Clin North Amer* 2012;41(1):57–87

2. McCall AL. Insulin pumps. In *Endocrine Essentials: Endocrine Update for General Medicine*, Bradley Anawalt, Ed. Endocrine Society, 2012, 109–119

3. Leinung MC, Thompson S, Luo M, Leykina L, Nardacci E. Use of insulin pump therapy in patients with type 2 diabetes after failure of multiple daily injections. *Endocr Pract* 2013;19(1):9–13

4. de la Peña A, Riddle M, Morrow LA, et al. Pharmacokinetics and pharmacodynamics of high-dose human regular U-500 insulin versus human regular U-100 insulin in healthy obese subjects. *Diabetes Care* 2011;34:2496–2501

Case 31

Difficulties in Managing Patients with Insulin Resistance: Alternatives to U-500 Insulin

Narmada Movva, MD;[1,2] Boby G. Theckedath, MD, FACE;[1,2] and Janice L. Gilden, MS, MD, FCP, FACE[1,2]

A 63-year-old Caucasian man was referred for management of uncontrolled type 2 diabetes (T2D) of 18 years' duration. He was taking glipizide 20 mg twice daily and pioglitazone 15 mg daily. Metformin was not given because of his stage 3 chronic kidney disease. Three months of pioglitazone therapy resulted in weight gain of 27 lb (278 lb; BMI 35.5 kg/m²), and a hemoglobin A1c (HbA$_{1c}$) of 7.7%.

Other medical problems included hypertension, dyslipidemia, and depression. Other medications included clonidine 0.3 mg/day patch, losartan 100 mg daily, clopidogrel 75 mg daily, gemfibrozil 600 mg b.i.d, simvastatin 40 mg, gabapentin 600 mg twice daily, and aripiprazole 2.5 mg daily.

Lifestyle modification and metformin is the preferred initial therapy for patients with T2D, unless there are contraindications. Further therapy depends on the individual patient and the HbA$_{1c}$.

With HbA$_{1c}$ <7.5%, monotherapy is recommended. If HbA$_{1c}$ >6.5% in 3 months, then a second drug should be added. If HbA$_{1c}$ ≥7.5%, therapy with metformin and a second drug (glucagon-like peptide 1 [GLP-1] RA, dipeptidylpeptidase [DPP]-4 inhibitor, thiazolidinedione [TZD], sodium-glucose cotransporter [SGLT]-2 inhibitor, basal insulin, colesevelam, bromocriptine, or α-glucosidase inhibitor) is recommended.[1] Triple therapy is suggested when A1C is not at goal. For HbA$_{1c}$ >9%, dual or triple therapy should be started unless symptomatic, in which case insulin with or without other agents is recommended.[2,3]

Glycemic control continued to worsen despite adherence to a diabetic diet and 30 min of daily moderate exercise. Pioglitazone was stopped because of continual weight gain. Therapy with glargine insulin (10 units at bedtime) was added to the glipizide.

For T2D with persistent hyperglycemia despite other antihyperglycemic agents, insulin may be added. A basal long-acting insulin (such as detemir or

---

[1]Endocrinology Division, Department of Medicine, Rosalind Franklin University of Medicine and Science/Chicago Medical School, North Chicago, IL. [2]Endocrinology Section, Department of Medicine, Captain James A. Lovell Federal Health Care Center, North Chicago, IL.

This research was supported in part by the Captain James A. Lovell Federal Health Care Center.

DOI: 10.2337/9781580405713.31

glargine) is a reasonable choice. Long-acting basal insulin tends to achieve similar improvements in glucose levels with less hypoglycemia than NPH.[4]

Blood glucose (BG) continued to increase despite 56 units glargine daily. Therefore, premeal short-acting insulin (4 units aspart) was started and glipizide therapy was stopped. BG remained uncontrolled with titration of insulin to 60 units of daily glargine and aspart 10 units with meals. Hence pioglitazone 15 mg daily was restarted. A continuous glucose monitoring (CGM) evaluation was done, which demonstrated persistent hyperglycemia throughout the day and postprandial BG elevation (Fig. 31.1).

Six months later, HbA$_{1c}$ increased to 9.6%. The total daily insulin dose was 125 units (80 units glargine; 15 units premeal aspart). All of the self-monitoring of blood glucose (SMBG) readings were >140 mg/dL (7.769 mmol/L) with a range of 162–501 mg/dL (8.9–27.8 mmol/L) and half were >250 mg/dL (13.9 mmol/L). Continuous subcutaneous insulin infusion (CSII) therapy was initiated (basal rate of 2.5 units/h, insulin-to-carbohydrate ratio = 1:8 and insulin sensitivity factor = 1:25). Pioglitazone was continued.

CSII can be useful for intensive insulin therapy in T2D. Despite limited data from randomized control studies, longitudinal data in actual use settings suggest that CSII may be preferred to multiple daily injections (MDI) in patients with T2D who have severe insulin resistance and poor glycemic

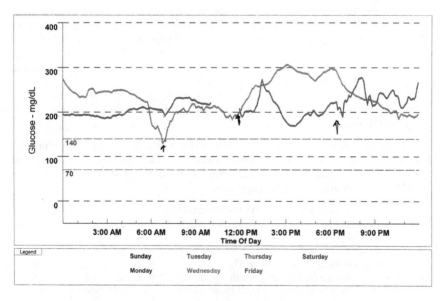

Figure 31.1—CGM study when patient was treated with basal and bolus insulin regimen (arrows indicate meals).

control, despite sufficient insulin titration and adherence to lifestyle recommendations.[5]

There was some improvement in BG after starting the insulin pump, as evidenced by an A1C decrease of 0.8% and 1.1% by 2 months and 8 months, respectively.

After 10 months of CSII (basal infusion rate of 4.5–5 units/h along with mealtime boluses), the total daily dose was 180 units. He also continued to gain weight (BMI 38 kg/m²; 293 lb). A trial of pramlintide before meals was started with titration to 120 micrograms/meal.

Pramlintide can be used as an adjunct to mealtime insulin in patients with type 1 diabetes (T1D) or T2D who are not able to achieve glycemic control despite optimal insulin therapy. For patients with T2D, pramlintide can be used as an adjunct to mealtime insulin with or without concurrent oral sulfonylurea agents or metformin.[6]

Secondary causes of insulin resistance, including acromegaly and Cushing's disease, were ruled out.

A repeat CGM study was done in October 2011, which showed persistent hyperglycemia throughout the day and less severe postprandial spikes (HbA$_{1c}$ 9.5%) (Fig. 31.2).

Switching insulin to U-500 was considered 22 months later, because the total daily dose was ~200 units. His pharmacy plan, however, did not approve this change.

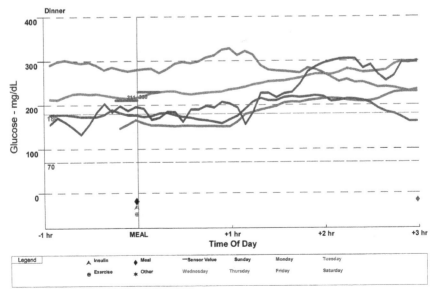

Figure 31.2—CGM study 10 months after starting CSII.

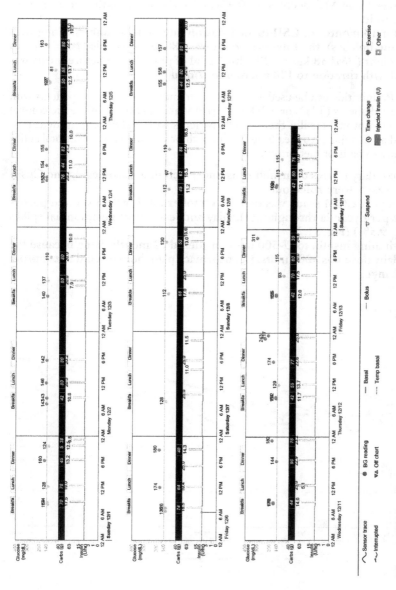

Figure 31.3—Overview of glycemic control 1 year after starting liraglutide.

The use of U-500 insulin is another treatment option for severely insulin-resistant patients with T2D. A trial of exenatide 5 mcg twice daily was prescribed in addition to CSII and pioglitazone therapy with some minimal improvement in BG, but this was discontinued after 1 month because of nausea and diarrhea.

A trial of liraglutide (0.6 mg daily) was then started, in addition to his usual insulin (total daily dose = 200 units of insulin; basal 65% and bolus 35%). This is an off-label use of a combination of prandial insulin with liraglutide, but the patient did not experience side effects even after 1.8 mg of liraglutide. BG decreased from 300s to 200s mg/dL (from 16.6 to 11.1 mmol/L) after 1 month of therapy and HbA$_{1c}$ of 7.7% after 2 months. Six months later, aripiprazole was stopped. Medications for depression were no longer required

The total daily dose of insulin remained about 200–220 units/day. By 1 year of CSII, pioglitazone and liraglutide, HbA$_{1c}$ improved to 6.6%; body weight was between 290 and 300 lb (Fig. 31.3).

GLP-1 analogs, a new class of pharmacologic agents, can improve glycemic control by promoting insulin secretion of pancreatic β-cells with improvement in β-cell sensitivity to glucose and suppression of glucagon secretion, thereby reducing hepatic glucose production, inhibiting gastric emptying, and promoting satiety with resulting weight loss. Studies have confirmed improvements in glycemic control and decreases in insulin doses when liraglutide is added to insulin for patients who are obese with T1D.[7] Thus, GLP-1 analogs can be used as an option for the management of diabetes with severe insulin resistance as observed in our patient. This case highlights the difficulty in managing a patient with T2D and extreme insulin resistance. Despite multiple therapeutic trials, BG control remained problematic until the addition of a GLP-1 analog.

REFERENCES

1. Inzucchi SE, Bergenstal RM, Buse JB, et al. Management of hyperglycemia in type 2 diabetes, 2015: a patient-centered approach: update to a position statement of the American Diabetes Association and the European Association for the Study of Diabetes. *Diabetes Care* 2015;38:140–149

2. American Diabetes Association. Standards of medical care in diabetes, 2015. *Diabetes Care* 2015;38(Suppl. 1):S1–S93

3. Garber AJ, Abrahamson MJ, Barzilay JI, Blonde L, Bloomgarden ZT, Bush MA, Dagogo-Jack S, Davidson MB, Einhorn D, Garvey WT, Grunberger G, Handelsman Y, Hirsch IB, Jellinger PS, McGill JB, Mechanick JI, Rosenblit PD, Umpierrez G, Davidson MH, American Association of Clinical Endocrinologists. AACE comprehensive diabetes management algorithm 2013. *Endocr Pract* 2013;19(2):327–336

4. Riddle MC, Rosenstock J, Gerich J, Insulin Glargine 4002 Study Investigators. The treat-to-target trial: randomized addition of glargine or human NPH insulin to oral therapy of type 2 diabetic patients. *Diabetes Care* 2003;26: 3080–3086

5. Reznik Y, Cohen O. Insulin pump for type 2 diabetes. *Diabetes Care* 2013;36(Suppl. 2):S219–S225

6. Pullman J, Darsow T, Frias JP. Pramlintide in the management of insulin-using patients with type 2 and type 1 diabetes. *Vasc Health Risk Manag* 2006;2(3): 203–212

7. Kuhadiya ND, Malik R, Bellini NJ, Patterson JL, Traina A, Makdissi A, Dandona P. Liraglutide as additional treatment to insulin in obese patients with type 1 diabetes mellitus. *Endocr Pract* 2013;19(6):963–967

Case 32

Management Issues in the Syndrome of Autoantibodies to the Insulin Receptor (Type B Insulin Resistance)

ELAINE COCHRAN, MSN, CRNP;[1] REBECCA BROWN, MD, MHSC;[1] AND PHILLIP GORDEN, MD[1]

A 29-year-old African American woman presented to her primary care provider (PCP). Over the preceding 6 months, she had experienced a dramatic change to her health, including development of insulin resistant diabetes, polycystic ovarian syndrome, hyperandrogenism (testosterone >900 ng/mL), and a 35–40 lb weight loss. She had seen three endocrinologists but did not receive a diagnosis. When seen by the PCP, she required 500–1,000 units/day of insulin, but continued to lose weight (current BMI 19.5 kg/m²) with increasing insulin requirements.

The PCP suspected type B insulin resistance, an extreme form of insulin resistance caused by autoantibodies to the insulin receptor. The PCP was unable to locate a laboratory to test for antibodies to the insulin receptor and could not find guidance on treatment. By searching www.clinicaltrials. gov, the PCP located our research team at the National Institutes of Health (NIH).

We advised the PCP to obtain blood tests, and within a week had the following results:

Cholesterol	165 mg/dL
Triglycerides	63 mg/dL
HDL	105 mg/dL
LDL	47mg/dL
Blood glucose	309 mg/dL
C-peptide	2.5 ng/mL
ANA (antinuclear antibody)	5 EU (normal <1)
ENA (extractable nuclear antibody)	120 EU (normal <20)
WBC (white blood cell)	3.22 K/µL
ANC (anti-neutrophil cytoplasmicantibody)	–930
Adiponectin	24 mg/L

The patient was enrolled in a treatment protocol at NIH. Her HbA$_{1c}$ was 13.9%, despite 3,000 units/day of concentrated U-500 insulin. Antibody testing was performed by a research laboratory; several weeks later, the patient's sample was confirmed to be strongly positive for autoantibodies to the insulin receptor.

[1]National Institutes of Health, National Institute of Diabetes, Digestive, and Kidney Diseases, Diabetes, Endocrine, and Obesity Branch, Bethesda, MD.

DOI: 10.2337/9781580405713.32

Before confirmation of autoantibodies to the insulin receptor, treatment was initiated based on the classic presentation of symptoms and conventional laboratory results.[1,2] The patient was an African American woman, with abrupt onset of severe insulin resistance associated with significant sudden weight loss, extremely high insulin requirements, and severe hyperandrogenism. Autoimmune screening showed positive ANA and ENA, and low WBC count with neutropenia. Despite her extreme insulin resistance, she had very low triglycerides, elevated HDL, and elevated adiponectin. Adiponectin >7 mg/L in severe insulin resistance has a 97% positive predictive value for disorders of the insulin receptor, whereas a level <5 mg/L has a 97% negative predictive value.

THERAPY

Conventional diabetes therapies are of no benefit in this extreme form of insulin resistance. Concentrated U-500 insulin has a temporizing role, ameliorating the extreme catabolic state when given in extraordinarily high doses (>10 units/kg/day).[3] Although this clinical syndrome was described 37 years ago,[1] it is only recently that a systematic therapeutic approach has been developed.[4] The goal of therapy is to eliminate the autoantibody. Temporary measures such as plasmapheresis have been used, but no long-term benefits have been seen. The current approach uses combination immunotherapy to eliminate the autoantibody while producing minimal toxicity.[4] The first agent is rituximab, which eliminates precursor β-cells. Simultaneously, pulsed steroids are administered to reduce antibody producing plasma β-cells. Intermittent steroids are preferred over daily therapy to minimize side effects. Finally, oral cyclophosphamide is given to inhibit helper T-cells related to antibody production; cyclosporine is used as an alternative if cyclophosphamide is not tolerated. CD19 counts are monitored monthly, and rituximab therapy is repeated only if the CD19 count is not suppressed and the patient continues to have severe insulin resistance. Steroid pulses are administered monthly until remission is achieved, defined by normalization of glucose (and testosterone, in women) and the discontinuation of exogenous insulin.

As treatment progresses, clinicians must be prepared to rapidly taper exogenous insulin as soon as the patient experiences hypoglycemia. After remission, daily cyclophosphamide is switched to azathioprine 50–100 mg daily. Hypoglycemia in the fasting or postprandial state is common after remission occurs, *even in the absence of exogenous insulin therapy*. This is due to the autoantibody acting as a partial agonist at the insulin receptor: It antagonizes insulin action in high titer, but stimulates insulin signaling at low titer.

The patient received 1 cycle of rituximab, defined as two 1-g doses given 14 days apart. With each rituximab dose, the patient received 40 mg of dexamethasone daily for 4 days. Oral cyclophosphamide, 100 mg daily, was initiated with the first rituximab dose. One month later, her CD19 count was 0, but she continued to have significant hyperglycemia despite 3,000 units/day of insulin. Monthly steroid pulses and cyclophosphamide were continued for the next 4 months. Because the CD19 count remained low,

rituximab was not repeated. Five months after the start of immunosuppression, the patient developed significant hypoglycemia. Exogenous insulin was stopped, cyclophosphamide was discontinued, and azathioprine was started. One additional steroid pulse was given, as her fasting insulin level, off exogenous insulin therapy, was elevated at 36 μIU/mL. After 2 months on azathioprine, her fasting insulin was 25 μIU/mL and her HbA_{1c} was 5.7%.

Type B insulin resistance results from an antibody against the cell surface insulin receptor and is representative of a class of diseases in which autoantibodies are produced against cell surface receptors. The condition usually occurs in the context of a collagen vascular disease, such as lupus or mixed connective tissue disease, or as a paraneoplastic syndrome, and is seen more commonly in women, particularly those of African descent. In this case, an astute primary care practitioner recognized an unusual presentation of diabetes. The key clinical features were a nonobese young woman, refractory to large doses of insulin, with severe insulin resistance and acanthosis nigricans.

Conventional laboratory tests can aid in making the diagnosis in the absence of confirmatory testing for antibodies in a research laboratory. In contrast to obesity-associated insulin resistance, these patients typically have normal or low triglycerides, and normal or high HDL. The absolute neutrophil count is often low, and immunologic markers consistent with lupus or mixed connective tissue disease are usually present. In addition, adiponectin, which is usually low in insulin resistance, is increased in disorders of the insulin receptor, including either autoantibodies or inherited mutations of the insulin receptor.

This patient had a completely curable form of extreme insulin resistance and resulting hyperglycemia, and achieved a complete remission of this disease.

REFERENCES

1. Kahn CR, Flier JS, Bar RS, Archer JA, Gorden P, Martin MM, et al. The syndromes of insulin resistance and acanthosis nigricans. Insulin-receptor disorders in man. *N Engl J Med* 1976;294:739–745

2. Arioglu E, Andewelt A, Diabo C, Bell M, Taylor SI, Gorden P. Clinical course of the syndrome of autoantibodies to the insulin receptor (type B insulin resistance): a 28-year perspective. *Medicine* 2002;81:87–100

3. Cochran E, Musso C, Gorden P. The use of U-500 in patients with extreme insulin resistance. *Diabetes Care* 2005;28:1240–1244

4. Malek R, Chong AY, Lupsa BC, Lungu AO, Cochran EK, Soos MA, et al. Treatment of type B insulin resistance: a novel approach to reduce insulin receptor autoantibodies. *J Clin Endocrinol Metab* 2010;95:3641–3647

Case 33

Type B Insulin Resistance

NISHA BINCENT JACOB, APN, FNP-C, CDE, MBA;[1] HILARY TREVINO, APN, FNP-C;[1] AND CHANHAENG RHEE, MD, MBA[1]

A 24-year-old African American woman with a history of sickle cell trait anemia presented to an outside hospital with complaints of fever, chills, myalgia, and arthralgia. She had been treated with olsetamivir and antibiotics without improvement. After lymph node and bone marrow biopsy and a lumber puncture, she was diagnosed with disseminated cytomegalovirus (CMV). With 12 days of ganciclovir treatment, her symptoms improved for only a short time. She developed an erythematous rash on her face, chest, arms, hands, back, and upper legs; oral ulcers; acute kidney injury; pericardial effusion; and pleural effusions with consolidation. Upon admission to our hospital, the patient's blood glucose (BG) was found to be >400 mg/dL (22.2 mmol/L) with a normal anion gap, and an HbA_{1c} of 8.1%. Her skin biopsy revealed erythema multiforme, and she was empirically started on prednisone (70 mg/day), resulting in rapid improvement. The patient did not have any history of diabetes.

Intravenous insulin infusion was initiated at 10–12 units/h with BG >400 mg/dL (22.2 mmol/L) and was uptitrated to 110 units/h (total daily dose [TDD] of insulin = 2,640 units).

Type B insulin resistance is a result of anti-insulin receptor antibodies, which inhibit insulin's ability to bind to insulin receptors. The number of insulin receptor binding sites decreases and insulin receptor function is impaired, causing insulin resistance.[1] This condition has been identified in patients with other autoimmune diseases, such as systemic lupus erythematosus (SLE) and less frequently with Sjogren's syndrome, alopecia, and vitiligo.[1] It is hypothesized that the same pathogenesis of SLE, characterized by the loss of normal immune regulation and self-tolerance, is responsible for the production of these autoantibodies, and that SLE exacerbation and severe insulin resistance occur concomitantly.[2]

The findings in this patient were suggestive of SLE, based on her anti-Smith, anti-U1-RNP, and +ANA, as well as the myalgia, arthralgia, adenopathy, rash, serositis, lymphopenia, and thrombocytopenia. An elevated serum creatinine and proteinuria were suggestive of lupus glomerulonephritis. The patient stayed on an insulin infusion for 6 days. The degree of persistent hyperglycemia and insulin resistance were consistent with type B insulin resistance.

[1]University of Texas Southwestern Medical Center, Department of Internal Medicine, Division of Endocrinology and Metabolism, Dallas, TX.

DOI: 10.2337/9781580405713.33

Unfortunately, we could not find a laboratory willing to perform a titer for insulin receptor autoantibodies. All antibiotics were discontinued, and she was started on hydroxychloroquine 200 mg by mouth twice daily and mycophenolate 500 mg daily, along with continuation of prednisone at 60 mg/day.

A review of 28 reported cases with "type B insulin resistance" presented to the National Institutes of Health over 30 years found the typical clinical presentation of these patients to be predominately female, of African American or Caribbean origin, with an average age of 39 years (range, 10–63 years). Patients presented with rapid-onset, rapidly progressing insulin-resistant diabetes requiring large amounts of insulin (5,100 units/day [range, 200–250,000 units]) and an autoimmune disease, such as SLE, which may have been accompanied by acanthosis nigricans, hyperandrogenism, and alopecia.[3] Many of these patients had proteinuria, likely related to lupus glomerulonephritis, an elevated testosterone level, and enlarged ovaries. Additionally, each patient was proven to have insulin receptor autoantibodies by assay.[4]

Various immunotherapies have been tried, including corticosteroids, plasmapharesis, cyclophosphamide, cyclosporine, azothiaprine, mycophenolate mofetil, and monoclonal antibodies.[5] Some patients experienced clinical remission in association with immunotherapy (within 6 weeks), and others experienced prolonged hyperglycemia or spontaneous remission without therapy.[1] Ultimately, remission was associated with a resolution of hyperglycemia and a disappearance in the insulin receptor antibody titer.[4,5]

The patient's high insulin requirement continued for 4 days after the initiation of immune therapy. Her insulin requirements eventually came down with the BG trending down to 130–150 mg/dL (7.2–8.3 mmol/L) while on insulin infusion. The patient recovered from the acute exacerbation phase with resolution of fevers, rashes, and arthralgia. She was transitioned to subcutaneous basal bolus insulin with a target TDD of 150 units, along with metformin 500 mg/day.

She was discharged home on insulin glargine 50 units in the morning and 25 units in the evening, insulin aspart 25 units with meals, a correction insulin scale, and prednisone 30 mg twice daily for 30 days.

At her 1-week follow-up, the patient had a BG range between 100 and 300 mg/dL (5.5–16.7 mmol/L). The patient was instructed to continue the discharge dose of glargine and prandial aspart and to slightly increase correction insulin and metformin (to 1,000 mg twice daily).

Shortly after follow-up, the patient started having episodes of hypoglycemia (30s–40s mg/dL or 1.7–2.2 mmol/L) and subsequently stopped taking insulin. A review of her home monitoring device showed BGs in the low 100s (5.5 mmol/L) or lower.

Several patients with type B insulin resistance have experienced severe hypoglycemia (BG <25 mg/dL or 1.4 mmol/L) after remission, requiring treatment with high-dose steroids, a high-carbohydrate diet, or scheduled eating every 3 h to keep the plasma glucose within a normal range. Of note, among the few reported cases in the literature, this diagnosis carries a high mortality rate (54%) even in patients who entered remission, with complications from intractable hypoglycemia being the major trend.[4]

On the second endocrinologist visit, she was instructed to stop metformin. HbA$_{1c}$ trended down to 6.2% 3 months after discharge, and 5.4% after 1 year. To date, the patient has been released from the care of an endocrinologist. She currently takes mycophenolate 1,000 mg twice daily along with periodic pulse dose steroids with no further episodes of hyperglycemia.

It is hypothesized that the anti-insulin receptor antibody production is stimulated by the active disease state of SLE. This is supported by co-occurrence of the two conditions, and the resolution and remission of hyperglycemia after treatment with immunosuppressive therapies.[2] Thus, future issues with glucose intolerance can be avoided through management and treatment of SLE.

REFERENCES

1. Ostwal V, Oak J. Type B insulin resistance in the systemic lupus erythematosus patient. *Int J Rheum Dis* 2009;12:174–176

2. Kawashiri S, Kawakami A, Fujikawa K, Iwamoto N, Aramaki T, Tamai M, Nakamura H, Origuchi T, Ida H, Eguchi K. Type B insulin resistance complicated with systemic lupus erythatosus. *Intern Med* 2010;49:487–490

3. Coll AP, Morgansterin D, Jaynet D, Soos MA, O'Rahilly S, Burke J. Successful treatment of type B insulin resistance in a patient with otherwise quiescent systemic lupus erythematosus. *Diabet Med* 2005;22:812–815

4. Arioglu E, Andewelt A, Diabo C, Bell M, Taylor S, Gorden P. Clinical course of the syndrome of autoantibodies to the insulin receptor (type B insulin resistance): a 28 year prospective. *Medicine* 2002;81:87–100

5. Bao S, Root C, Jagasia S. Type B insulin resistance syndrome associated with systemic lupus erythematosus. *Endocr Pract* 2007;13(1):51–55

Case 34

Adhering or Not? That Is the Question: A Case of Glucolipotoxicity and Concentrated Insulin

Sanaa Deshmukh, MD;[1] Rino Buzzola, MD;[1] Mariana Touza, MD;[1] Michael Gardner, MD;[1] and James R. Sowers, MD[1]

The patient is a 57-year-old woman with past medical history significant for obesity, stage 3 chronic kidney disease (with polycystic kidney disease), hypertension, and hyperlipidemia. She presented to the clinic for follow-up of uncontrolled type 2 diabetes, diagnosed 3 years prior. Her medical regimen consisted of liraglutide 0.6 mg subcutaneously daily, insulin aspart 50 units three times a day with meals (a combination used off-label), and insulin glargine 75 units two times per day. On this regimen, she reported experiencing low blood glucose approximately two times per month, usually in the evenings before bedtime. She reported not checking her blood glucose because she had misplaced her home glucose monitoring. Labs obtained during that visit were significant for the following:

HbA$_{1c}$	9.6%
eGFR	17.56 mL/min
Total cholesterol	235 mg/dL
Triglycerides	345 mg/dL
LDL	102 mg/dL

She was advised to return 2 weeks later with blood glucose recordings as a guide to determine an appropriate U-500 insulin regimen.

Given that this patient had a total daily requirement of 300 units/day of insulin, in combination with uncontrolled diabetes (despite being on a large dose of total daily insulin), the decision to place her on U-500 insulin was appropriate. U-500 insulin has been shown to significantly improve glycemic control in patients with highly insulin resistant type 2 diabetes, as evidenced by a marked reduction in HbA$_{1c}$ levels after initiation of therapy on this more concentrated form of insulin.[1] U-500 insulin has been especially helpful in obese patients (such as this one) with particularly resistant type 2 diabetes requiring ≥200 units/day of U-100 insulin.[2]

The patient returned 2 weeks later, at which time she was transitioned to U-500 insulin. Review of her home blood glucose recordings revealed results ranging from 150 to 190 mg/dL (8.3–10.6 mmol/L), with fasting

[1]Division of Endocrinology, Diabetes and Metabolism, Department of Medicine, University of Missouri, Columbia, MO.

DOI: 10.2337/9781580405713.34

blood glucose levels in the range of ≥150 mg/dL (8.3 mmol/L) or more. She was placed on a three-time per day regimen with instructions to take 0.24 mL (120 units) of U-500 with breakfast, and 0.18 mL (90 units) of U-500 with lunch and supper. Her liraglutide, insulin glargine, and insulin aspart were discontinued at that time, and she was advised to return to the clinic 2 weeks later for follow-up (an appointment for which the patient did not present).

For patients requiring 300 units/day of insulin, U-500 insulin can be administered three to four times per day.[1,2] This also eliminates the need for additional basal insulin, given the prolonged length of action of U-500 insulin in comparison to U-100 insulin.[2]

Four weeks later, she presented to the emergency department because of a syncopal episode while shopping at the supermarket. Fingerstick glucose was 27 mg/dL (1.5 mmol/L) for which she was given 50 cc of 50% dextrose before presenting to the emergency room. She was admitted and placed on a 10% dextrose infusion. Blood glucose slowly returned to normal. Review of her home glucose records showed a downward trend in her glucose levels, with hypoglycemia present the week before admission. She continued to take her insulin U-500 as prescribed, however. The remainder of her hospitalization remained uneventful, and she was eventually discharged home on insulin glargine 10 units at bedtime with insulin aspart 3 units before each meal, a total daily dose of 19 units/day (one-fifteenth of her total dose on admission). Her blood glucose levels ranged from 80 to 170 mg/dL (4.4 to 9.4 mmol/L) per review of her home records during her follow-up appointment 2 weeks after discharge.

This patient continued to take the same initial dose of U-500 insulin despite hypoglycemia on the regimen. Her blood glucose levels likely decreased before of increased insulin sensitivity in association with insulin therapy.[3] Several studies have shown that in the acute setting, exogenous glucose enters the pancreatic β-cell via GLUT2 transporters to stimulate the production of insulin by pancreatic β-cells.[4] In chronic hyperglycemia, there is decreased β-cell function (i.e., decreased glucose sensitivity) due to β-cell exhaustion (depletion of insulin sources) and β-cell desensitization (the cell is refractory to further stimulation and thus unable to release more insulin). Chronic hyperglycemia decreases β-cell proliferation and differentiation, and increases proapoptotic signals (resulting in β-cell death).[4] Decreased sensitivity is reversible with insulin therapy, while apoptosis is irreversible.[3,5]

The other factor worth considering in this patient was her obesity, or in other words, her presumed exposure to free fatty acids, a concept known as lipotoxicity. β-Cell function has been shown to decrease with the build-up of reactive oxidative species within the islet cells as a result of free fatty acid metabolism.[3] Several studies also exist that suggest the negative effects of free fatty acid metabolite accumulation can occur only in the presence of prolonged hyperglycemia (both of which were the case in this patient).[3]

Patients not requiring U-500 after initial therapy with U-500 are not entirely unheard of, as reports exist showing some patients can be transitioned back to U-100 insulin once their blood glucose levels have become better controlled with U-500 therapy.[2] Although many may question her adherence to her regimen before starting U-500 therapy, her euglycemia just before the change in regimen stands testament to her increased needs at that time. Both her weight and renal function remained stable during this clinical course, and therefore they were not contributing factors toward decreased insulin resistance. Her eventual hypoglycemia on U-500 points toward treatment of glucolipotoxicity, resulting in improved insulin sensitivity.

REFERENCES

1. Dailey AM, Tannock LR. Extreme insulin resistance: indications and approaches to the use of U-500 insulin in type 2 diabetes mellitus. *Curr Diab Rep* 2011;11:77–82

2. Jones P, Idris I. The use of U-500 regular insulin in the management of patients with obesity and insulin resistance. *Diabetes Obes Metab* 2013;15:882–887

3. Cernea S, Dobreanu M. Diabetes and beta cell function: from mechanisms to evaluation and clinical implications. *Biochem Med* 2013;23(3):266–280

4. Bensellam M, Laybutt DR, Jonas JC. The molecular mechanisms of pancreatic β-cell glucotoxicity: recent findings and future research directions. *Mol Cell Endocrinol* 2012;364:1–27

5. Banerji MA. Impaired beta-cell and alpha-cell function in African-American children with type 2 diabetes mellitus—"Flatbush diabetes." *J Pediatr Endocrinol Metab* 2002;15(Suppl. 1):493–501

Case 35

Cosecreting Adrenal Tumor Causing Severe Insulin Resistance

Kathya Rivera, MD;[1] Kenneth Cusi, MD;[1,2] and Catherine Edwards, MD[1]

A 38-year-old Caucasian woman was referred to our care with a presumed diagnosis of primary hyperaldosteronism and an associated large adrenal mass. She was found by her primary care physician (PCP) to have severe hypokalemia on routine lab work although she was completely asymptomatic.

Past medical history included osteoporosis, hyperlipidemia, meningioma, seizure disorder, and hypothyroidism. Family history included type 2 diabetes (T2D), hypertension, dyslipidemia, and coronary heart disease. Medications at the time of endocrine evaluation included KCl 40 mEq p.o. q.i.d., diltiazem 60 mg p.o. q.i.d., losartan 25 mg p.o. daily, spirinolactone 50 mg p.o. daily, insulin glargine 45 units subcutaneously b.i.d., insulin aspart 26 units subcutaneously before meals, and a correction scale and pioglitazone 15 mg daily. On examination, blood pressure was 177/90 mmHg and pulse was 112 bpm. She was 4' 9" tall, weighed 36 kg and had a BMI of 17.2 kg/m². Physical examination revealed a young female with a round face, bilateral clavicular fullness, and proximal muscle wasting of the extremities but no acanthosis nigricans, facial plethora, acne, bruises, hirsutism, central obesity, or purple striae.

Review of prior records indicated that on presentation to her PCP, plasma potassium had been 1.4 mEq/L and plasma glucose was 324 mg/dL. Additional work-up included a low plasma renin activity of 0.39 ng/mL/h (normal, upright: 0.5–4.0 ng/mL/h), elevated aldosterone of 181.9 ng/dL (normal, upright: 4.0–31.0 ng/dL), and A/R ratio of 466. An abdominal computed tomography (CT) scan with contrast revealed a 10 cm heterogeneous left suprarenal mass with tumor thrombus extending from this mass into the inferior vena cava (IVC), concerning for carcinoma (Fig. 35.1). Upon arrival to our facility, laboratory data included the following:

Sodium	141 mmol/L
Potassium	4.4 mmol/L
Magnesium	2.4 mg/dL
Phosphorus	3.5 mg/dL
Fasting glucose	170 mg/dL
A1C	7.9% (normal: 4.1–6.1%)

[1]Division of Endocrinology, Diabetes and Metabolism, University of Florida, Gainesville, FL. [2]Division of Endocrinology, Diabetes and Metabolism, Malcom Randall VAMC, Gainesville, FL.

          DOI: 10.2337/9781580405713.35

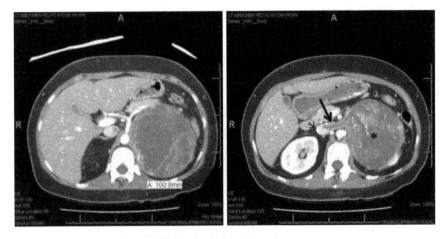

Figure 35.1 — CT scan of the abdomen and pelvis with IV contrast showed (*left*) a heterogeneous 10 cm left suprarenal region mass with (*right*) tumor thrombus (large arrow) extending from the mass (*) into the IVC (small arrow).

Given the patient's clinical history of new-onset hypertension and hypokalemia, with history and physical findings suggestive of Cushing's syndrome (CS) in the setting of a large adrenal mass, she was suspected to have an aldosterone-producing adrenocortical carcinoma with possible cosecretion of cortisol. A low dose dexamethasone suppression test was performed, which did not suppress (cortisol 21.7 µg/dL).

Adrenal masses can be functional or nonfunctional, and either malignant or benign. Adrenocortical carcinomas are rare (1–2 cases per million) with approximately 60% being functional.[1] Unlike benign functional adenomas, adrenocortical carcinomas often cosecrete multiple hormones. Solitary hypercortisolism is seen in 30–40% of cases and hyperaldosteronism has been reported in 2.5% of cases.

The clinical manifestations of hypercortisolism are well recognized, although the majority of signs and symptoms are nonspecific. One such finding is the impairment of glucose metabolism. Most patients with hypercortisolism have impaired glucose metabolism and many patients with undiagnosed CS have hyperglycemia often attributed to T2D. Despite its role in contributing to morbidity and mortality in patients with CS,[2] the available data do not support the cost-effectiveness of screening in patients with T2D.[3]

During her hospitalization, the patient's blood glucose (BG) levels remained elevated. She was continued on pioglitazone, insulin glargine was increased to 50 units b.i.d., and insulin was increased aspart to 30 units before meals. Before surgery, BG levels improved and ranged between 90 and 160 mg/dL (3.3–8.9 mmol/L) (Fig. 35.2).

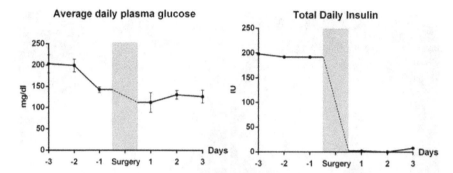

Figure 35.2—Graphic representation of the patient's average daily plasma glucose and total daily insulin doses in the perioperative period. Standard deviation for each average daily plasma glucose levels is also shown.

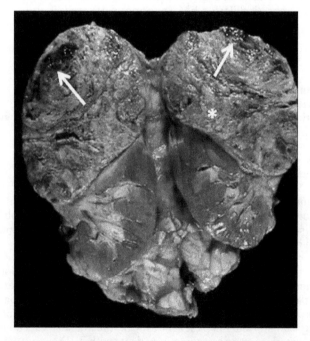

Figure 35.3A—The gross picture shows a bivalved kidney with a large (12.0 x 10.0 x 8.0 cm), well-circumscribed, white-tan mass, compressing the superior pole of the kidney. The mass is diffusely necrotic (*) and focally hemorrhagic (arrows). Images courtesy of Jennifer Loch, D.O., Department of Pathology, University of Florida.

The predominant mechanisms underlying the impairment of glucose metabolism in CS involve the development of liver, muscle, and adipose tissue insulin resistance.[4] Steroid-induced hepatic insulin resistance stimulates hepatic glucose production through increased glycogenolysis and gluconeogenesis, which becomes more evident during the postprandial period. Corticosteroids have been reported to impair insulin secretion.[4] At the level of skeletal muscle, glucocorticoids alter postreceptor insulin signaling, inhibiting insulin receptor substrate (IRS-1), phosphatidylinositol 3-kinase, protein kinase B (Akt), and other key signaling steps and worsening insulin resistance. In adipose tissue, glucocorticoids also impair insulin action, leading to excessive lipolysis.

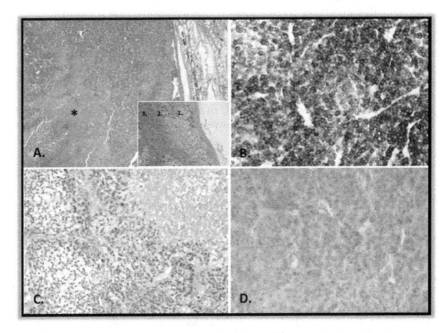

Figure 35.3B—Low-power view (4x) of the adrenocortical tumor shows the diffuse architecture of the tumor with confluent necrosis (*) on H&E stain (*A*). In comparison, a low-power view (4x, H&E) of a normal adrenal cortex (right lower corner, *A*) shows the distribution of the 3 anatomical zones: the zona glomerulosa (1), zona fasciculata (2), and zona reticularis (3). Immunohistochemical studies show the tumor is strongly positive for inhibin stain (10x, *B*), focally positive for melan-A stain (10x, *C*), and negative for chromogranin stain (10x, *D*) supporting the diagnosis of an adrenocortical neoplasm. Images courtesy of Jennifer Loch, D.O., Department of Pathology, University of Florida.

This increases free fatty acid flux to the liver contributing to hepatic insulin resistance and the development of fatty liver. Glucocorticoids also influence the synthesis and release of adipokines, causing subclinical inflammation and contributing to the development of systemic insulin resistance.[5]

Five days after admission, her potassium levels had remained stable, her blood pressure and glucose levels were better controlled, and she underwent radical left nephrectomy with adrenalectomy and infrahepatic IVC thrombectomy (Fig. 35.3A). Histopathology confirmed an adrenocortical carcinoma (Fig. 35.3B). Immunohistochemistry revealed that the tumor was diffusely immunoreactive for inhibin, focally immunoreactive for melan-A, and negative for chromogranin, S100, cytokeratin AE1/AE3, and calretinin (Fig. 35.3B), supporting the diagnosis of an adrenocortical neoplasm.

Postoperatively, she was empirically started on hydrocortisone 50 mg every 8 h anticipating suppression of endogenous cortisol production by the remaining adrenal gland. Over the following 48–72 h hydrocortisone was decreased to a maintenance dose of 15 mg every morning (QAM) and 5 mg every evening with close monitoring of BG levels. Insulin requirements decreased from almost 200 units/day to requiring only 2–4 units/day of correctional insulin to maintain BG levels of 100–130 mg/dL (5.6–7.2 mmol/L) (Fig. 35.3). This was despite supraphysiological doses of corticosteroids immediately postoperatively.

In patients with hypercortisolism caused by functioning adrenal carcinomas, adrenalectomy is the therapeutic gold standard.[1] The impairment of glucose metabolism generally resolves with normalization of cortisol levels. Metabolic abnormalities, such as hypertension and insulin resistance are likely multifactorial, however, and may not resolve entirely despite surgical resection.[1] Therefore, antidiabetic drugs should be carefully adjusted in the perioperative period to avoid hypoglycemia. Close outpatient follow-up should be established to monitor for subsequent increase in BG levels especially if normalization of cortisol secretion does not occur.

On postoperative day 10, she was discharged with good glycemic control on insulin glargine 10 units QAM and metformin 500 mg orally b.i.d. with meals. The patient continues to follow up with her local endocrinologist, who reports adequate glycemic control, but insulin requirements have progressively increased in the 6 months postoperatively. Her most recent HbA$_{1c}$ is 7% on her current regimen of basal bolus insulin glargine and aspart, which has increased to more than 3 units/kg/day. Unfortunately, this progressive insulin resistance is suspicious for residual or metastatic adrenocortical carcinoma. She has established care with a local oncologist and will undergo further evaluation with positron emission tomography–CT scan.

REFERENCES

1. Allolio B, Fassnacht M. Clinical review: adrenocortical carcinoma: clinical update. *J Clin Endocrinol Metab* 2006;91:2027–2037

2. Nieman LK, Biller BM, Findling JW, Newell-Price J, Savage MO, Stewart PM, Montori VM. The diagnosis of Cushing's syndrome: an Endocrine Society Clinical Practice Guideline. *J Clin Endocrinol Metab* 2008;93:1526–1540

3. Mullan K, Black N, Thiraviaraj A, Bell PM, Burgess C, Hunter SJ, McCance DR, Leslie H, Sheridan B, Atkinson AB. Is there value in routine screening for Cushing's syndrome in patients with diabetes? *J Clin Endocrinol Metab* 2010;95:2262–2265

4. Yuen KC, Chong LE, Riddle MC. Influence of glucocorticoids and growth hormone on insulin sensitivity in humans. *Diabet Med* 2013;30:651–663

5. Pivonello R, De Leo M, Vitale P, Cozzolino A, Simeoli C, De Martino MC, Lombardi G, Colao A. Pathophysiology of diabetes mellitus in Cushing's syndrome. *Neuroendocrinology* 2010;92(Suppl. 1):77–81

Management of Severe Insulin Resistance in a Pregnant Patient with Type 2 Diabetes: The Use of U-500 Regular Insulin via Continuous Subcutaneous Infusion

Tiffany Hor, MD,[1] and David Baldwin, MD[1]

A 33-year-old woman with type 2 diabetes presented for management of uncontrolled blood glucose. She was diagnosed with diabetes at age 25 years. Her BMI was 35.5 kg/m². Her father and older brother also have type 2 diabetes. She was initially managed with insulin glargine once a day, insulin lispro with meals, and metformin 1,000 mg b.i.d. She was subsequently switched to lispro insulin by continuous subcutaneous insulin infusion (CSII) because of suboptimal glycemic control. She required about 225–250 units/day of insulin, but HbA$_{1c}$ remained 8–9%. She was disappointed with her results and was frustrated with the need to change her insulin cartridges almost daily. She was concerned about her glycemic control since she was planning to get pregnant within the next year. She wanted to know options for improving her diabetes control.

Patients with diabetes who require >200 units/day of insulin are considered to have insulin resistance.[1] These patients require large volumes of insulin to achieve good glycemic control. Administration of large volumes of insulin can lead to complications, such as injection site discomfort, leakage of insulin, and reduced insulin absorption.[2] Furthermore, these patients may require 4–8 injections/day since the largest insulin syringes only hold 100 units of insulin and insulin pens only dial up to 60–80 units at one time. These extra injections of insulin can lead to poor medication adherence and further limit glycemic control.[1] The largest reservoirs in CSII pumps only hold 300 units of insulin; thus, patients with significant insulin resistance require frequent cartridge changes.

U-500 regular (U-500 R) insulin (500 units/mL) is fivefold more concentrated than U-100 regular (U-100 R) insulin (100 units/mL), which allows administration of the same dose of insulin at 20% of the volume of U-100 R insulin.[2] Reduction in insulin volume with the use of U-500 R insulin results in fewer injections, less discomfort, improved insulin absorption, and better medication adherence.[1] In a study evaluating the pharmacodynamics of U-500 R insulin in patients with type 2 diabetes and significant insulin resistance, subcutaneous administration of 100 units resulted in an onset of action of 30 min and duration of at least 7 h. This is similar to that of U-100 NPH insulin.[3] U-500 R insulin can be given twice a day, three times a day, or four times a day or via CSII. U-500 R insulin is sometimes combined with rapid-acting U-100

[1]Division of Endocrinology, Rush University, Chicago, IL.

 DOI: 10.2337/9781580405713.36

insulin analogs or U-100 basal insulin, depending on individual patient characteristics.[1]

A recent meta-analysis of 310 patients found that multiple daily injections of U-500 R insulin resulted in a significant increase in the total daily dose of insulin (TDD) by 51.9 units as compared to U-100 R insulin, with a 1.59% reduction in HbA$_{1c}$. There was a significant weight gain of 4.38 kg, however. The delivery of U-500 R insulin via CSII resulted in a similar reduction of HbA$_{1c}$ by 1.64%, but there was no difference in weight or TDD as compared to U-100 R insulin. The use of U-500 R insulin was associated with significant increase in the frequency of mild hypoglycemia, ranging from 13 to 42%, but no increase in severe hypoglycemia.[1]

U-500 R insulin is labeled category B by the U.S. Food and Drug Administration for use during pregnancy. The use of U-500 R insulin via multiple daily injections (MDI) or CSII during pregnancy has been reported.[4,5]

Initially, HbA$_{1c}$ was 8.2% while on CSII with lispro insulin using a Medtronic insulin pump. The TDD was 225 units/day. Fasting blood glucose was 170–220 mg/dL (9.4–12.2 mmol/L) and 2 h postprandial blood glucose was 180–250 mg/dL (10–13.9 mmol/L). She was switched to U-500 R insulin via CSII. The initial basal rate for U-500 R insulin was determined by dividing half of the TDD by 24 and further dividing by 5 to achieve a setting of U-500 R 0.95 "pump units/hour." The carbohydrate-to-insulin ratio for meals of 2 grams : 1 unit of lispro insulin was multiplied by 5 to get a ratio of 10 to 1; indicating 10 grams : 1 "pump unit" of U-500 R insulin. The insulin sensitivity factor was multiplied by 5 to get 35 mg/dL (1.9 mmol/L) per "pump unit" of U-500 R insulin. The active insulin time was increased to 6 h, and the target blood glucose was set at 80–120 mg/dL (4.4–6.7 mmol/L). On the basis of the pharmacodynamics of U-500 R insulin, the patient was instructed to check her glucose and bolus insulin 30–60 min before eating.

The change to U-500 R insulin reduced the total volume of insulin, allowing the patient to change her reservoir every 3 days instead of daily. Her pump settings were adjusted every 1 to 2 weeks. Six months after starting U-500 R insulin via CSII, HbA$_{1c}$ decreased to 7.5%, and 3 months later it was 7.1%. She became pregnant 9 months later. She was followed closely with frequent insulin titration, and HbA$_{1c}$ was 6–7% during pregnancy. She required 25% more insulin during pregnancy. She had a second successful pregnancy 4 years later while continuing U-500 R insulin using CSII. She did not have significant hypoglycemia with the exception of several overnight episodes, blood glucose 40–60 mg/dL (2.2–3.3 mmol/L), during the last 2 weeks of both pregnancies. Suspension of basal insulin infusion overnight eliminated further episodes. Liraglutide 1.8 mg/day and metformin 1,000 mg b.i.d. were added to her regimen between pregnancies, and reduced her insulin requirement by ~25%.

Glycemic control poses significant challenges during pregnancy, especially in patients with significant insulin resistance. The use of U-500 R insulin with MDI or CSII is a safe and effective option. With careful titration, good glycemic control can be achieved with a limited risk of hypoglycemia.

REFERENCES

1. Reutrakul S, Wroblewski K, Brown RL. Clinical use of U-500 regular insulin: review and meta-analysis. *J Diabetes Sci Technol* 2012;6(2):412–420

2. Dailey AM, Tannock LR. Extreme insulin resistance: indications and approaches to the use of U-500 insulin in type 2 diabetes mellitus. *Curr Diab Rep* 2011;11(2):77–82

3. Davidson MB, Navar MD, Echeverry D, Duran P. U-500 regular insulin: clinical experience and pharmacokinetics in obese, severely insulin-resistant type 2 diabetic patients. *Diabetes Care* 2010;33(2):281–283

4. Hatipoglu B, Soni S, Espinosa V. Glycemic control with continuous subcutaneous insulin infusion with use of U-500 insulin in a pregnant patient. *Endocr Pract* 2006;12(5):542–544

5. Reutrakul S, Brown RL, Koh CK, Hor TK, Baldwin D. Use of U-500 regular insulin via continuous subcutaneous insulin infusion: clinical practice experience. *J Diabetes Sci Technol* 2011;5(4):1025–1026

Case 37
Diabetes in Hereditary Hemochromatosis

DONALD A. MCCLAIN, MD, PHD[1]

A 58-year-old Caucasian man was referred to the University Diabetes Center after unsuccessful attempts to achieve adequate glycemic control with a sulfonylurea and metformin. His diabetes had been diagnosed 8 months earlier by fasting glucose and confirmed by HbA$_{1c}$ at a routine visit to his primary care provider. There was a family history of diabetes in an older brother and his father. The patient was moderately overweight (BMI 28 kg/m^2), but the physical exam was otherwise completely normal. Prior laboratory testing had revealed an HbA$_{1c}$ of 8.2% on therapy, with normal electrolytes, renal function, and liver function tests.

It is important to consider that diabetes presenting in older adults is not always typical type 2 diabetes. Type 1 diabetes and late autoimmune diabetes of adults (LADA) are not uncommon, accounting for up to 10% of cases. In addition, certain medications and other conditions, such as Cushing's syndrome, pancreatitis, cystic fibrosis, and hereditary hemochromatosis, may cause diabetes through defined mechanisms. It is important to consider these in every new case of diabetes because treatment strategies for LADA and so-called secondary diabetes may differ (e.g., surgery for Cushing's and early use of insulin rather than oral agents in type 1 diabetes) and the predisposing conditions themselves may carry other comorbidities that need to be investigated and addressed. These considerations are especially important for those whose phenotype or history is not typical of type 2 diabetes, including individuals who are not obese, individuals with family histories of type 1 diabetes or other autoimmune disorders, or individuals with other comorbidities or laboratory results that might suggest another process or syndrome.

The patient was not obese and did not have hypertension or other stigmata of Cushing's syndrome. He did not use alcohol and had not had any recent weight loss to suggest malabsorption. Anti-GAD antibodies were negative, and the C-peptide was low (0.9 ng/mL). Because he was of Northern European extraction and was not obese, he was screened for hemochromatosis by determining his transferrin saturation, which was elevated (54%). This triggered gene testing for hereditary hemochromatosis (HH). He was found to be

[1]Department of Internal Medicine, University of Utah School of Medicine, Salt Lake City, UT.

DOI: 10.2337/9781580405713.37

homozygous for the C282Y mutation of the *HFE* gene. Serum ferritin was elevated at 544.

HH is characterized by tissue iron overloading secondary to increased dietary absorption that is transmitted as an autosomal recessive trait and occurs in ~5 per 1,000 Caucasians of Northern European descent. Most patients with hemochromatosis are homozygous for a mutation (C282Y) in the hemochromatosis gene (*HFE*); a second mutation, H63D, is seen in other populations, such as Hispanics. H63D homozygosity has a milder phenotype and in many cases is not associated with significant iron overload. Mutations in other genes required for normal iron sensing and regulation occur more infrequently and generally cause a more severe phenotype (Table 37.1). Normal HFE is required for iron stimulation of hepcidin, and failure to induce hepcidin results in unregulated iron entry into the circulation from the gastrointestinal tract and macrophages.[1]

HH was originally described as a triad of diabetes, cirrhosis, and skin pigmentation. Other morbidities including arthritis, dilated cardiomyopathy, and hypogonadotrophic hypogonadism also occur. There is significant controversy about the frequency and mechanism of morbidity that accompanies HH, although recent studies suggest even in clinically unselected probands (i.e., without the selection bias of having sought medical care) that the prevalence of liver fibrosis and diabetes is significant.[2]

Table 37.1—Genetic Forms of Hereditary Hemochromatosis

Gene	Gene function	Inheritance and phenotype
HFE	Receptor involved in hepatic iron sensing and stimulation of hepcidin secretion	Recessive, variable penetrance, generally after the fifth decade
TFR2	Transferrin receptor 2, interacts with *HFE* and other hepatic receptors to sense iron	Recessive, symptoms generally appearing in the third or fourth decades
HAMP	Hepcidin, the peptide secreted by the liver in response to *HFE* and inflammatory signaling that down regulated iron channels, limiting iron uptake from the gut	Recessive, presentation in second or third decade, often with amenorrhea in females and sexual dysfunction or delayed puberty in males
SLC40A1	Ferroportin, the export channel that releases iron into the circulation from cells such as gut epithelia and macrophages	Dominant, onset and clinical picture similar to *HFE*
HFE2	Hemojuvelin, a coreceptor for bone morphogenetic proteins that regulate hepcidin levels	Recessive, presentation in second or third decade, often with amenorrhea in females and sexual dysfunction or delayed puberty in males

Many of the classic comorbidities of HH are seen only with higher levels of ferritin; hypogonadism and dilated cardiomyopathy, for example, are rarely seen in individuals with ferritin below 1,000. Recent evidence suggests that even high-normal ferritin levels are associated with increased risk for typical type 2 diabetes in individuals without HH,[3] so it is reasonable to assume that similar levels of iron overload in HH also will be associated with diabetes.

Screening has been recommended to Caucasians with diabetes, especially in combination with other stigmata of HH. Controversy exists regarding the cost effectiveness of screening. Recent studies show the prevalence of diabetes to be 13–22% and impaired glucose tolerance to be 18–30%. Of note, HH is largely a disease of individuals of Northern European descent, wherein the background prevalence rate of diabetes is only ~5–10%. Given a prevalence of HH of 5/1,000, if 20% of those adults have diabetes, and the prevalence of diabetes in a Northern European population is 100/1000, then approximately 1% of Caucasians diagnosed with type 2 diabetes have hemochromatosis.

Insulin therapy was initiated and ultimately adjusted to 16 units nightly of insulin glargine, which resulted in good control of fasting and postprandial glycemia. Phlebotomy therapy was initiated, and with a loss of 9 units of blood over a period of 6 months, ferritin levels decreased to 52.

The pathophysiology of diabetes associated with HH is controversial, with evidence for both insulin deficiency and insulin resistance as contributing factors. In one study of HH subjects with prediabetes, subjects differed significantly from controls only in terms of insulin secretory capacity and had a trend toward *increased* insulin sensitivity. Subjects with overt diabetes exhibited insulin resistance, but most (80%) were also obese. These data suggest that HH is diabetogenic mainly because of decreased insulin secretion, and diabetes usually results when insulin resistance from an independent mechanism such as obesity intervenes, wherein the individuals with HH cannot respond with increased insulin secretion because of primary pathology in the β-cells. Consistent with this hypothesis, insulin secretory abnormalities but not insulin sensitivity of HH improve with phlebotomy therapy.[4,5] In this case, the successful treatment with a relatively low dose of basal but no prandial insulin reflects the partial loss of insulin secretory capacity and the relative insulin sensitivity of these patients. Later presentation with higher iron loads can result in increased insulin requirements, including the need for multiple insulin injection dosing.

The optimal targets for phlebotomy therapy are not established with regard to diabetes outcomes. Of note, while phlebotomy is in progress, the HbA_{1c} cannot be used to follow diabetes status.

REFERENCES

1. Nemeth E, Tuttle MS, Powelson J, et al. Hepcidin regulates cellular iron efflux by binding to ferroportin and inducing its internalization. *Science* 2004;306:2090–2093

2. Bulaj ZJ, Ajioka RS, Phillips JD, et al. Disease-related conditions in relatives of patients with hemochromatosis. *N Engl J Med* 2000;343:1529–1535

3. Simcox JA, McClain DA. Iron and diabetes risk. *Cell Metab* 2013;17:329–341

4. Abraham D, Rogers J, Gault P, et al. Increased insulin secretory capacity but decreased insulin sensitivity after correction of iron overload by phlebotomy in hereditary haemochromatosis. *Diabetologia* 2006;49:2546–2551

5. Hatunic M, Finucane FM, Norris S, et al. Glucose metabolism after normalization of markers of iron overload by venesection in subjects with hereditary hemochromatosis. *Metabolism* 2010;59:1811–1815

Case 38

Challenging Insights from Albuminuria Early in the Course of Disease

Cem Demirci, MD;[1] Vered Lewy-Weiss, MD;[2] and Mark A. Sperling, MBBS, FRACP[2]

CASE A

The patient was a Caucasian woman diagnosed with type 1 diabetes (T1D) at the age 11 years when she presented in mild DKA, pH of 7.20, and hemoglobin A1c (HbA$_{1c}$) 11.5%. Testing for the presence of islet cell antibodies was not performed. She responded well to treatment, initially consisting of basal and bolus injections, and after 2 years, using insulin pump therapy, she maintained excellent metabolic control with all HbA$_{1c}$ values <6.5% after stabilization (Fig. 38.1). Her HbA$_{1c}$ values were still in the near normal range at 5.8% (N = 4.3–6.1%) several years after diagnosis, and total daily insulin varied from 0.5 to 0.7 units/kg/day. Her general health was excellent with normal systolic and diastolic blood pressures; height was at the 50th percentile, weight was at the 90th percentile with BMI in 95–97th percentile. Annual tests of thyroid function and lipid profile were normal. Because "dipstick" urine for protein was positive 3 years after diagnosis, she provided an overnight urine collection for measurement of albumin excretion rate, which was 156.8 μg/min (normal = <21 μg/min). A split day-night urine collection showed that albumin excretion was 143 mg/dL during the day and 10.6 mg/dL at night. Normal nocturnal albumin excretion is up to 1.9 mg/dL, so the nocturnal albumin excretion was increased. Her albumin-to-creatinine ratio was 1,254.4 mg/g during the day and 87.6 mg/g at night, with a normal range being 15–37 mg/g. These findings were consistent with both daytime macroalbuminuria and nighttime microalbuminuria.

In an adolescent with persistent near-normal HbA$_{1c}$ of <6.5%, requiring relatively low insulin doses despite being overweight, and maintaining excellent metabolic control over a period of years, the early development of albuminuria within 3 years of diagnosis suggested an unusual form of diabetes rather than the usual pattern observed in patients with typical T1D.

Albuminuria is rare after only 3 years of diabetes and generally is related to the degree of metabolic control.[1] An attempt to find a unifying hypothesis led to the consideration of maturity-onset diabetes of the young (MODY-5), and the discovery of a novel change in intron 2 of the TCF2 gene, at a location that was

[1]Department of Endocrinology, Connecticut Children's Medical Center, Hartford, CT.
[2]Children's Hospital of Pittsburgh of UPMC, Pittsburgh, PA.
DOI: 10.2337/9781580405713.38

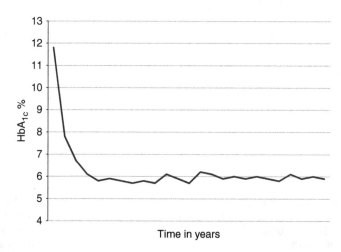

Figure 38.1—HbA$_{1c}$ values for patient A. Maintaining excellent metabolic control with all HbA$_{1c}$<6.5% after initial stabilization.

considered likely to alter a splice site resulting in an altered protein product. The family tree of the patient and the sequence variant resulting in the amino acid change in intron 2 of the hepatocyte nuclear factor 1, homeobox B (HNF-1β) gene is shown in Fig. 38.2. Periodic evaluation in our nephrology department showed there consistently was a greater protein excretion during daytime hours than during sleep. She was prescribed an angiotensin II receptor blocker.

HNF-1β (also known as TCF2) encodes transcription factor 2, a liver-specific factor of the homeobox-containing basic helix-turn-helix family. The TCF2 protein is believed to form heterodimers with another liver-specific member of this transcription factor family, TCF1. Depending on the TCF2 isoform, the result may be to activate or inhibit transcription of target genes. Mutations of TCF2 that disrupt normal function have been identified as the cause of MODY-5.[2] It is known that HNF-1β relates to and regulates HNF-4α, thereby providing a potential link between MODY-5 and MODY-1. MODY-5 is characterized by renal cysts, vaginal-uterine malformations, abnormal liver function, and nondiabetic renal disease; >40 mutations have been described for HNF-1β.[2]

Careful monitoring and investigations of our patient did not reveal evidence of renal cysts or deterioration in renal function. Therefore, no specific intervention for a renal disease was performed. Because of the unusual intronic site of the novel sequence, and our uncertainty as to its significance, we sequenced the mother because of the family history of "diabetes" in the maternal grandfather (Fig. 38.2). The mother has the same sequence variant in intron 2 as that described for her daughter but without any evidence of hyperglycemia, abnormal HbA$_{1c}$, or albuminuria. Thus, we concluded that this sequence variant is not pathological, although we cannot exclude this possibility completely. Nevertheless, this case illustrates the importance of fully investigating albuminuria when it appears early in the course of an otherwise exceptionally well-controlled

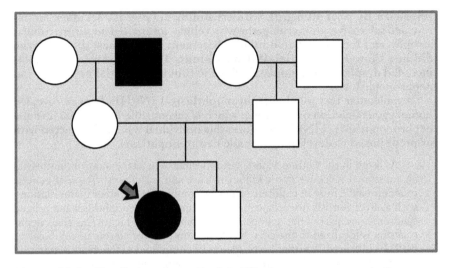

Figure 38.2—Family tree for patient A. Filled square represents the affected male with diabetes. Filled circle represents the affected female index case with diabetes. Arrow indicates documentation of a novel variant sequence c.544+14T.C resulting in an amino acid change CGA>CAA in intron 2 of the HNF-1β gene.

patient with T1D. T1D was subsequently confirmed at age 18 years by demonstrating positive GAD65 antibodies (>30 units) as well as ICA512 antibodies of 4.4 units; C-peptide was negligible at <0.1 ng/ml despite the near-normal metabolic control. An overriding lesson is that a sequence variant in a gene is not synonymous with disease causing mutation.

CASE B

This boy was diagnosed with T1D at age 6 years and 5 months, was treated initially with multiple daily insulin injections, and later was switched to an insulin pump. At diagnosis, his creatinine values were normal at 0.5 mg/dL; albumin was not detected in his urine. For 5 years, HbA$_{1c}$ was in the mid-6–7% range; thereafter, HbA$_{1c}$ was 89%. At age 14 years, weight was at the 30th percentile, height was in the 29th percentile, and BMI was in the 35th percentile. He displayed poor growth despite going through puberty. At age 15 years and 3 months, weight was at the 12th percentile, height was in the 17th percentile, and BMI was in the 21st percentile; he was Tanner stage 4 in puberty. Blood pressure was normal at 110/62 mmHg. Examination of the urine revealed an albumin of 2+ without glucose or ketones. Lipid profile and thyroid function tests were normal, but a basic metabolic profile revealed a BUN of 40 mg/dL with creatinine 2.5 mg/dL. A kidney biopsy revealed sclerosing glomerulopathy with tubulo-interstitial nephritis, tubular atrophy, and focal lamellated tubular basement membranes; the glomeruli did not show Kimmelstiel-Wilson lesions. The differential diagnosis included dysplasia or hypoplasia, chronic tubulointerstitial nephritis, and nephronophthisis.

A molecular test for the nephronophthisis-1 (NPHP-1) gene revealed homozygous deletion of this gene, which is responsible for familial juvenile nephronophthisis (FJN).[3] Therefore, this individual was likely affected with or predisposed to developing juvenile nephronophthisis.

As listed in the Online Mendelian Inheritance in Man, nephronophthisis is an autosomal recessive cystic kidney disease and is the most frequent genetic cause of renal failure in children. It may be combined with other manifestations, such as liver fibrosis or cardiac malformations. Nephronophthisis and related syndromes are part of the "ciliopathies" because the product of this gene, nephrocystin, is localized to the cilia. Nephrocystin may play a role in cell polarity. NPHP1 is caused by either homozygous or compound heterozygous mutation or, as in this case, deletion of the gene encoding nephrocystin; the gene is located on chromosome 2q13.

The patient underwent a living donor related renal transplant with significant improvement in renal function (BUN 25 mg/dL; creatinine 1.4 mg/dL). There has been a significant improvement in growth since the successful renal transplant; weight increased to the 31st percentile and height to the 22nd percentile. Persistent albuminuria in a child with T1D requires periodic evaluation of renal function.

REFERENCES

1. Stone ML, Craig ME, Chan AK, et al. Natural history and risk factors for microalbuminuria in adolescents with type 1 diabetes: a longitudinal study. *Diabetes Care* 2006;2072–2077

2. Edghill EL, Bingham C, Ellard S, Hattersley AT. Mutations in hepatocyte nuclear factor-1beta and their related phenotypes. *J Med Genet* 2006;43:84–90

3. Simms RJ, Eley L, Sayer JA. Nephronophthisis. *Eur J Hum Genet* 2009;17: 406–416

Case 39

Copresentation of Addison's Disease and Type 1 Diabetes in a 9-Year-Old Boy

Shideh Majidi, MD,[1] and Jennifer Raymond, MD, MCR[2]

A 9-year-old boy presented to the emergency room (ED) on May 3, 2013, after his brothers noted he was acting confused, "walking funny," and "ignoring them." In the ED, he was hypotensive to 87/41 mmHg. He responded to questions, but slower than usual. Past medical history was significant for seizures, which resolved 3 years ago. Over the past few months, he developed darker skin pigmentation, abdominal pain, and salt craving. He has had poor growth and poor weight gain. Family history was significant for maternal grandmother with hypothyroidism. Labs in the ED were significant for the following:

Sodium	127 mmol/L
Potassium	7.0 mmol/L
Bicarbonate	14 mmol/L
Glucose	55 mg/dL (with repeat glucose of 47 mg/dL)

He received a D25 bolus and normal saline bolus, and he was transferred to a pediatric hospital.

This patient's presentation with hyponatremia, hyperkalemia, and hypoglycemia along with abdominal pain, darkening skin pigmentation, and salt craving are concerning for cortisol deficiency. Cortisol deficiency occurs when a portion of an individual's hypothalamic-pituitary-adrenal (HPA) axis is deficient. This can be from a central (secondary) deficiency (abnormality in the hypothalamus or pituitary gland) or peripheral (primary) deficiency (abnormality in the adrenal gland). Central deficiency does not result in hyponatremia and hyperkalemia, as the mineralocorticoid axis in the adrenal gland is not affected. This patient's symptoms and labs indicate a peripheral deficiency (primary adrenal insufficiency). The most common etiologies of primary adrenal insufficiency are congenital adrenal hyperplasia, Addison's disease, and adrenoleukodystrophy.[1] Obtaining a cortisol and ACTH level and starting immediate treatment with stress-dose steroids would be appropriate in this case, as the patient is acutely ill. Evaluation for Addison's disease also could

[1]Pediatric Endocrinology Fellow, University of Colorado Denver, Aurora, CO. [2]Assistant Professor, Pediatric Endocrinology, Barbara Davis Center for Diabetes, University of Colorado Denver, Aurora, CO.

DOI: 10.2337/9781580405713.39

include an ACTH stimulation test (using 250 mcg cosyntropin), renin level, and 21-hydroxylase antibodies. In our patient, ACTH stimulation testing and labs were obtained before starting specific treatment for adrenal insufficiency.

After labs were obtained, he was started on stress dose hydrocortisone (50 mg/m²/day) and fludrocortisone 0.1 mg/day. His electrolytes improved, and hydrocortisone was decreased to maintenance dose 24 h later.

A peak post-ACTH cortisol level was low, 0.34 mcg/dL (cortisol peak level ≥15–18 is considered normal). Renin level was elevated at 31 ng/mL/h (range 0.9–2.9 ng/mL/h). He had a thyroid-stimulating hormone (TSH) of 11 mIU/mL (range 0.7–5.7 mIU/mL) and total T4 of 6.1 mcg/dL (range 4.7–12.4 mcg/dL). Repeat thyroid labs were normal. Cortisol normally inhibits TSH release, and TSH levels are often high at initial diagnosis of cortisol deficiency. If there is no underlying thyroid disease, TSH returns to normal once hydrocortisone is started.[2] The patient's 21-hydroxylase antibodies were positive, diagnostic of Addison's disease.

Autoimmune Addison's disease is a disorder characterized by serum antibodies against specific steroidogenic enzymes, including 21-hydroxylase, which is necessary for aldosterone and cortisol production. Symptoms are often nonspecific, including fatigue, nausea, vomiting, and weight loss. As the illness progresses, skin hyperpigmentation, salt craving, hypoglycemia, electrolyte abnormalities, and hypotension can develop. Treatment includes glucocorticoid and mineralocorticoid replacement. Hydrocortisone dosing is based on the patient's body surface area, and higher doses are recommended during illness to mimic the body's normal cortisol increase during stress.[3]

As the patient improved, he became hyperglycemic to the 300s–600s mg/dL (Table 39.1) even after dextrose fluids were discontinued and hydrocortisone decreased to maintenance dosing (8.5 mg/m²/day). His hemoglobin A1c was 6.1%. He received 1 unit of lispro. He was discharged with a blood glucose meter, and he had evening blood glucose in the 500s mg/dL. He was subsequently started on glargine and lispro. Additional testing revealed positive IA-2 and ZNT8RW antibodies (Table 39.2).

Addison's disease often presents with hypoglycemia, which is secondary to lack of cortisol. Glucocorticoids stimulate phenlethanolamine-N-methyl transferase, which leads to an increase in epinephrine, a counterregulatory

Table 39.1—Glucose Trend

Date/ Time	5/3 1646	5/4 0820	5/4 1600	5/5 0545	5/5 1200	5/5 1645	5/5 2000	5/6 fasting A.M.
Glucose (mg/dL)	47	162	216	385	500	582	602—Lispro 1 unit given	158

Table 39.2—Autoantibodies

Autoantibody	Result
GADA	0
mIAA	−0.001
IA-2	**97**
ZNT8RW	**0.395**
21 hydroxylase	**0.733**
Anti-thyroid peroxidase antibody	<1.0

Boldface results are positive.

hormone that results in inhibition of insulin release from β-cells and stimulates glycogenolysis and glycolysis.[3,4] Glucocorticoids also stimulate gluconeogenesis. Cortisol deficiency, therefore, results in decreased gluconeogenesis and impairment of epinephrine production and secretion. Once his cortisol deficiency was treated, hyperglycemia was noted and the patients' diabetes was unmasked.

Patients who have one autoimmune disorder are at risk of developing other autoimmune disorders as well. Addison's disease is present in two syndromes composed of multiple autoimmune disorders—autoimmune polyglanduar syndrome type 1 and type 2 (APS-1 and APS-2). APS-1 is a rare autosomal recessive disorder and is diagnosed when two of the following are present: mucocutaneous candidiasis, hypoparathyroidism, or Addison's disease. Mucocutaneous candidiasis usually manifests first, often in infancy. Addison's disease typically presents in the second decade of life. APS-2 is a multifactorial syndrome and susceptibility is determined by genetics and interaction with environmental factors. HLA haplotypes seen in APS-2 include HLA-A1, HLA-B8, HLA DR3, DQA1*0501, and DQB1*0201. APS-2 is diagnosed when two of the following are present: Addison's disease, type 1 diabetes (T1D), or autoimmune thyroid disease. T1D already exists, subclinically, in about 20% of patients with APS-2 in cases in which Addison's disease is diagnosed first.[2] Therefore, as in this patient, when a diagnosis of Addison's disease is made, it is important to investigate whether symptoms of T1D are present, and obtain urinalysis, glucose, or A1C, if needed. It is important to consider T1D even if the patient presents with hypoglycemia. In the literature, there is one case report of a patient copresenting with T1D and Addison's disease. In this case, a 12-year-old female presented similarly to our patient and was found to have elevated renin and ACTH and failed an ACTH stimulation test. Once on hydrocortisone, she developed hyperglycemia and was found to have an A1C of 6.1% and positive T1D autoantibodies.[4]

The risk of Addison's disease in patients with existing T1D is 0.5%.[5] Currently, there are no guidelines for monitoring for Addison's disease in patients with T1D. Our current practice is to screen patients with T1D for

21-hydroxylase antibodies at onset, and subsequently if symptoms present, although some providers regularly screen every 2 years.

The patient is doing well on hydrocortisone, fludrocortisone, glargine, and lispro. His thyroid peroxidase antibody, which checks for autoimmune thyroid dysfunction, is negative at this time.

REFERENCES

1. Perry R, Kecha O, Paquette J, Huot C, Van Vliet G, Deal C. Primary adrenal insufficiency in children: twenty years experience at the Sainte-Justine Hospital, Montreal. *J Clin Endocrinol Metab* 2005;90(6):3243–3250

2. Owen CJ, Cheetham TD. Diagnosis and management of polyendocrinopathy syndromes. *Endocrinol Metab Clin N Am* 2009;38:419–436

3. Sperling M. *Pediatric endocrinology*. Philadelphia, W.B. Saunders, 2008, 430–431

4. Aijaz NJ, Blanco E, Lane AH, Wilson TA. Type 1 diabetes mellitus masked by primary adrenal insufficiency in a child with autoimmune polyglandular syndrome type 2. *Clin Pediatr* 2003;42:75–77

5. Barker JM, Yu J, Yu L, Wang J, Miao D, Bao F, Hoffenberg E, Nelson JC, Gottlieb PA, Rewers M, Eisenbarth GS. Autoantibody "subspecificity" in type 1 diabetes. *Diabetes Care* 2005;28:850–855

Diagnosis of Addison's Disease and Type 1 Diabetes in Twin Boys

Andrea Dann Urban, MSN, PNP-BC, CDE,[1] and
William V. Tamborlane, MD[2]

A 3-year-old Caucasian twin boy (A) presented to the emergency department (ED) because of lethargy, nausea, and vomiting for 3 days. He had a 2-week history of polyuria, polydipsia, and 11 lb weight loss. His past medical history was significant for prematurity (27 weeks estimated gestational age), apnea of prematurity, gastro-esophageal reflux, constipation, and excessive salt craving. Family history was positive for type 1 diabetes (T1D) in a maternal cousin.

On arrival to the ED, the patient was lethargic and moderately dehydrated; his pulse was 134, blood pressure was 80/48 mmHg, RR 30. The skin was slightly tan in color. Physical exam was normal. Labs showed the following:

Blood glucose	323 mg/dL (17.9 mmol/L)
Sodium	114 mmol/L
Bicarbonate	12 mmol/L
K	6.7 mmol/L

There were ketones present in urine. Venous blood gas showed pH 7.34 and CO_2 25 mmHg. The patient was given aggressive fluid resuscitation with normal saline (NS) and started on an intravenous (i.v.) regular insulin drip at 0.1 unit/kg/h. He continued to receive NS at 1.5 times maintenance requirements without potassium. Insulin was transitioned from i.v. to subcutaneous (SQ) after resolution of the acidosis and when able to resume oral intake. The serum sodium remained 125–129 mmol/L despite i.v. NS and it decreased to 124 mm/L after discontinuing NS. The urine sodium was 79 mmol/L, urine potassium was 14.8 mmol/L, urine osmolarity was 356 mOsm/kg, and serum osmolality was 279 mOsm/kg.

Persistent hyponatremia in this patient, even after resolution of the hyperglycemia and acidosis, warranted a renal consult. The nephrologists suggested SIADH due to high urine osmolarity in a setting of low serum osmolality.

[1]Yale Children's Diabetes Program, Associate Clinical Faculty, Yale University School of Nursing, New Haven, CT. [2]Professor of Pediatrics, Department of Pediatrics, Chief, Pediatric Endocrinology, Deputy Director, Yale Center for Clinical Investigation, Director, Children's Diabetes Program, Yale School of Medicine, New Haven, CT.

DOI: 10.2337/9781580405713.40

While the results of the laboratory studies for workup of adrenal insufficiency were pending, fluid restriction at two-thirds maintenance was begun.

Baseline plasma cortisol at 8 A.M. was in normal range at 15 µg/dL, but cortisol levels failed to increase after administration of 250 mcg of Cortrosyn. The serum ACTH was 280 pg/mL (reference 6–48 pg/mL), plasma renin was 42.9 ng/mL/h (<10), serum aldosterone was 1 ng/dL (2–37), and antiadrenal antibodies were positive. ICA 512 antibody 18 units/mL (normal <1.0), and anti-insulin antibody 32 µU/mL (normal 0–5) were also positive, but anti-GAD antibodies were <0.5 unit/mL. The TSH level was 0.14 and antitransglutaminase antibodies for celiac disease was 4 (0–20). These findings in combination with persistent hyponatremia confirmed the diagnosis of Addison's disease (AD), and the child was started on hydrocortisone 12 mg/m²/day and fludrocortisone 0.1 mg/day. The parents began education for diabetes management and adrenal insufficiency.

The incidence of T1D in the U.S. is 1 in 300 individuals, and the prevalence of T1D in the U.S. for children <20 years of age has risen by 23% between 2001 and 2009.[1] T1D also is associated with other autoimmune diseases, including autoimmune thyroid disease, celiac disease, and AD.[2] The early detection of other autoimmune diseases is critical to preventing morbidity related to unrecognized disorders.[3] The American Diabetes Association (ADA) and the International Society of Pediatric and Adolescent Diabetes (ISPAD) have guidelines for screening T1D patients for thyroid and celiac disease. Autoimmune hypothyroidism has been reported in 3–18% of patients with T1D and 25–30% develop thyroid antibodies.[4] The guidelines suggest obtaining TSH and thyroid antibodies at the diagnosis of T1D and TSH every 1–2 years or sooner if symptomatic. Celiac disease is an immune-mediated disorder and is reported in 1–16% of patients with T1D, compared with 0.3–1% in the general population.[5] The current ADA guideline suggests obtaining an IgA antitissue transglutaminase (TTG) antibody at the time of diabetes diagnosis and every 2 years or sooner, if the patient is symptomatic.

The association of AD with T1D is seen in autoimmune polyglandular syndromes (APS). APS are disorders that involve two or more organ-specific autoimmune dysfunctions. APS II is the most common of the syndromes and includes T1D, AD, and thyroid autoimmune disease. APS II is associated with many HLA alleles. The current ADA guidelines do not recommend routine screening for AD in youth with T1D because its low prevalence makes the screening cost ineffective. Screening should be reserved for those with a high risk of developing the disease, such as those who have a first-degree relative with AD and having clinical signs of AD.

This patient was started on an insulin infusion pump at 5 years of age using aspart insulin. The two most recent HbA$_{1c}$ levels were 8.3% and 8.9%. Pump settings are as follows, basal rates (units/h): 12 A.M. 0.65, 3 A.M. 0.725, 6:30 A.M. 0.675, 9 A.M. 0.7, 12 P.M. 0.65, 3 P.M. 0.95, and 9 P.M. 0.85. Insulin-to-carbohydrate ratios were as follows: 12 A.M. 32, 6 A.M. 11, 11 A.M. 18, 3 P.M. 11 (gm/unit). Insulin sensitivity: 12 A.M. 165, 6 A.M. 145. Oral medications included the following: hydrocortisone at 5 mg t.i.d. and fludrocortisones

0.1 mg at bedtime. The patient's blood glucose levels often increase dramatically to >400 mg/dL after doses of hydrocortisone. There are also periods of unexplained hypoglycemia to <40 mg/d, but no episodes of severe hypoglycemia or diabetic ketoacidosis. He did have one admission for Addisionian crisis following an episode of dehydration. The mother contacts the diabetes clinic weekly by phone to review blood glucose levels and make changes to the pump settings.

Because of the increased prevalence of T1D (50%) in twins, the patient's identical twin brother (B) was closely monitored by his pediatrician for signs or symptoms of T1D and AD and other autoimmune diseases. At 6 years of age, the previously healthy twin presented to a local hospital with 4 days of vomiting, one episode of diarrhea, and a single episode of fever to 103°F. Labs showed hyponatremia, hyperkalemia, and a cortisol level of 6.8 μg/dL, but normal glucose levels. He was hemodynamically stable and promptly started on hydrocortisone. He was also enrolled in the TrialNet Natural History study, in which diabetes autoimmune markers were tested annually. At 8 years of age, the twin brother's (B's) diabetes autoimmune markers became elevated, with no signs or symptoms of the disease. Parents opted for no treatment through the Natural History Study at that time. The AD was well controlled in this patient and review of systems continued to be negative.

At 9 years old, twin B presented to endocrine clinic for routine monitoring of AD, being treated with hydrocortisone 7.5 mg q.i.d. A.M., and 5 mg in the afternoon, and 5 mg in the evening, along with florinef 0.1 mg q.i.d. P.M. During this visit, the mother reported that the patient was experiencing increased thirst and urine output and had lost several pounds of weight. Review of systems was otherwise negative. A urinalysis and HbA$_{1c}$ was sent in clinic. Laboratory processing showed the HbA$_{1c}$ to be 10.7 %. The urine specimen was positive for glycosuria, but ketones were negative. The sibling was started on 1 unit/kg/day of insulin, divided into three injections daily. Because his twin had been on an insulin pump for several years, the parents decided it would be best to transition the brother to an insulin pump as soon as possible. At ~3 weeks after the diagnosis of T1D, insulin pump therapy was initiated.

The child was seen for follow-up after pump therapy at approximately 8 weeks postdiagnosis with T1D. His HbA$_{1c}$ at that time was 6.9%. He was in the honeymoon phase and blood glucose levels were well controlled in the 80–150 mg/dL range. Twin B was beginning to perform some boluses with the supervision of parents and school nurse. He had become adept at carbohydrate counting and blood glucose monitoring.

We found it interesting that the parents of twin B did not recognize the signs and symptoms of diabetes, nor test his blood glucose levels at the first signs and symptoms of diabetes, despite knowing that the T1D antibodies were positive for >1 year. This was most likely due to denial of the fact that their other child could develop the same two life-threatening conditions that had affected their other son. It also may explain why twin A consistently had HbA$_{1c}$ levels that have been well above the target level recommended by ISPAD of <7.5%.

REFERENCES

1. NIDDK. Diabetes [Internet]. Available from niddknih.gov/dmpubs/statistics/index:htm#i_youngpeople

2. Barker JM. Clinical review: type 1 diabetes–associated autoimmunity: natural history, genetic associations, and screening. *J Clin Endocrinol Metab* 2006;91:1210–1217

3. Triolo T, Armstrong T, McFann K, Yu L, Rewers M, Klingensmith G, Eisenbarth G, Barker J. Additional autoimmune disease found in 33% of patients at type 1 diabetes onset. *Diabetes Care* 2011;34(5):1211–1213

4. Roldan MB, Alonso M, Barrio R. Thyroid auto-immunity in children and adolescents with type 1 diabetes mellitus. *Diabetes Nutr Metab* 1999;12:27–31

5. Holmes GK. Screening for celiac disease in type 1 diabetes. *Arch Dis Child* 2002;87:495–498

Case 41

New-Onset Type 1 Diabetes, Addison's Disease, and Hypothyroidism: A Case of Autoimmune Polyendocrine Syndrome Type 2

Lauren Golden, MD,[1] and Robin Goland, MD[2]

A 49-year-old obese Caucasian woman with a 2-year history of alopecia totalis presented to the emergency department (ED) complaining of profound weakness, polyuria, polydipsia, nausea, abdominal pain, and near-syncope. She described a 2-year history of abdominal pain and weight loss of 50–70 lb. Multiple workups, including an inpatient evaluation for severe abdominal pain, had been unrevealing except for unexplained eosinophilia. She was treated for presumptive "gastritis" with antacids and histamine blockers without relief and was referred for psychiatric evaluation.

The week prior to admission, she noted worsening weakness, polyuria, blurred vision, and nausea. In the ED she was found to be hypotensive (systolic blood pressure 60 mmHg) with hyperglycemia (glucose 500 mg/dL or 27.8 mmol/L), an elevated anion gap, acidosis, and elevated serum ketones. A diagnosis of new-onset diabetes with diabetic ketoacidosis (DKA) was made. She was started on intravenous insulin and fluids and admitted to the medical intensive care unit. Blood pressure was unresponsive to fluids.

This adult patient with a history of autoimmune alopecia totalis initially had a subacute presentation with nonspecific complaints of abdominal pain, weight loss, and eosinophilia. These symptoms were misdiagnosed as gastritis, the treatment of which had little effect on her symptoms. Given the lack of response to gastrointestinal-directed therapy, her history of autoimmunity, and the presence of unexplained eosinophilia, the differential diagnosis should have included autoimmune adrenalitis, or Addison's disease. As in this case, adults may have an insidious onset of symptoms of adrenal insufficiency. If left untreated, however, they may progress to frank adrenal crisis, particularly in the context of coexisting illness or physical stress, such as the coincident presentation with diabetes as seen in this case.

This new diagnosis of diabetes, with hyperglycemia and an elevated anion gap, is consistent with DKA. In light of her presentation with DKA, and her history of autoimmunity, the diagnosis of type 1 diabetes (T1D) becomes more likely. It is notable that T1D may present at any age, with peaks at ages 5–12 years, 20–39 years, and 50–69 years. Suspicion for T1D should be heightened in the presence of a personal or family history of autoimmunity. This is regardless

[1]Assistant Professor Clinical Medicine, Naomi Berrie Diabetes Center, Columbia University Medical Center, New York, NY. [2]J. Merrill Eastman Professor of Clinical Diabetes, Columbia University Medical Center, New York, NY.

DOI: 10.2337/9781580405713.41

149

of the age of onset of hyperglycemia and is not excluded by presence of obesity, which increases with age.

Because of the continued hypotension despite fluid resuscitation, a diagnosis of hypoadrenalism was considered. A plasma cortisol was measured, was low at 1 µg/dL, and failed to respond to Cotrosyn stimulation. The patient was diagnosed with Addison's disease. Stress dose hydrocortisone was initiated with rapid improvement in the patient's blood pressure. Once stable, this was titrated to replacement dosing of 20 mg in the morning and 10 mg in the evening. Her gastrointestinal symptoms resolved completely with hydrocortisone replacement therapy. Thyroid function was later assessed. TSH was elevated with a low free thyroxine of 0.7. Thyroid antibodies were negative. Replacement dosing of levothyroxine 50 mcg was initiated after adrenal replacement. Screening for celiac disease was negative. A diagnosis of autoimmune polyendocrine syndrome type 2 (APS2) was made. Upon further questioning, there was a strong family history of autoimmune disorders, including Crohn's disease in her father and brother, and thyroid disease (Graves' disease) in her brother.

The autoimmune polyendocrine syndromes are diverse disorders, including multiple endocrine disorders, as well as nonendocrine autoimmunity. APS2 occurs more commonly than type 1 (Table 41.1). Onset may occur over a broad age range from infancy to adulthood. As compared with APS1, which is monogenic in origin (AIRE gene), APS2 is polygenic in inheritance. Associated genotypes include HLA-DQ2 and HLA-DQ8; HLA-DRB1*0404.[1] Although relatively rare, this diagnosis must be considered in a patient with multiple endocrine deficiencies, particularly in the context of a strong family history of autoimmunity, as in this case. Such patients, and their relatives, are at increased risk for multiple autoimmune disorders, and prompt screening should be performed as indicated.[2]

The most common clinical phenotype of APS2 includes adrenal insufficiency, T1D, and chronic thyroiditis. T1D occurs in up to 20% of cases. Nonendocrine manifestations include vitiligo, alopecia, pernicious anemia, rheumatoid arthritis, and myasthenia gravis. As distinct from APS1, APS2 does not include autoimmune hypoparathyroidism. Addison's disease may present simultaneously with autoimmune thyroid disease or T1D, as in the case here, or may follow those diagnoses.

Once her DKA resolved, she was transitioned to multiple daily injections of insulin and discharged with a regimen of glargine 10 units in the evening and aspart 2–4 units with meals. Two months later she presented to the diabetes center for evaluation. She reported frequent hypoglycemia to the 30 mg/dL range (1.7 mmol/L), particularly overnight, as well as variable postprandial blood glucose in the 164–288 mg/dL range (9.1–16 mmol/L). HbA$_{1c}$ was 7.5%. She met with a diabetes educator and was taught carbohydrate counting, starting with a carbohydrate ratio of 1:30 g, and a correction dose of 1:100 mg/dL (5.5 mmol/L) >120 mg/dL (6.7 mmol/L). The glargine dose was reduced to 8 units. Over the following 3 weeks, her dosing was titrated to a carbohydrate ratio of 1:20 g and a correction dose

Table 41.1—Features of Autoimmune Polyendocrine Syndromes Type 1 and Type 2

APS1	APS2
Major clinical features (order of prevalence)	
Endocrine	**Endocrine**
Hypoparathyroidism	*Adrenal insufficiency*
Chronic mucocutaneous candidiasis (immunodeficiency)	*Autoimmune thyroid disease*
Adrenal insufficiency	*Type 1 diabetes*
Primary hypogonadism	Primary hypogonadism
Hypothyroidism	Hypophysitis/diabetes insipidus
Type 1 diabetes	
Nonendocrine	**Nonendocrine**
IgA deficiency	Vitiligo
Malabsorption syndromes	*Alopecia*
Alopecia totalis or areata	Pernicious anemia
Pernicious anemia	Myasthenia gravis
Vitiligo	ITP
	RA
Time of onset	
Infancy	Infancy through adulthood
Genetics	
AIRE (chromosome 21, recessive)	Polygenic

of 1:75 mg/dL (4.2 mmol/L). She was educated about the risks of hypoglycemia and avoidance strategies as related to increased activity, alcohol consumption, and Addison's disease.

Patients with new-onset T1D demonstrate improved insulin sensitivity in the weeks following diagnosis as their glucose toxicity resolves. It is vital to provide prompt diabetes education to patients with new-onset diabetes and to transition them to more physiologic insulin dosing regimens. Patients should be advised to be proactive and should inform their clinical team of reduced insulin requirements before frank hypoglycemia occurs.

Patients with Addison's disease are likewise at increased risk of hypoglycemia because of a partial failure in the counterregulatory response to hypoglycemia.[3,4] In this case, the patient's glargine dose was reduced 20%, and blood glucose correction target was adjusted to a target of >120 mg/dL (6.7 mmol/L) to reduce hypoglycemia.

Five months later, she was able to go on vacation for the first time in years. Upon her return, she transitioned to an insulin pump with further improvement in her HbA$_{1c}$ to 6.6% with less frequent hypoglycemia.

REFERENCES

1. Eisenbarth G, Gottlieb P. Autoimmune polyendocrine syndromes. *N Engl J Med* 2004;350:2068–2079

2. Husebye ES, Allolio B, Badenhoop K, Bensing S, Betterle C, Falorni A, Gan EH, Hulting AL, Kasperlik-Zaluska A, Kampe O, Lovas K, Meyer G, Pierce SH. Consensus statement on the diagnosis, treatment and follow-up of patients with primary adrenal insufficiency. *J Int Med* 2014;275:104–115

3. Cryer P, Davis S, Shamoon H. Hypoglycemia in diabetes. *Diabetes Care* 2003;26:1902–1912

4. Gerich J, Cryer P, Rizza R. Hormonal mechanisms in acute glucose counter-regulation: the relative roles of glucagon, epinephrine, norepinephrine, growth hormone, and cortisol. *Metabolism* 1980;29:1164–1175

Case 42

The Slow Progression of Type 1 Diabetes as Part of Autoimmune Polyendocrine Syndrome Type 2

Natalia Pertzeva, MD,[1] and Boris Mankovsky, MD, PhD[2]

Patient was a 53-year-old white woman admitted to the hospital for diabetes control. She was diagnosed with autoimmune thyroiditis and hypothyroidism in 1996 (17 years before the current admission) and was taking L-thyroxin 150 mcg daily.

Eleven years after the diagnosis of hypothyroidism (at the age of 46 years), she developed hyperglycemia and was diagnosed with type 2 diabetes. She was prescribed metformin and glibenclamide. During the 5 years following her diagnosis of diabetes, she lost 40 kg and was switched to insulin. Now she takes basal bolus insulin therapy: glargine 36 units at night and glulisine 10–12 units three times daily immediately before meals. Her diabetes is characterized by frequent and severe swings of glycemia, including severe hypoglycemia.

Three years ago, the patient developed skin hyperpigmentation, fatigue, and hypotension and adrenal failure (Addison's disease) was diagnosed. She was placed on hydrocortisone orally, 45 mg total daily dose, and mineralocorticoid fludrocortisone 0.1 mg daily. Despite this replacement therapy, she developed Addisonian crisis in 2010.

Other past medical history was remarkable for five gastrointestinal polypectomies (five anal polyps and one gastric polyp). All removed polyps were benign. Family history was unremarkable, with no endocrine diseases reported.

Her exam revealed the following:

BMI	26 kg/m^2
Pulse	80 bpm
Blood pressure	130/85 mmHg
HbA$_{1c}$	13.1%

Typical blood glucose levels during the day were: 17.8–20.4–15.4 mmol/L (320–367–277 mg/dL). Thyroid-stimulating hormone (TSH) level was low (0.066 µU/ml) and ACTH level was elevated (34 pg/mL). All other laboratory tests (including plasma sodium and potassium levels) were normal.

[1]Dnepropetrovsk Medical Academy, Dnepropetrovsk, Ukraine. [2]National Medical Academy for Postgraduate Education, Kiev, Ukraine.

DOI: 10.2337/9781580405713.42

The basal and prandial insulin doses were titrated up to bring glucose levels <10 mmol/L (180 mg/dL) during the day. The dose of L-thyroxin was decreased to 125 mcg daily.

This patient has the full clinical picture of autoimmune polyendocrine syndrome (APS) type 2 (Schmidt syndrome). The complete triad of Addison's disease, thyroid autoimmune disease, and type 1 diabetes is also termed Carpenter's syndrome. Her gastrointestinal polyposis appears unrelated as no association with APS has been reported.

The prevalence of APS type 2 has been estimated at 1.4 to 4.5 per 100,000.[1,2] It can occur at any age but most commonly occurs in patients 30–40 years of age. Women are affected three times more often than men.[3] In ~50% of cases, adrenocortical insufficiency is the initial endocrine abnormality.[4] While approximately half of patients have relatives with autoimmune disorders,[5] the close relatives of our patient showed no indication of the presence of autoimmune disease. It is presumed that the development of this syndrome is the result of the complex interaction between non-HLA loci and environmental factors.[5]

Although type 1 diabetes does not always present as part of this syndrome, Addison's disease is required for the diagnosis.[1] The presence of type 1 diabetes was reported to range from 23 to 52%, while the presence of all three autoimmune diseases was noted in 11.6% cases. Diabetes usually is diagnosed at age 20 years or older in 85% of cases.

We believe this patient has type 1 diabetes or possibly its late autoimmune diabetes in adults (LADA) variation. She was diagnosed at age 46 years, is only mildly overweight (BMI 26 kg/m²), and suffers from frequent hypoglycemia and brittle diabetes. Most important, the association with two other typical autoimmune endocrine disorders, such as autoimmune thyroiditis and Addison's disease, strongly suggests the autoimmune genesis of diabetes. Unfortunately, we do not have information on C-peptide levels or diabetes-associated antibodies, such as GAD.

This patient's diabetes progressed rather slowly, and no typical clinical or laboratory features of type 1 diabetes were observed within the first few years after the diabetes diagnosis. This initial course of diabetes led to the erroneous diagnosis of type 2 diabetes. The significant weight loss and poor glycemic control, which gradually occurred after the initial diagnosis of diabetes, and the association with Addison's disease required reconsidering the diagnosis and changing it to type 1 diabetes.

REFERENCES

1. Betterle C, Dal Pra C, Mantero F, Zanchetta R. Autoimmune adrenal insufficiency and autoimmune polyendocrine syndromes: autoantibodies, autoantigens, and their applicability in diagnosis and disease prediction. *Endocr Rev* 2002;23:327–364

2. Chen QY, Kukreja A, Maclaren NK. The autoimmune polyglandular syndromes. In De Groot LJ, Jameson JL, editors. *Endocrinology*. 4. Philadelphia: W.B. Saunders, 2001, p. 587–599

3. Schatz DA, Winter WE. Autoimmune polyglandular syndrome. II: Clinical syndrome and treatment. *Endocrinol Metab Clin North Am* 2002;31:339–352

4. Majeroni BA, Patel P. Autoimmune polyglandular syndrome, type II. *Am Fam Physician* 2007;75:667–670

5. Robles DT, Fain PR, Gottleib PA, Eisenbarth GS. The genetics of autoimmune polyendocrine syndrome type II. *Endocrinol Metab Clin North Am* 2002;31:353–368

Case 43

Atypical Type 2 Diabetes with Profound Dyslipidemia

Jeremy H. Pettus, MD,[1] and Robert R. Henry, MD[2]

A 30-year-old otherwise-healthy African American man presented to his health care provider after recently being discharged from the military to establish care. At that time, he was complaining of rapid, unintentional weight loss (roughly 100 lb in the past 9 months) with a current BMI of 27 kg/m², polyuria, polydipsia, blurred vision, and numbness in his extremities. Blood work obtained showed the following:

Fasting glucose	430 mg/dL (23.9 mmol/L)
Urinary ketones	2+
Anion gap	19
A1C	>17% (above upper limit of detection)
Total cholesterol	991 mg/dL
HDL	103 mg/dL
Triglycerides	6,940 mg/dL
GAD	negative
Insulin antibodies	negative
C-peptide level	2.80 ng/dL
Concurrent glucose	248 mg/dL (13.8 mmol/L)

The patient was started on metformin 1,000 mg twice a day and 10 units of glargine insulin daily and was referred to the outpatient diabetes clinic.

At the time of presentation, the patient had several clinical questions that needed to be addressed: *1)* What form of diabetes did he have? *2)* What would be the best way to treat him both acutely and in the long term? and *3)* How should we approach his dramatic dyslipidemia?

The patient was given a diagnosis of atypical ketosis-prone type 2 diabetes (T2D) and rapidly uptitrated on multiple daily injections with glargine and aspart insulin plus metformin. Given his blurry vision, the patient was given insulin pens to rely on the clicking mechanism to assist with dosing. Over

---

[1]Endocrinology Fellow, Division of Endocrinology and Metabolism, University of California, San Diego, CA. [2]Professor of Medicine, Division of Endocrinology and Metabolism, University of California, San Diego, CA; Chief, Section of Diabetes, Endocrinology and Metabolism; Director, Center for Metabolic Research, VA San Diego Healthcare System, San Diego, CA.

          DOI: 10.2337/9781580405713.43

several weeks, he was titrated up to 40 units of glargine at night, 12 units of aspart at each meal with a correctional factor, plus 1 g of metformin twice a day. On this regimen, his glucose values decreased dramatically to near euglycemia with values rarely exceeding 150 mg/dL (8.3 mmol/L).

In 1987, Winter et al. reported in the *New England Journal of Medicine* a small cohort of African American patients who presented with severe hyperglycemia, but who subsequently were found to be autoantibody negative and had an insulin secretion profile somewhere between healthy subjects and those with type 1 diabetes.[1] They termed this new condition "atypical diabetes." Since that time, the condition has been given many names, including type 1b, atypical type 1 diabetes, type 1.5, ketosis-prone T2D, and Flatbush diabetes (named after Flatbush, New York, where many of the patients lived). Regardless of the name, the condition is an underrecognized and increasing form of diabetes that can be confused with type 1 diabetes or late autoimmune diabetes of adulthood with an estimated prevalence of 20–50% in patients who have been newly diagnosed with T2D and who have diabetic ketoacidosis (DKA). In this atypical form of diabetes, however, there is no evidence for an autoimmune insult, typical type 1 HLA genetic associations are not seen, and endogenous insulin production returns, with many patients being able to maintain control on oral agents alone. Patients are typically obese with a family history of T2D and presentation most commonly is seen in African Americans, Hispanics, and Asians. Insulin resistance and insulinopenia both are thought to play a role, as is the resulting glucotoxicity that can lead to profound metabolic derangements and frank DKA. Initial treatment requires aggressive insulin therapy to relieve glucose toxicity and to allow for endogenous β-cell function to recover. Inpatient management is frequently required for aggressive hydration, intravenous insulin therapy, and intensive diabetic education on insulin injections and blood glucose monitoring. After normalization of blood glucose values, the majority of patients are able to come off insulin therapy entirely with frequent normalization of blood glucose levels that occurs in weeks to months. However, in one cohort of patients that was followed for 10 years, although the majority came off of insulin initially, 60% of patients ultimately required insulin at the end of the follow-up period.[2] In this way, acute remission is frequently followed by repeated "exacerbations" or recurrence over time.

The patient followed a classic course for atypical T2D in that his glucose profile rapidly normalized, but he was not able to come off insulin therapy entirely. He was successfully transitioned off mealtime insulin and placed on the glucagon-like peptide-1 (GLP-1) agonist, liraglutide, in its place and titrated up to 1.8 mg daily. He continued, however, to require basal insulin. His A1C improved quickly to 8.6%, but his weight increased dramatically with a >60 lb weight gain in only 5 months. Additionally, without specific lipid therapy, his cholesterol profile essentially normalized. These parameters are all shown in Table 43.1.

The patient's cholesterol profile serves as a dramatic representation of diabetic dyslipidemia. In the setting of severe insulin resistance or decreased

Table 43.1—Patient Parameters

	WEIGHT (lb)	BMI	TOTAL CHOLES-TEROL (mg/dL)	LDL (mg/dL)	HDL (mg/dL)	TRIGLYC-ERIDES (mg/dL)	A1C (%)
AT DIAGNOSIS	216	27.0	991	N/A	103	6940	>17
1 MONTH LATER	239.5	30.0	384	229	36	593	>17
2 MONTHS LATER	253.7	31.8	—	—	—		
5 MONTHS LATER	280.0	35.0	174	81	42	255	8.6

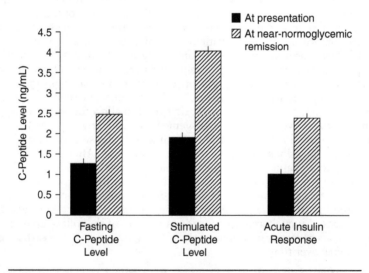

Insulin secretion was assessed 1 day after resolution of diabetic ketoacidosis (at presentation) and after 10 weeks of follow-up. Data are expressed as means and SDs. Acute insulin response to glucagon is the incremental change in C-peptide level over the baseline level. To convert values to nmol/L, multiply by 0.333.

Figure 43.1—Insulin secretion is blunted initially but dramatically increases 10 weeks after presentation in patients with atypical type 2 diabetes.

Source: Adapted from Umpierrez.[4]

secretion, hormone sensitive lipase (HSL) in adipose cells acts in an unrestricted manner to break down triglycerides (TGs) into free fatty acids (FFA). FFAs are then re-esterified in the liver back to TGs and ultimately VLDL. Without insulin activity, lipoprotein lipase (LPL) present on endothelial cells has blunted activity and is unable to "clear" VLDL. The result is markedly elevated TG levels and high VLDL as seen in this patient.[3] With insulin therapy, HSL is inhibited, TGs are no longer released by the adipose tissue, and LPL activity is restored, thus enabling active clearance of VLDL. As seen in this patient, this can result in rapid normalization or near-normalization of the lipid panel.

The ultimate cause of β-cell dysfunction in ketosis-prone T2D is not known. Studies have shown that the dysfunction appears to be temporary with rapid improvement in insulin secretion after only 10 weeks of follow-up (as shown in Fig. 43.1).[4] Both glucotoxicty and lipotoxicity have been implicated as potential causes given that both chronic hyperglycemia and FFA exposure are known to be toxic to β-cells. In this regard, the patient's lipid panel becomes even more interesting in that the lipid derangements may not only represent a result of the β-cell failure, but also may contribute to or compound the underlying *cause* as well.

The decision to place the patient on a GLP-1 agonist was made on the basis of helping to offset his weight gain and as a potential therapy to help maintain his β-function and cell mass. This particular class of agents has shown some effect in helping β-cells reduce apoptosis in the setting of multiple insults, including lipotoxicity.[5]

REFERENCES

1. Maturity-onset diabetes in young black Americans. *New Eng J Med* 1987;317(6):380–382

2. Mauvais-Jarvis F, et al. Ketosis-prone type 2 diabetes in patients of sub-Saharan African origin: clinical pathophysiology and natural history of beta-cell dysfunction and insulin resistance. *Diabetes* 2004;53(3):645–653

3. Mooradian AD. Dyslipidemia in type 2 diabetes mellitus. Nature clinical practice. *Endocrinol Metab* 2009;5(3):150–159

4. Umpierrez GE, Smiley D, Kitabchi AE. Narrative review: ketosis-prone type 2 diabetes mellitus. *Ann Intern Med* 2006;144(5):350–357

5. Buteau J, et al. Glucagon-like peptide-1 prevents beta cell glucolipotoxicity. *Diabetologia* 2004;47(5):806–815

Case 44

Patient with Diabetes Who Has Hemiballismus

Miriam Padilla, MD, CDE,[1] and Jorge Mestman, MD[2]

A 70-year-old Hispanic woman with a past medical history of type 2 diabetes, diabetic retinopathy, dementia, chronic kidney disease, depression, hyperlipidemia, and hypertension was brought into the emergency department by her family for multiple falls. Per the family, the patient was experiencing general lack of coordination, difficulty walking, difficulty speaking, and worsening confusion. It was noted that the patient had not taken her insulin for a few days before this presentation. The patient's exam showed the following:

Blood pressure	221/96 mmHg
Heart rate	82 bpm
Oxygen saturation	97% on room air
Sodium	115 mEq/L
Potassium	5.2 mEq/L
Carbon dioxide	19 mEq/L
Glucose	1,250 mg/dL (69.4 mmol/L)
Creatinine	2.56 mg/dL
Troponin	0.01 ng/mL
Hemoglobin	9.1 g/dL
Urine analysis	negative for ketones
Venous pH	7.31

Computed tomography of the head showed no intracranial mass, shift, or bleed. The patient was transferred to the medical intensive care unit (MICU) and was started on normal saline at 200 cc/h as well as continuous insulin infusion for hyperosmolar hyperglycemic syndrome.

The day after admission, the patient was transferred out of the MICU to a general medicine ward. Her chemistry panel at this point showed glucose of 170 mg/dL (9.4 mmol/L) and sodium of 133 mEq/L. She was started on NPH 14 units in the morning, NPH 7 units in the evening, regular insulin

[1]Fellow, Department of Endocrinology and Diabetes at University of Southern California. [2]Professor of Clinical Medicine in the Department of Endocrinology and Diabetes at University of Southern California, Professor of Clinical Medicine in the Department of Obstetrics and Gynecology at University of Southern California.

DOI: 10.2337/9781580405713.44

6 units in the morning, and regular insulin 5 units in the evening. Her blood work revealed the following:

HbA_{1c}	17.8%
Total cholesterol	152 mg/dL
Triglycerides	199 mg/dL
HDL	30 mg/dL
LDL	82 mg/dL

Three days after admission, the patient developed acute onset of involuntary movements of the left side of the face and left arm, which included flinging her arm laterally. On exam, the patient was alert and oriented but noted to have intermittent nonrhythmic movement of the left side of the face, more on the lower part of the face, as well as of the left arm. Neurology was consulted and diagnosed her with hemichorea-hemiballismus (HHH) resulting from nonketotic hyperglycemia (see Table 44.1).

Table 44.1 — Differential Diagnosis of Acute Hemichorea-Hemiballismus

Differential diagnosis	Example
Medications	Metoclopramide Levodopa
Metabolic	Thyrotoxicosis Hyperglycemia Hyponatremia
Ischemic	Small infarcts or hemorrhages in the vicinity of the subthalamic nucleus or in contralateral caudate nucleus Lacunar infarcts in basal ganglia Hypoxic encephalopathy
Infectious	Granulomatous disease Post-streptococcal Sydenham's chorea Borreilosis HIV/AIDS Rheumatic fever Cerebral toxoplasmosis
Malignancy	Brain tumors — lesions affecting the subthalamic fasciculus and the head of the caudate nucleus
Genetic	Wilson's disease Huntington's chorea Neural acanthocytosis
Chemical	Carbon monoxide poisoning Cocaine use
Autoimmune	Antiphospholipid syndrome Systemic lupus erythematosus

Hemiballismus usually is characterized by involuntary wide amplitude motion of the extremities that can involve proximal and/or distal muscles on one side of the body. In cases of HIHH the mean age of onset is 72 years old, but the age of onset can range from 50 to 80 years old. Women are affected 1.8 to 5-fold more commonly than men.[3] This possibly could be related to postmenopausal alterations of the gamma amino butyric acid (GABA) or dopamine receptors.[2] In HIHH, serum glucose levels also are elevated, in the range of 400–1,000 mg/dL.[2] This hyperglycemia and hyperviscocity can cause perfusion changes in the contralateral striatum, which then can result in excessive inhibition of the subthalamic nucleus.[1]

The subthalamic nucleus normally uses glutamate to excite the medial part of the globus pallidus, which then uses GABA to inhibit the activity of the ventrolateral thalamus. Damage to the subthalamic nucleus thus results in an increase of the thalamic excitation of the motor and premotor cortex resulting in involuntary movements.[2]

Magnetic resonance imaging (MRI) of the brain showed diffuse cerebral and cerebellar volume loss with mild periventricular and deep white matter hyperintense T2/fluid-attenuated inversion recovery signal. Magnetic resonance angiogram of the head showed normal flow of bilateral high cervical, petrous, cavernous, and supraclinoid internal carotid arteries with no evidence of significant stenosis.

Case reports have documented that in patients with nonketotic HHH, the MRI of the brain often shows hyperintense caudate or putaminal lesions on T1 weighted images and hypointensities in the basal ganglia on T2.[2] CT scan of brain typically shows an area of hyperdensity in the basal ganglia without mass effect.[1] Computed tomography (CT) and single-photon emission computed tomography (SPECT) studies indicate decreased perfusion in the basal ganglia consistent with ischemia.[4] Interestingly, positron emission tomography (PET) scans have shown decreased basal ganglia glucose metabolism.[4] Clinical and radiological signs usually resolve within 6 months following correction of hyperglycemia, but some case reports have documented resolution of hemiballistic movements as soon as 24–48 h after the correction of hyperglycemia.[4]

In our patient, neurology recommended clonazepam 0.5 mg by mouth every night for symptomatic relief (see Table 44.2). Hemiballistic movements initially improved but then worsened, interfering with eating. Clonazepam was increased to 0.5 mg t.i.d. to help with symptoms. Four days after starting this dose, hemiballistic movements resolved. The patient was discharged home with a plan to take clonazepam 0.5 mg t.i.d. by mouth for 6 weeks. She also was discharged home with NPH 18 units in the morning and 6 units in the evening, as well as regular insulin 7 units in the morning and 2 units in the evening. Four weeks after discharge, the patient presented to a different hospital complaining of worsening hemiballistic movements. The hospital stopped clonazepam and started diazepam 5 mg every 8 h and divalproex 250 mg q.i.d. every 8 h. Two weeks later she presented to our clinic still complaining of worsening movements. Divalproex was increased to 500 mg every 8 h and diazepam was continued at 5 mg every 8 h.

Table 44.2 — Possible Treatments for Hemichorea-Hemiballismus

Tetrabenazine
Clonazepam
Reserpine
Aggressive glycemic control
Dopamine blocking agents –Haloperidol –Risperidone
Anticonvulsants –Topiramate

Two weeks later, the patient was seen in the neurology clinic still having constant large and small amplitude involuntary movements of the left upper and lower extremities. Neurology believed the patient's hemiballistic movements could have been caused by a small lacunar stroke in the right basal ganglia, given her sudden onset of dramatic hemichorea, which was exacerbated by her poorly controlled blood glucose. They recommended tapering and discontinuing diazepam and giving quetiapine 50 mg at night.

Preexisting basal ganglia disease, such as focal small vessel ischemia, may be present in patients with HHH.[4] Hyperglycemia then triggers cellular dysfunction. This causes hypoperfusion and GABA depletion in the basal ganglia as a result of anaerobic metabolism, resulting in hemiballistic movements.[4] Most cases of HHH resolve 24–48 h after correction of hyperglycemia, but some cases can last up to 6 months.

REFERENCES

1. Padmanabhan S, Zadami A, Poynten A. A case of hemichorea-hemiballismus due to nonketotic hyperglycemia. *Diabetes Care* 2013;36:e55–e56

2. Ifergane G, Masalha R, Herishanu YO. Transient hemichorea/hemiballismus associated with new onset hyperglycemia. *Can J Neurol Sci* 2001;28:365–368

3. Narayanan S. Hyperglycemia-induced hemiballismus hemichorea: a case report and brief review of literature. *J Emerg Med* 2012;43(3):442–444

4. Cheema H, Federman D, Kam A. Hemichorea-hemiballismus in non-ketotic hyperglycemia. *J Clin Neurosci* 2011;18:293–294

5. Piccolo I, Defanti C, Soliveri P, Volonte M, Cislaghi G, Girotti F. Cause and course in a series of patients with sporadic chorea. *J Neurol* 2003;250:429–435

Case 45

A Case of Diabetic Myonecrosis

Umal Azmat, MD;[1] Jason E. Payne, MD;[2] Kathleen Dungan, MD;[1] and Steven W. Ing, MD[1]

A 27-year-old African American man with type 1 diabetes since age 10 years old and multiple complications, including stage 5 chronic kidney disease, severe neuropathic pain, retinopathy, gastroparesis, and hypertension, as well as a recent left below-the-knee amputation for osteomyelitis, was being transferred to an inpatient rehabilitation hospital. He had a history of longstanding poor glycemic control but recent improvement with intensive insulin therapy in the inpatient setting. Three days before transfer, he was ambulating with a new orthotic device under supervision when he noted sudden onset of right thigh pain. The pain worsened over the next few days requiring addition of narcotics but with minimal effect.

He was afebrile with normal heart and respiratory rate and mild hypertension at 142/76 mmHg. His pain was 5/10 at rest and 10/10 pain with active or passive movement of right hip. A patent arteriovenous fistula was present in the left upper extremity. Radial pulses were 2+ bilaterally. Hands were warm and well perfused. The right lower extremity showed 1+ pitting edema. There was no tenderness of the right lower leg, foot, or ankle; however, flexion of the right knee was limited by pain, and substantial tenderness to palpation was noted in the right lateral thigh. Right dorsalis pedis pulse was 1+. Skin examination showed an area of tenderness, erythema, and warmth over the anterior lateral right thigh. A right great toe ingrown toenail showed some pustular discharge. Monofilament exam showed absent sensation from the right foot to the mid-shin. Site of left below-the-knee amputation showed good granulation tissue without infection. The remainder of his exam was unremarkable. Laboratory values were remarkable for the following:

Blood urea nitrogen	52 mg/dL
Creatinine	6.01 mg/dL
Creatine kinase	434 units/L
Fasting glucose	131 mg/dL
A1C	9.8% (11.9% 2 months previously)

[1]Division of Endocrinology, Diabetes and Metabolism, Ohio State University Wexner Medical Center, Columbus, OH. [2]Division of Radiology, Ohio State University Wexner Medical Center, Columbus, OH.

DOI: 10.2337/9781580405713.45

Magnetic resonance imaging (MRI) of the right thigh showed extensive subcutaneous and muscular edema diffusely throughout the thigh and significant loss of architecture of the mid- and distal aspects of the vastus medialis, rectus femoris, and (to a lesser extent) the vastus lateralis. Patchy edema was noted within the adductor and hamstring musculature. Contrast was not administered in the setting of his chronic kidney disease. These findings were consistent with diabetic myonecrosis with myositis.

Diabetic myonecrosis was first described by Angervall and Stener in 1965[1] and is a rare end-organ complication of diabetes. It is often seen in patients with poorly controlled, longstanding diabetes >15 years with end-organ damage, including retinopathy (71%), nephropathy (57%), and neuropathy (55%).[2] Although the exact pathophysiology has yet to be clarified, it is hypothesized to result from atherosclerotic and diabetic microangiopathy leading to muscle infarction. The most common presentation is the abrupt onset of nontraumatic pain and swelling of the affected muscle, sometimes accompanied by a palpable mass and fever. The average age of presentation is 40 years. It is slightly more common in women and patients with type 1 diabetes. Areas most commonly affected are the quadriceps (60–65%), hip adductors (13%), hamstrings (8%), and hip flexors (2%).[3] Less commonly reported are cases involving the upper limb or both upper and lower limb muscle groups.

The diagnosis necessitates exclusion of other potential causes, including deep vein thrombosis, pyomyositis, necrotizing fasciitis, hematoma, abscess, rhabdomyolysis, compartment syndrome, trauma, osteomyelitis, and neuropathy. Although muscle biopsy is the gold standard for diagnosis, it is avoided because of the risk for complications of delayed healing, hematoma formation, and superimposed infections. MRI is very helpful in making the diagnosis and ruling out other etiologies. A presumptive diagnosis of diabetic myonecrosis can be made on the basis of history, physical examination, high clinical suspicion, and characteristic MRI findings. Typical MRI findings include marked edema and mass-like enlargement of the involved muscles (see Fig. 45.1, perifascicular fluid on T2-weighted, inversion recovery, and gadolinium-enhanced images, and isointense or hypointense areas on T1 weighted images).[4] Gadolinium is typically helpful in acute diabetic myonecrosis. In chronic cases, the T2 hyperintensity is usually not present, corresponding to areas of nonenhancement (Fig. 45.2*B*). Gadolinium may reveal regions of myonecrosis, which usually demonstrate rim enhancement or central nonenhancing tissue (Fig. 45.3). Gadolinium, however, is often contraindicated in this population because of chronic kidney disease, as in this patient.

On the basis of the clinical picture and imaging results, the patient was managed symptomatically with narcotic analgesia, bed rest, and optimized glycemic control. Unfortunately, 2 days after diagnosis, the patient developed acute left arm pain, lost consciousness, and died. The etiology of the left arm pain could not be determined. The cause of death based on autopsy was determined to be a fatal cardiac arrhythmia in the setting of previously unrecognized dilated cardiomyopathy with a code panel potassium of 6.9 mmol/L (despite normal potassium the previous day).

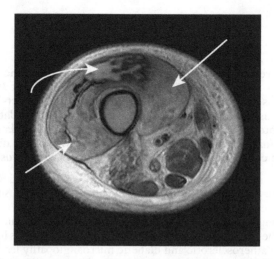

Figure 45.1—Case patient image without gadolinium contrast. Axial T2-weighted image at the level of the distal femur demonstrates diffuse edema within the vastus medialis and vastus lateralis (arrows) and subcutaneous tissues. An irregular fluid collection is seen anteriorly (curved arrow) compatible with myonecrosis.

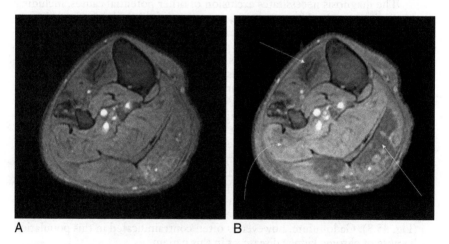

A   B

Figure 45.2—*A:* Pregadolinium image (not the case patient). Axial T1 fat-saturated image at the level of the midcalf. *B:* Postgadolinium image. Axial T1 fat-saturated postgadolinium image at the level of the midcalf shows irregular areas of nonenhancing muscle (arrows) involving primarily the anterior tibialis and gastrocnemius muscles compatible with chronic diabetic myonecrosis. Diffuse enhancement within the remaining musculature (curved arrow) is nonspecific but likely represents acute areas of involvement.

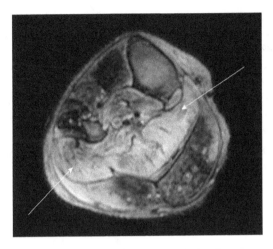

Figure 45.3—Axial stir image. Axial short-tau inversion recovery at the level of the midcalf shows edema (arrows) in the distribution of the enhancement described in Fig. 45.2. The nonenhancing areas demonstrate decreased signal on stir sequences.

   No guidelines have been established for treatment of diabetic myonecrosis and no randomized controlled trials have evaluated treatment modalities. Recent studies have shown that early mobilization and physical therapy may actually aggravate necrotic muscle, increasing hemorrhage and prolonging recovery.[5] The leading treatment modality at this time is supportive care. Patients generally are advised to maintain bed rest with limb elevation and non-weight-bearing status for at least 3–7 days. Most require initiation of opioid medications. Given significant debility and care requirements, some patients require temporary skilled nursing placement with 24 h supervision. Tight glycemic control has not been shown to reduce the duration of an episode in the acute and resolving setting. Patients should be educated on diet, glucose control, and insulin management to prevent future complications, with a goal of good glycemic control. Diabetic myonecrosis resolves in 3–31 days with an average duration of 2 weeks, with minimal long-term impairment. The likelihood of recurrence in the same muscle or contralateral limb is >29–71%, with as many as 1 to 2 episodes per year after the initial event. Patient prognosis is poor as most patients have severe microvascular disease at the time of diagnosis. Studies indicate 2-year mortality rates ranging from 4 to 29%.[5] Given this high degree of mortality, intensive monitoring of clinical and metabolic status should be undertaken, particularly if the patient requires inpatient treatment.

REFERENCES

1. Angervall L, Stener B. Tumoriform focal muscular degeneration in two diabetic patients. *Diabetologia* 1965;1:39–42

2. Choudhury BK, Saikia UK, Sarma D, Saikia M, Choudhury SD, Bhuyan D. Diabetic myonecrosis: an underreported complication of diabetes mellitus. *Indian J Endocrinol Metab* 2011;15(Suppl. 1):S58–S61

3. Rashidi A, Bahrani O. Diabetic myonecrosis of the thigh. *J Clin Endocrinol Metab* 2011;96(8):2310–2311

4. Jelinek JS, Murphey MD, Aboulafia AJ, Dussault RG, Kaplan PA, Snearly WN. Muscle infarction in patients with diabetes mellitus: MR imaging findings. *Radiology* 1999;211:241–247

5. Kapur S, McKendry RJ. Treatment and outcomes of diabetic muscle infarction. *J Clin Rheumatol* 2005;11:8–12

Case 46

A Case of Stiff Person Syndrome in a Patient with Type 1 Diabetes

MATTHEW P. GILBERT, DO, MPH,[1] AND MURIEL H. NATHAN, MD, PHD[1]

The patient, a 45-year-old woman with type 1 diabetes, presented to her endocrinologist with the complaint of pain and stiffness in her back. She noticed that the discomfort was worse during stressful situations, such as giving presentations at work. The back pain and stiffness made it difficult to walk, and she reported frequent falls. She could no longer stand for an extended period of time and had difficulty bending over to tie her shoes. She had been seeing a chiropractor and was participating in physical therapy without improvement. The patient was also seen in consultation by a rheumatologist and an extensive evaluation did not reveal an etiology for the patient's symptoms. Initial laboratory testing, including a complete blood count, metabolic panel, and thyrotropin, was normal. Anti-GAD56 antibody was found to be significantly elevated at 1,041 nmol/L (normal <0.02 nmol/L). The patient was referred to neurology with concern for possible stiff person syndrome (SPS).

SPS is a rare disorder characterized by fluctuating rigidity and stiffness of the axial and proximal lower limb muscles, with painful spasms and continuous motor unit activity on electromyography.[1] The exact prevalence of SPS is unknown. The most recent clinical criteria for SPS were published by Dalakas in 2009 and can be found in Table 46.1.[2] Symptoms can range from mild to severe and can result in significant morbidity. It is estimated that ~65% of patients with SPS cannot independently perform activities of daily living.[2]

SPS typically presents in adulthood and is more common in women. Rigidity and stiffness of the axial muscles and subsequent back pain are the earliest symptoms. Paraspinal rigidity often progresses, causing development of a hyperlordosis of the lumbar spine. The muscle rigidity may progress to the proximal lower limb muscles causing gait disturbances. The gait of patients with SPS typically is described as wide and slow to help maintain balance. Patients with severe SPS may become unable to ambulate. Muscle spasms are initially intermittent and are often precipitated by noise, touch, sudden movements, or emotional stress. Hypertonia and the superimposed spasms can lead to a loss of postural reflexes resulting in falls. Patients with SPS frequently have coexisting psychiatric symptoms, such as task-specific phobias (i.e., crossing the

[1]Department of Medicine, Division of Endocrinology and Diabetes, University of Vermont College of Medicine, Burlington, VT.

DOI: 10.2337/9781580405713.46

Table 46.1 — The Clinical Criteria for the Diagnosis of Stiff Person Syndrome[2]

- Stiffness in the axial muscles, prominently in the abdominal and thoracolumbar paraspinal muscle leading to a fixed deformity (hyperlordosis)
- Superimposed painful spasms precipitated by unexpected noises, emotional stress, and tactile stimuli
- Confirmation of the continuous motor unit activity in agonist and antagonist muscles by electromyography
- Absence of neurologic or cognitive impairments that could explain stiffness
- Positive serology for GAD65 autoantibodies, assessed by immunocytochemistry, western blot, or radioimmunoassay
- Response to diazepam

street, stairs, or walking alone without assistance), depression, and anxiety. The psychiatric features can be prominent, and the presence of these associated symptoms can complicate the diagnosis, leading to increased suspicion of malingering in patients who do not have a definitive diagnosis of SPS.[1]

Electromyography was ordered. This showed normal right tibial and sural conductions, but increased firing in the paraspinal musculature, rectus muscles, gluteus maximus, and tensor fascia lata. The patient attempted to relax, but this did not change the increased firing. There was an increased startle response to clapping with needle placement in the paraspinal musculature.

Solimena et al. were the first to identify a link between SPS and type 1 diabetes (T1D). Their studies suggested that antibodies against GAD, an enzyme found both in the pancreatic islets and the central nervous system, play an important role in the connection between the two diseases.[3] GAD is responsible for the synthesis of γ-aminobutyric acid (GABA), an inhibitory neurotransmitter in the brain and spinal cord. GABAergic pathways serve as an inhibitory pathway by which spinal interneurons coordinate motor function by inhibiting spontaneous discharges from spinal motor neurons. Impairment of these inhibitory pathways by GAD autoantibodies leads to the continuous firing of spinal motor neurons and fluctuating muscle rigidity. Approximately 60–80% of patients with SPS have autoantibodies against GAD. GAD65 is the main target for GAD autoantibodies in both SPS and T1D.[1] The authors of a 2012 observation study found that 43% of patients with SPS also had T1D.[4] The onset of diabetes predated SPS by a median of 5 years (range, 1–33 years).[4]

GAD antibodies are detected in the majority of patients with SPS and strongly support the diagnosis. The absence of GAD antibodies does not exclude the condition. Electromyography is an important diagnostic tool in the evaluation of possible SPS. Patients with SPS have findings on electromyography consistent with continuous motor unit activity in agonist and antagonist muscles.

The patient was initially started on oral valium for symptom management. She had an initial positive response to treatment, reporting less stiffness and improvement in her gait. After several months of treatment, however, her symptoms returned. She was placed on a combination of

valium and baclofen and was subsequently given several treatments of intra-venous immunoglobulin (IVIG) with symptomatic relief. She is currently maintained on valium twice a day. She continues to struggle with gait instability and frequent falls.

The available treatments for SPS are aimed at relieving symptoms or modulation of the underlying immune process. The low prevalence of SPS has limited the available clinical trial data to guide treatment. Benzodiazepines augment GABA-dependent pathways and generally are considered to be an effective first-line therapy for symptom management. Diazepam is the most commonly used benzodiazepine. Patients who are unresponsive to diazepam are often prescribed baclofen, a GABA-B agonist that is used to treat spasticity. Over time, patients often need increasing doses of diazepam or baclofen leading to troublesome side effects.[1] Corticosteroids are used in patients refractory or intolerant to benzodiazepines or baclofen. IVIG is a second-line agent for the treatment of SPS. Dalakas et al.[5] conducted a randomized, double-blinded, placebo-controlled, crossover trial of monthly IVIG that showed a significant decrease in stiffness. Patients treated with IVIG also had improvement in their ability to perform activities of daily living.[5] Treatment of SPS with intravenous methocarbamol, vigabatrin, sodium valproate, azathioprine, botulinum toxin A, propofol, plasmapharesis, and rituximab also have been reported in the literature.

REFERENCES

1. Hadavi S, Noyce AJ, Leslie RD, Giovannoni G. Stiff person syndrome. *Practical Neurology* 2011;11:272–282

2. Dalakas MC. Stiff person syndrome: advances in pathogenesis and therapeutic interventions. *Curr Treat Options Neurol* 2009;11:102–110

3. Solimena M, Folli F, Denis-Donini S, Comi GC, Pozza G, De Camilli P, Vicari AM. Autoantibodies to glutamic acid decarboxylase in a patient with stiff-man syndrome, epilepsy, and type 1 diabetes mellitus. *N Engl J Med* 1988;318:1012–1020

4. McKeon A, Robinson MT, McEvoy KM, Matsumoto JY, Lennon VA, Ahlskog E, Pittock SJ. Stiff-man syndrome and variants. *Arch Neuro* 2012;69:230–238

5. Dalakas MC, Fujii M, Li M, Lutfi B, Kyhos J, McElroy B. High-dose intravenous immune globulin for stiff-person syndrome. *N Engl J Med* 2001;345:1870–1876

Case 47

Stiff Person Syndrome in a Patient with Multiple Autoimmune Diseases

Jing Hughes, MD, PhD,[1] and Janet B. McGill, MD[1]

G. T. is a 56-year-old woman with an extensive past medical history of autoimmune disorders who complained of right leg stiffness at a follow-up office visit. Her first autoimmune disease was ulcerative colitis with onset during her teen years, which prompted a total colectomy at age 19 years. She was subsequently diagnosed with Graves' disease at age 25 years, which was treated with subtotal thyroidectomy. She developed type 1 diabetes (T1D) at age 32 years, and despite insulin pump use had an HbA$_{1c}$ of 9.8%. Celiac disease was diagnosed at age 55 years, but it may have been present for >10 years. Her symptoms of painful spasms of her right leg began ~10 months prior to the visit and were gradually progressive. She described leg stiffness that extended from hip to ankle and felt like "general weakness with periodic spasms." The spasms were so severe that she was not able to bend her knee or fully extend or flex her hip, causing impaired balance and several falls. She noted that these spastic episodes were exacerbated by cold weather as well as emotional stress and anxiety, as when she was being observed. On exam, she was noted to have a markedly abnormal gait, characterized by swinging of the right leg and overcompensation of the trunk. She was unable to perform tandem walk and had impaired balance with movement but negative Romberg. Thigh palpation revealed muscle tightness. No sensory deficits were identified. The symptoms had escalated and were now debilitating.

The differential of unilateral leg weakness is broad and includes several categories: neuropathy, vasculopathy, or myopathy. Specific to the T1D population, however, the most likely defect lies in the peripheral nervous system, for example, a motor neuropathy that manifests as focal weakness. In our patient, poorly controlled diabetes certainly could have led to the development of a focal peripheral polyneuropathy, although the lack of sensory deficits makes this diagnosis less likely. The waxing and waning nature of her leg spasms, as well as their association with emotional triggers, also point to an unusual cause.

The patient underwent neuromuscular evaluation. Nerve conduction studies showed no evidence of large fiber neuropathy, but electromyogram

---

[1]Professor of Medicine, Director, Fellowship in Endocrinology, Diabetes and Metabolism, Division of Endocrinology, Metabolism and Lipid Research, Washington University School of Medicine, St. Louis, MO.

 DOI: 10.2337/9781580405713.47

(EMG) showed continuous motor unit potentials in the tibialis anterior muscle, consistent with stiffness and spasticity. Serum anti-GAD antibody level was elevated above the threshold of the assay (>30 units/mL). Given the clinical history, exam, EMG results, and markedly high anti-GAD titer, the patient was diagnosed with stiff person syndrome (SPS). Out of concern for her osteoporosis and diabetes, the treatment team elected against using steroids in the treatment. Also, because of a history of benzodiazepine intolerance in her family, the patient was not given diazepam but instead was trialed on low-dose Baclofen for the management of her muscle spasms. Meanwhile, intravenous immunoglobulin (IVIG) was initiated as an immune-modulating therapy.

SPS is a rare and fascinating neurologic disease characterized by progressive muscle rigidity and superimposed spasms.[1] The disease has a female predominance and often occurs in conjunction with other autoimmune conditions, such as type 1 diabetes, thyroiditis, vitiligo, and pernicious anemia. Elevation in the anti-GAD antibody titer is not only a marker for the disease but also the likely source for the neuropathy itself, as GAD antibodies target γ-aminobutyric acid (GABA)-ergic neurons and their nerve terminals. Because these antibodies also recognize pancreatic β-cells, there is an intriguing link between SPS and type 1 diabetes, although in the latter case, anti-GAD autoantibodies are not necessarily pathogenic.

The diagnosis of SPS is based on both clinical and neurophysiologic features. EMG usually shows abnormal contractions of antagonistic muscles and continuous motor unit activity, which can be abolished by diazepam, sleep, and anesthesia.[2] Notable differential diagnoses include tetany, restless leg syndrome, startle disease, and progressive encephalomyelitis with rigidity and myoclonus. In addition, because of the strong emotional component in SPS attacks and the fact that these patients often suffer psychiatric comorbidities, including anxiety and depression, SPS is unfortunately sometimes misdiagnosed as a factitious disorder, conversion disorder, or even malingering.

Treatment for SPS is twofold: symptomatic control with antispasmodics and immunosuppressive therapy. Diazepam has long been used in the management of SPS, as benzodiazepines can potentiate GABA activity. Baclofen is another GABA-modulating drug that can be used with or instead of benzodiazepines. When the disease is severe, immunosuppressive therapy is also considered, generally high-dose glucocorticoids or IVIG. Plasmapheresis is reserved for patients with respiratory compromise. Anecdotal use of the β-cell depleting agent rituximab has been reported with some success.[3]

Two weeks after treatment with 2 g/kg loading dose of IVIG, the patient reported clinical improvement. She has residual tightness in her back and groin but much less stiffness in her right leg. The frequency of her leg spasms declined, resulting in improved stability and no falls. Meanwhile, during her comprehensive workup for this condition, magnetic resonance imaging of the abdomen revealed a 1.2 × 1.2 cm mildly T2 hyperintense solitary liver nodule, the etiology of which remains unclear as the workup continues. A paraneoplastic panel is also pending.

Although the majority of SPS cases are autoimmune in nature, other subtypes exist, including the paraneoplastic and idiopathic variants. Paraneoplastic markers, such as antiamphiphysin antibodies, can be seen in SPS, predominantly in patients with carcinoma.[4,5] The discovery of the liver nodule in our patient prompts evaluations to rule out a neoplasm, as her history of autoimmune hepatitis does infer a small increased risk for cholangiocarcinoma and hepatocellular carcinoma.

The treatment plan for our patient is to continue IVIG infusions, titrating the interval according to her reported symptoms. After the initial loading dose of 2 g/kg IVIG, subsequent doses will likely be reduced to 1 g/kg for maintenance. The muscle relaxant Baclofen had minimal benefit, so a cautious trial of benzodiazepines may be considered for symptomatic relief in the future.

This patient provides a reminder that patients with T1D are at risk for many other autoimmune diseases, which can continue to present through their lifetime.

REFERENCES

1. Saiz A, Blanco Y, Sabater L, et al. Spectrum of neurological syndromes associated with glutamic acid decarboxylase antibodies: diagnostic clues for this association. *Brain* 2008;131(10):2553–2563

2. Lorish TR, Thorsteinsson G, Howard FM Jr. Stiff-man syndrome updated. *Mayo Clin Proc* 1989;64(6):629–636

3. Baker MR, Das M, Isaacs J, Fawcett PRW, Bates D. Treatment of stiff person syndrome with rituximab. *J Neurol Neurosurg Psychiatry* 2005;76(7):999–1001

4. Murinson BB, Guarnaccia JB. Stiff-person syndrome with amphiphysin antibodies: distinctive features of a rare disease. *Neurology* 2008;71(24):1955–1958

5. McKeon A, Robinson MT, McEvoy KM, et al. Stiff-man syndrome and variants: clinical course, treatments, and outcomes. *Arch Neurol* 2012;69(2):230–238

Case 48

Glycogenic Hepatopathy in an Adolescent with Type 1 Diabetes

Nehama Zuckerman-Levin, MD;[1] Oz Mordechai, MD;[1]
and Naim Shehadeh, MD[1]

A 13-year-old adolescent with type 1 diabetes (T1D) was admitted to the hospital with fatigue, vomiting, and weight loss. He was a second twin, born after an uneventful pregnancy, with a birth weight of 1,900 g. His family history included a twin brother with bronchial asthma, and a grandmother with type 2 diabetes (T2D).

T1D was diagnosed at the age of 9 years. No diabetic ketoacidosis (DKA) was noted at diagnosis. He had positive anti-GAD and anti-islet cell antibodies (ICA). He used an insulin pump for 2 years, but because of recurrent severe hypoglycemic episodes, his treatment was changed to multiple daily injections (MDI). On MDI, his blood glucose levels were high, and he developed repeated episodes of DKA. Recently, his DKA episodes were noted on a monthly basis. His glycemic control was very poor, with glycosylated hemoglobin levels between 8.5 and 13%. His height and weight curves were noted to follow the growth chart normally.

On admission, history revealed a weight loss of 5 kg, fatigue, nausea, vomiting, and night sweats. On physical examination, abdominal obesity and upper abdominal tenderness were noted, and hepatomegaly was detected with the left liver edge palpated 4 cm below the costal margin. His spleen was not palpable. His height and weight were noted to be within normal limits. Laboratory tests demonstrated the following:

WBC	6,380
Hb	14.5
Plt	285,000
HbA$_{1c}$	12.1%
Lactic acid	9.1 mmol/L (normal range 0.5–2.4 mmol/L)

High lactate levels were documented during his DKA episode and even after achieving near-normal glucose levels.

Total bilirubin level	0.46 mg/dL
Aspartate aminotransferase	358 units/L
Alanine transaminase	429 units/L

[1]Department of Pediatrics, Pediatric Diabetes and Obesity Clinic, Rambam Health Care Campus, Bruce Rappaport Faculty of Medicine, Technion, Haifa, Israel.

DOI: 10.2337/9781580405713.48

γ-Glutamyl transpeptidase	82 units/L
Alkaline phosphatase	277 units/L
Lactate dehydrogenase	319 units/L
Total protein	6.6 g/dL
Albumin	3.3 g/dL
γ-Globulins	normal
Prothrombin time	normal (international normalized ratio 0.93)
Cholesterol	149 mg/dL
Triglycerides	407 mg/dL
Ceruloplasmin levels	normal

Serology showed the following:

Hepatitis B and C	negative
CMV	negative
EBV	positive
Antinuclear antibodies	negative
Antisaccharomyces cerevisiae antibodies	negative
Celiac antibodies	negative
Thyroid function tests	within normal limits

Urine analysis showed high levels of lactic acid and ketones (3-hydroxybutirate and acetoacetate), high methylglutaconic acid, and hydroxyl methylglutaric acid. Sonography and abdominal computed tomography (CT) revealed hepatomegaly, mainly in the left lobe. Liver length 20 cm, with hyperechogenicity and appearance consistent with fatty liver. The patient's liver biopsy showed macrovesicular steatosis and glycogen storage in cytoplasm of hepatocytes. On follow-up, the patient was treated with intensive insulin regimen and very tight metabolic control. His blood glucose levels decreased to almost within the normal range. Resolution of the hepatomegaly and elevated liver enzymes were observed within several weeks.

DISCUSSION

Several years after introducing insulin as a treatment modality in T1D, Mauriac[i] described patients with T1D who had growth retardation, delayed puberty, cushingoid features, hepatomegaly, and elevated liver enzymes. Those patients had uncontrolled diabetes.

Since Mauriac's first description, the involvement of the liver in T1D has been described in several case reports, with different clinical symptoms and signs. The common signs are hepatomegaly and elevated liver enzymes . Liver involvement in this condition is due to hepatocellular glycogen accumulation (Fig. 48.1). Terms such as "liver glycogen storage," "liver glycogenosis," and lately "glycogenic hepatopathy" have been used to describe this clinical picture.

Despite advanced monitoring and treatment modalities in T1D, liver involvement as described by Mauriac still occurs. It is described both with MDI and continuous subcutaneous insulin infusion (CSII).

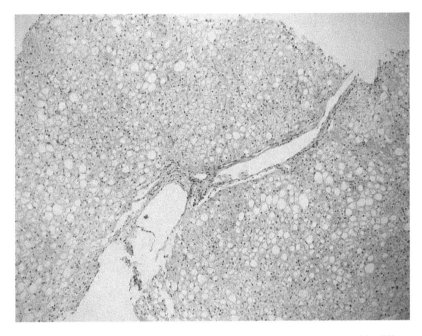

Figure 48.1—The histology demonstrates normal architecture with diffuse hepatocellular change characterized by pale hepatocytes with cytoplasmic rarefaction and accentuation of the cell membranes. Few glycogenated nuclei are noted. There is no inflammation.

The pathophysiology behind glycogenic hepatopathy is explained by recurrent episodes of hyperglycemia, followed by insulin overdosage, alternating with hypoglycemia treated with glucose. Also important is the contribution of counterregulatory hormones.

Hyperglycemia in uncontrolled T1D is followed by entrance of glucose into the hepatocytes, inducing glycogen synthesis. The high rate of hepatic glycogen synthesis in this condition is due to combined stimulation of glycogen synthase and inhibition of glycogen phosphorylase.[2] The clinical picture of hepatic glycogenosis includes the following: abdominal pain, nausea, and vomiting. Hepatomegaly is a predominant finding, but splenomegaly and ascites are not common. Mildly to moderately elevated liver enzymes with normal synthetic function are the main biochemical findings.[3-5] Hepatic glycogenosis can occur at any age.

Imaging techniques can demonstrate hepatomegaly, but cannot differentiate between excessive glycogen storage (such as in glycogenosis) and fatty liver (with steatosis). The latter is part of nonalcoholic fatty liver disease (NAFLD), another form of liver disease commonly associated with diabetes mellitus. Liver biopsy is the examination of choice in this clinical setting. The histology reveals large hepatocytes with excess glycogen in the cytoplasm,

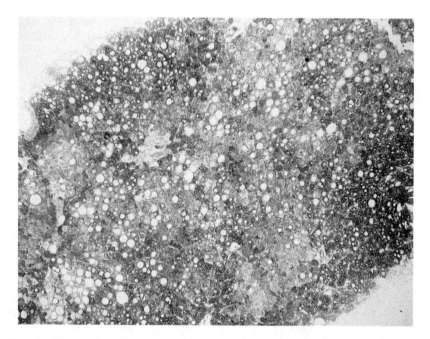

Figure 48.2—Abundant cytoplasmic glycogen deposits can be demonstrated by PAS stains, which disappear after digestion with diastase.

and glycogenated nuclei without significant fatty change, inflammation, and lobular spotty necrosis. Elevated liver enzymes are presumed to be caused by hepatocellular injury and enzyme "leakage" and not by cell death.[1] Some patients may demonstrate mild fibrosis and inflammation.[3] Periodic acid–Schiff staining is strongly positive (Fig. 48.2). Liver histology is diagnostic and may help the clinician reassure the patient about the benign nature of liver involvement. Hepatic glycogenosis, in contrast to primary glycogen storage disease and NAFLD, may be transient.

Several weeks of better glycemic control can cause the hepatic derangements to resolve. Liver enzymes normalize and the liver returns to its normal size. Hepatic glycogenosis must be considered in any patient with uncontrolled T1D, and awareness of this phenomenon can prevent delay in diagnosis and result in a favorable outcome.

REFERENCES

1. Mauriac P. Gros ventre, hepatomegalie, troubles de las croissance chez les enfants diabetiques traits depuis plusieurs annes par l'insuline. *Gax Hebdo Med Bordeaux* 1930;26:402–410

2. Petersen KF, Laurent D, Rothman DL, Cline GW, Shulman GI. Mechanism by which glucose and insulin inhibit net hepatic glycogenolysis in humans. *J Clin Invest* 1998;101:1203–1209

3. van den brand M, Elving LD, Drenth JP, van Krieken JH. Glycogenic hepatopathy: a rare cause of elevated serum transaminases in diabetes mellitus. *Neth J Med* 2009;67(11):394–396

4. Cha JH, Ra SH, Park YM, Ji YK, et al. Three cases of glycogenic hepatopathy mimicking acute and relapsing hepatitis in type I diabetes mellitus. *Clin Mol Hepatol* 2013;19(4):421–425

5. Fitzpatrick E, Cotoi C, Quaglia A, Sakellariou S, Ford-Adams ME, Hadzic N. Hepatopathy of Mauriac syndrome: a retrospective review from a tertiary liver center. *Arch Dis Child* 2014;99:354–357

Case 49

Glycemic Control in a Child with Type 1 Diabetes and Autoimmune Hepatitis

SANDRO MUNTONI, MD, PHD,[1] AND MAURO CONGIA, MD[2]

A 5-year-old girl was brought to our clinic in July 2009 for increased values of liver transaminases. She was naturally born at the 40th week of gestation and breast-fed for 6 months. At the 10th month of age after the last mandatory vaccine dose, she developed type 1 diabetes (T1D), a frequent autoimmune disorder in Sardinian children[1,2] because of a strong genetic predisposition.[3] Because in the past 8 months she showed abnormal liver serum transaminase levels, the patient was admitted in the hospital where serological and instrumental tests were performed. Virological (hepatitis B virus, hepatitis C virus, human immunodeficiency virus, *Toxoplasma gondii*, rubella, cytomegalovirus and herpes simplex virus, human herpes virus 6, parvovirus B19), metabolic (α-1-antitrypsin, ceruloplasmin, plasmatic, and urinary copper), celiac disease (CD) screening tests, and thyroid autoimmunity analysis were all in the normal range. Genetic screening for the most common Sardinian autoimmune regulator gene mutations was also normal. On the other hand, immunoglobulin G (IgG)/γ-globulin levels, antinuclear antibodies (ANA), antismooth muscle antibody (ASMA), F-actin, and soluble liver antigen (SLA), all markers for autoimmune hepatitis (AIH), were increased. No liver ultrasonographic abnormalities or liver fibrosis by fibroscan were found. The HLA DRB1*0301 was found in homozygosis. The diagnosis of AIH was suspected, and a liver biopsy was requested and corticosteroid therapy planned. The parents refused liver biopsy and corticosteroid treatment, however, in fear of the procedural risks and potential for worsening glycemic control. After more than 3 years of stable liver function tests, they suddenly became quite high (Fig. 49.1). Corticosteroid treatment was promptly started and liver biopsy planned. A complete normalization of transaminases, γ-glutamyltransferase (GGT), alkaline phosphatase and autoantibodies in about 3 months was observed.

T1D may be associated with autoimmune thyroid disease, CD, Addison's disease, and other autoimmune diseases, such as AIH, as reported here. The diagnosis of AIH should be considered when more common causes of liver

[1]Department of Biomedical Sciences, University School of Cagliari and Centre for Metabolic Diseases and Atherosclerosis, The ME.DI.CO Association, Cagliari, Italy.
[2]Pediatric Gastroenterologic Unity, Microcitemic Hospital, ASL 8, Cagliari, Italy.

DOI: 10.2337/9781580405713.49

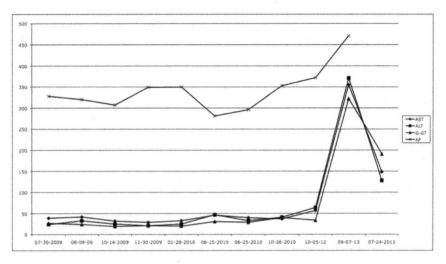

Figure 49.1 — Transaminase, GGT, and alkaline phosphatase variation in T1D-AIH Sardinian patient.

disease have been ruled out. Autoantibodies can help delineate the type of AIH. Three types of AIH are described: type 1 showing positivity for antismooth muscle antibody ASMA and frequently also for ANA; type 2 with the antibody positivity to liver/kidney microsomes type 1 and liver cytosol type 1; type 3 mainly characterized by anti-SLA/liver-pancreas antibodies positivity. It is more frequent in females and shows a strong association with some HLA class II genotypes (HLA-DR3-DQ2 and -DR4-DQ8 for type 1 and HLA-DR3-DQ2 and -DR7-DQ2 for type 2). The mode of presentation of AIH in childhood is variable. The course may be fluctuating, with flares and spontaneous remissions, a pattern that may result in delayed diagnosis as in the present case. The majority of the children on physical examination present clinical signs of an underlying chronic liver disease, including cutaneous stigmata (spider nevi, palmar erythema, leukonychia, and striae), firm liver with splenomegaly, and parenchymal alteration on ultrasonography or fibroscan. On the contrary, in our case, no clinical signs or ultrasonographic abnormalities were detected.

Compatible clinical signs and symptoms, laboratory abnormalities, serological and histological findings, and the exclusion of other conditions that can cause chronic hepatitis are the mainstays for the diagnosis that is based on the following: *1)* evaluation by diagnostic scoring systems (Table 49.1; see also http://napervillegi.com/contrivances/aihcalc.html); *2)* other serological markers (anti-SLA and atypical perinuclear antineutrophil cytoplasmic antibody); *3)* exclusion of the autoimmune polyendocrinopathy candidiasis ectodermal dystrophy (APECED) syndrome by testing for typical mutations in patients with AIH and multiple endocrine disorders;[4] *4)* classification of autoimmune hepatitis as type 1 or type 2; and *5)* nuclear magnetic resonance–cholangiography to exclude primary sclerosing cholangitis.

Table 49.1—Scoring System for the Diagnosis of Autoimmune Hepatitis

Sex	Female	+2	HLA	DR3 or DR4	+1
AP:AST (or ALT) ratio	>3 <1.5	−2 +2	Immune disease	Thyroiditis, colitis, others	+2
γ-globulin or IgG level above normal	>2.0 1.5–2.0 1.0–1.5 <1.0	+3 +2 +1 0	Other markers	Anti-SLA, anti-actin, anti LC1, pANCA	+2
ANA, SMA, or anti-LKM1 titers	>1:80 1:80 1:40 <1:40	+3 +2 +1 0	Histological features	Interface hepatitis Plasmacytic Rosettes None of above Biliary changes Other features Complete Relapse	+3 +1 +1 −5 −3 −3 +2 +3
AMA	Positive	−4	Treatment response		
Viral markers	Positive Negative	−3 +3			
Drugs	Yes No	−4 +1	Pretreatment aggregate score: Definite diagnosis >15 Probable diagnosis 10-15		
Alcohol	<25 g/day >60 g/day	+2 −2	Posttreatment aggregate score: Definite diagnosis >17 Probable diagnosis 12-17		

AMA, antimitochondrial antibody; anti-LC1, antibody to liver cytosol type 1; anti-LKM1, antibody to liver/kidney microsomes type 1; anti-SLA, antibody to soluble liver antigen; ANA, antinuclear antibody; AP:AST (or ALT) ratio, ratio of alkaline phosphatase level to aspartate or alanine aminotransferase level; HLA, human leukocyte antigen; IgG, immunoglobulin G; pANCA, perinuclear anti neutrophil cytoplasmic antibody; SMA, smooth muscle antibody.

Source: Reprinted with permission from Manns.[5]

THERAPY

Treatment in children should be instituted with prednisone (1–2 mg/kg daily; maximum dose 60 mg daily) in combination with azathioprine (1–2 mg/kg daily) or 6-mercaptopurine (1.5 mg/kg daily). In our case, the parents' concerns about biopsy and corticosteroid therapy delayed diagnosis and therapy. The sharp increase of transaminases, γ-GT, alkaline phosphatase, and γ-globulins associated with increment of end-stage renal disease and C-reactive protein and the appearance of fatigue, arthralgias, and anorexia finally compelled prompt corticosteroid administration and liver biopsy.

Insulin therapy was increased from 23 units of insulin glargine to 33 units in the morning; insulin aspart before breakfast, lunch, and dinner was modified according to the glycemia, adjusting the total requirement to about 3 units/kg with 30 mg/day of prednisone.

At present, the patient has completely normalized transaminases; γ-GT values as well as the other liver parameters and IgG/γ-globulin levels have decreased from 41 to 23%. She is tapering down prednisone and recently has introduced azathioprine at the initial dosage of 1 mg/kg/day. In the following weeks, prednisone will be decreased further until reaching the dosage of 5 mg/day and will be maintained at this level for at least 1 year; azathioprine will be increased to 1.5–2 mg/kg/day.

This case shows that in children with diabetes, especially those with a very early onset, other autoimmune diseases (such as AIH) may appear. These patients should have a complete assessment, including the exclusion of rare diseases, such as APECED or Wilson disease. The diagnosis of AIH is based on both a scoring system and the liver biopsy. Finally, T1D is not a reason to delay or avoid corticosteroid administration.

REFERENCES

1. Muntoni S, Stabilini L, Stabilini M, et al. Steadily high IDDM incidence over 4 years in Sardinia. *Diabetes Care* 1995;18:1600–1601

2. Muntoni S, Fonte MT, Stoduto S, et al. Incidence of insulin-dependent diabetes mellitus among Sardinian-heritage children born in Lazio region, Italy. *Lancet* 1997;349:160–162

3. Motzo C, Contu D, Cordell HJ, et al. Heterogeneity in the magnitude of the insulin gene effect on HLA risk in type 1 diabetes. *Diabetes* 2004;53:3286–3291

4. Meloni A, Willcox N, Meager A, et al. Autoimmune polyendocrine syndrome type 1: an extensive longitudinal study in Sardinian patients. *J Clin Endocrinol Metab* 2012;97:1114–1124

5. Manns MP, Czaja AJ, Gorham JD, et al. Diagnosis and management of autoimmune hepatitis. *Hepatology* 2010;51:2193–2213

Case 50

Dizziness, Lightheadedness, and Syncope in a Patient with Type 2 Diabetes

Shalini Paturi, MD,[1,2] and Janice L. Gilden, MS, MD, FCP, FACE[1,2]

A 57-year-old man with type 2 diabetes (T2D) for 7 years and peripheral neuropathy was referred in 2008 for evaluation of episodic "hypoglycemic" symptoms (lightheadedness, dizziness, shakiness, sweating, headaches, tremors, and pallor), unrelated to position or meals, resulting in one episode of syncope and a fall. The episodes resolved with ingestion of glucose tablets or meals. These symptoms started 10 years ago, after an ablation for Wolff-Parkinson-White syndrome, and gradually increased in frequency.

Symptoms of hypoglycemia, mediated by the autonomic nervous system, are nonspecific. Neurogenic symptoms, such as tremors, palpitations, and anxiety, are catecholamine mediated; and other symptoms, like sweating, hunger, and paresthesia, are cholinergic mediated. Neuroglycopenic symptoms include cognitive impairment, behavioral changes, and psychomotor abnormalities.[1]

Past medical history was significant for panic disorder, posttraumatic stress disorder, fibromyalgia, hypertension, sleep apnea, and hyperlipidemia. Current medications for T2D were metformin 1,000 mg twice daily and pioglitazone 30 mg daily. Discontinuation of these medications did not reduce the occurrence of these episodes. Diet included three meals and two snacks daily, sometimes consisting of high calories and carbohydrates. Physical examination showed the following:

BMI	30 kg/m²
Blood pressure	145/80 mmHg supine
	120/90 mmHg standing

He was unable to stand >3 min because of lightheadedness and sweating. Blood pressure decreased by 25 mmHg during bedside tilt. Electrocardiogram, corrected Q and T waves (QTc) was 498 mm, and monofilament sensation was decreased.

[1]Endocrinology Division, Department of Medicine, Rosalind Franklin University of Medicine and Science/Chicago Medical School, North Chicago, IL. [2]Endocrinology Section, Department of Medicine, Captain James A. Lovell Federal Health Care Center, North Chicago, IL.

This research was supported in part by the Captain James A. Lovell Federal Health Care Center.

 DOI: 10.2337/9781580405713.50

Neurogenic orthostatic hypotension (NOH) can result from diabetic autonomic neuropathy (DAN) and is defined by a fall in systolic blood pressure ≥20 mmHg or diastolic blood pressure of ≥10 mmHg, accompanied by symptoms similar to hypoglycemia.[2] This autonomic imbalance can shift hypoglycemic symptoms thresholds to higher glucose levels.

Fasting and premeal self-monitored blood glucose (SMBG) ranged from 120 to 180 mg/dL (6.6–10 mmol/L), and postmeal SMBG ranged from 160 to 210 mg/dL (8.8–11.6 mmol/L).

Blood glucose (BG) values at which hypoglycemia occurs are variable. In people without diabetes, the secretion of insulin decreases as BG declines to 65 to 70 mg/dL (3.6 to 3.9 mmol/L) and counterregulatory hormones, glucagon, and epinephrine are released. In T2D, hypoglycemia occurs at levels ≤70 mg/dL (3.9 mmol/L).[1]

This patient's symptoms of lightheadedness, shaking, sweating, and tremors and relief of symptoms with meals and glucose tablets suggested hypoglycemia. Both the SMBG and BG, however, did not display values <70 mg/dL (3.9 mmol/L). In September 2008, hemoglobin A1c (HbA$_{1c}$) was 6.8%. A continuous glucose monitoring (CGM) study was performed.

CGM study involves interstitial glucose measurements every 5 min measured by a subcutaneous sensor. The information is transmitted to a wireless monitor. Capillary fingerstick glucose measurements are used to verify accuracy. Currently available CGM devices measure interstitial glucose, whereas fingerstick devices measure capillary BG. Because of a physiologic lag in equilibration between these two compartments, an increase or decrease in glucose levels will first be apparent in the blood, and then in the interstitial fluid. Clinical guidelines from the Endocrine Society recommend professional CGM studies in adult patients to detect situations suspicious for nocturnal hypoglycemia, the dawn phenomenon, and postprandial hyperglycemia.[3]

CGM study (Fig. 50.1) showed sensor glucose values between 72 and 208 mg/dL (4–11.5 mMol/L) with postmeal glycemic surges. The patient experienced symptoms at BG 140–150 mg/dL (7.7–8.3 mmol/L). Because the symptoms persisted, were inconsistent with meals, and no BG <70 mg/dL (3.9 mmol/L), we considered other causes for presyncope, flushing, and tremors.

Patients who experience symptoms of autonomic activity (tremors, palpitations, anxiety, sweating, hunger), but BG >70 mg/dL (3.9 mmol/L) may have other disorders, such as NOH, postprandial syndrome, cardiac disease (arrhythmia, valvular heart disease), medication complications, psychiatric disease, hyperthyroidism, or pheochromocytomoa.

Other laboratory tests ruled out carcinoid syndrome, pheochromocytomoa, thyroid dysfunction, cardiac disease, cerebrovascular disease, seizure disorder, and hypogonadism. Because of persistent early satiety and bloating sensation, a gastric emptying study was done. Results confirmed delayed emptying in all times (1 h = 26%, 2 h = 49%, 3 h = 71% emptying of stomach). Gastroparesis, NOH, and the prolonged QT interval of 498 mm were consistent with DAN.

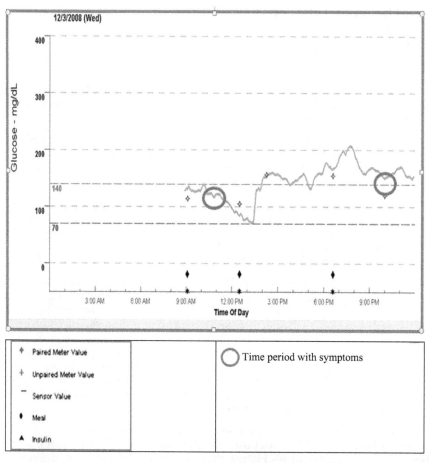

Figure 50.1 — CGM study from 2008, sample days with symptomatic
time periods noted. Average BG was 149 mg/dL
(8.2 mmol/L), ranged from 72 to 207 mg/dL (4–11.5 mmol/L).

Patients with T2D for ≥5 years who have symptoms of early satiety and bloating warrant evaluation for gastroparesis. This condition is known to be a complication of DAN and also can be associated with changes in glucoregulation.[4]

The patient had stopped taking his pioglitazone because of his fear of hypoglycemia. He was started on sitagliptin 50 mg daily (HbA$_{1c}$ 7%). He continued to complain of these episodes. In April 2010, the patient's SMBG showed fluctuating values between 120 and 220 mg/dL (6.6–12.2 mmol/L) with continued "hypoglycemic symptoms" at BG of 150 mg/dL (8.3 mmol/L). Therefore, acarbose 25 mg with breakfast was started. We also recommended

A

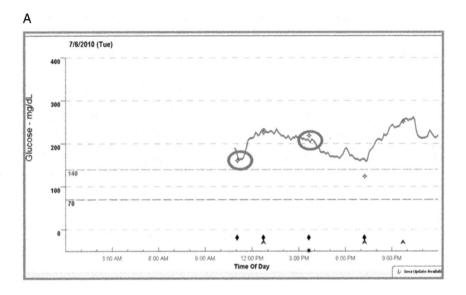

B

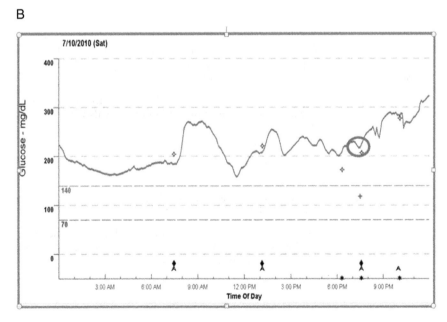

Figure 50.2—CGM study from 2010. *A:* Average BG was 219 mg/dL
(12.1 mmol/L) and ranged from 142 to 333 mg/dL
(7.8–18.5 mmol/L). *B:* CGM study from 2010.

dietary management with low-carbohydrate, high-protein regular meals and snacks.

Diet and α-glucosidase inhibitors, like acarbose, are often used to treat postprandial glucose fluctuations.[5]

In May 2010, he was started on glargine 5 units at bedtime in addition to acarbose 25 mg three times a day with meals, metformin 1,000 mg twice daily, and sitaglipitin 50 mg. CGM study in 2010 showed an average BG 219 mg/dL (12.1 mmol/L; range = 142–333 mg/dL, 7.8–18.5 mmol/L). Symptoms documented during the CGM study did not correlate with low BG readings (Figs. 50.2*A* and *B*). A1C remained between 6.2 and 7.1%.

Three years later, the patient returned to the endocrine clinic for reevaluation. He reported that whenever he did not follow the diet and forgot to take acarbose, he developed the "hypoglycemic symptoms," regardless of any other diabetes medication changes.

This case emphasizes the importance of recognizing multiple etiologies for syncope, lightheadedness, and dizziness, with symptoms similar to hypoglycemia in a patient with diabetes.

REFERENCES

1. Towler DA, Havlin CE, Craft S, Cryer P. Mechanism of awareness of hypoglycemia. Perception of neurogenic (predominantly cholinergic) rather than neuroglycopenic symptoms. *Diabetes* 1993;42:1791–1798

2. Maser RE, Mitchell BD, Vinik AI, Freeman R. The association between cardiovascular autonomic neuropathy and mortality in individuals with diabetes: a meta-analysis. *Diabetes Care* 2003;26:1895–1901

3. Klonoff DC, Buckingham B, Christiansen JS, et al. Continuous glucose monitoring: an Endocrine Society Clinical Practice Guideline. *J Clin Endocrinol Metab* 2011;96:2968–2979

4. Jones KL, Russo A, Stevens JE, et al. Predictors of delayed gastric emptying in diabetes. *Diabetes Care* 2001;24:1264–1269

5. Holman RR, Cull CA, Turner RC. A randomized double-blind trial of acarbose in type 2 diabetes shows improved glycemic control over 3 years (U.K. Prospective Diabetes Study 44). *Diabetes Care* 1999;22:960–964

Case 51

Growth Hormone Excess-Induced Diabetic Ketoacidosis

Andrew P. Demidowich, MD;[1] Maya Lodish, MD;[2] and
Kristina I. Rother, MD, MHSc[1]

A 17-year-old boy presented to a local emergency department with severe abdominal pain, nausea, and vomiting starting earlier that morning. He reported being in good health all his life, but he had not seen a physician since moving with his family from Korea 10 years prior. Upon prompting, he mentioned experiencing excessive thirst, frequent urination, and decreased energy for the preceding 6 months. On admission his glucose was 443 mg/dL (24.6 mmol/L), sodium 125 mmol/L, chloride 90 mmol/L, bicarbonate 15.0 mmol/L, urine ketones ≥150 mg/dL, and pH 7.27. The patient was diagnosed with diabetic ketoacidosis (DKA), and intravenous rehydration and insulin infusion were initiated.

DKA is a medical emergency and frequently presents with a constellation of symptoms, including abdominal pain, nausea, vomiting, dehydration, tachycardia, malaise, altered mental status, and, in severe cases, coma or even death. A ketotic or "fruity" breath odor may be present, and patients may exhibit tachypnea with deep or Kussmaul respirations. Classically DKA is associated with type 1 diabetes (T1D), because individuals are unable to produce sufficient insulin to prevent lipolysis and subsequent ketone formation.[1] DKA is frequently the inciting event that brings patients to medical attention.

DKA is diagnosed on the basis of hyperglycemia, acidosis, the presence of an anion gap, and ketones in the blood or urine. The immediate treatment for DKA is rehydration with intravenous fluids, potassium repletion, and insulin administration.

Over the next several days, the patient was successfully transitioned from intravenous (i.v.) infusion to a subcutaneous basal-bolus insulin regimen. However, the patient continued to experience hyperglycemia >300 mg/dL (16.7 mmol/L) despite receiving more than 0.9 units/kg/day of insulin. His hemoglobin A1C was 16.8%. The endocrinology service was consulted for further assistance.

On examination, the patient's height was 206 cm (6'9"), and he weighed 132 kg (BMI 31.1 kg/m²). He had a deep voice, prominent soft tissue swelling of the hands and feet, a shoe size of 18EEE, and multiple skin tags. He reported always being taller than his peers. Furthermore, his father's height

[1]Section on Pediatric Diabetes and Metabolism, Diabetes, Endocrinology, and Obesity Branch, NIDDK, National Institutes of Health, Bethesda, MD. [2]Heritable Disorders Branch, NICHD, National Institutes of Health, Bethesda, MD.

DOI: 10.2337/9781580405713.51

was 170 cm (5'7") and his mother's was 165 cm (5'5"). He reported profuse diaphoresis with minimal exertion, loud snoring, and recurrent headaches.

Growth hormone (GH) and insulin-like growth factor 1 (IGF-1) concentrations were elevated at 69 ng/mL (normal: 0–2.9 ng/mL) and 792 ng/mL (151–521 ng/mL), respectively, supporting the diagnosis of acromegaly. A pituitary magnetic resonance imaging revealed a macroadenoma measuring 2.5 cm in diameter.

GH affects multiple systems in the body, including bone, soft tissue, respiratory, cardiac, and energy regulation. GH is normally secreted in a pulsatile fashion, most prominently during slow-wave sleep,[2] and its secretion is tightly regulated. It is stimulated by GH-releasing hormone (GHRH) and ghrelin. It is negatively regulated by somatostatin, as well as by feedback inhibition from IGF-1 and GH itself.

Insulin and GH play different, but complementary, roles with respect to metabolic regulation. Insulin is secreted in periods of energy excess when glucose levels are elevated, whereas during energy restriction, insulin levels are suppressed, and GH is more abundantly released. GH promotes a switch from glucose to free fatty acids as the body's main source of energy by creating a temporary insulin-resistant state. Evolutionarily, these effects were advantageous, enabling the conservation of sparse glucose stores and decreasing the body's reliance on amino acids for fuel.[3]

In states of dysregulated GH production, however, these effects become deleterious. In children and adolescents, whose growth plates have not yet closed, GH excess exaggerates long-bone growth, leading to gigantism. In adults, GH excess more prominently affects joints, skull, and soft tissue, leading to acromegaly.[4]

Metabolic dysregulation is common in individuals with acromegaly: 19–56% have overt diabetes, 16–46% have impaired glucose tolerance, and up to 79% have diminished insulin sensitivity.[5] In some patients, insulin resistance can be profound, and maximal endogenous insulin secretion may not be adequate to suppress lipolysis, and DKA ensues.

The patient's insulin dose was uptitrated to 60 units of glargine twice daily and 22 units of insulin aspart with each meal, totaling 1.5 units/kg/day. His blood glucose, however, remained in the 200–300 mg/dL range (11.1–16.7 mmol/L). Upon confirming the diagnosis of acromegaly, he was started on octreotide 50 mcg by intramuscular injection three times daily, with improvement in glycemic control. Insulin requirements remained high, however, and the patient was switched from basal-bolus to U-500 insulin.

Surgical removal of the GH-producing adenoma is the first-line therapy in most patients with acromegaly and may result in complete resolution of hyperglycemia and insulin resistance. In patients unable or unwilling to undergo surgery, or in whom surgery is unsuccessful, somatostatin analogs are often started to suppress GH. Additionally, somatostatin analogs may be used initially to shrink the macroadenoma, particularly if it is close to vital structures, such as the optic chiasm or cavernous sinus.

Somatostatin analogs, such as octreotide or lanreotide, mimic the physiological inhibitory effects of somatostatin on GH-secreting pituitary adenomas by binding to somatostatin receptors 2 and 5. Long-term treatment can improve insulin resistance but may reduce β-cell secretory capacity.

Despite treatment with a somatostatin analog, subjects may remain profoundly resistant to insulin. As subcutaneous insulin depends on local blood flow dynamics for absorption, large doses may exhibit significant variability in rate of absorption and duration of action. U-500 may be an appropriate choice in this situation, as it facilitates larger doses of insulin in smaller volumes. This concentrated form of insulin has a longer half-life than regular insulin and is given without concomitant basal insulin. We converted the patient's total daily insulin dose of 186 units/day to 60 units (12 volume or syringe units) of U-500 three times daily. After achieving adequate glycemic control, the patient underwent transsphenoidal surgery, but surgical cure was not possible because of the tumor burden and invasion into the cavernous sinuses. His glycemia is currently well-controlled on octreotide and 75 units of U-500 (15 volume units) before each meal. Ultimately, the patient likely will require cranial radiation to achieve remission.

REFERENCES

1. Kitabchi AE, et al. Hyperglycemic crises in adult patients with diabetes. *Diabetes Care* 2009;32(7):1335–1343

2. Moller N, Jorgensen JO. Effects of growth hormone on glucose, lipid, and protein metabolism in human subjects. *Endocr Rev* 2009;30(2):152–177

3. Colao A, et al. Medical consequences of acromegaly: what are the effects of biochemical control? *Rev Endocr Metab Disord* 2008;9(1):21–31

4. Yoshida N, et al. Ketoacidosis as the initial clinical condition in nine patients with acromegaly: a review of 860 cases at a single institute. *Eur J Endocrinol* 2013;169(1):127–132

5. Katznelson L, et al. American Association of Clinical Endocrinologists medical guidelines for clinical practice for the diagnosis and treatment of acromegaly—2011 update. *Endocr Pract* 2011;17(Suppl. 4):1–44

Case 52

Refractory Angina in a Patient with Type 2 Diabetes

Mikhail Kosiborod, MD[1]

A 76-year-old man presents for a routine outpatient cardiology visit. He has a 15-year history of type 2 diabetes, with several diabetes-related microvascular complications, including stage III chronic kidney disease and mild peripheral neuropathy. He is currently on a combination of metformin and sulfonylurea (SU; sustained release glipizide) for glucose control, with last hemoglobin A1c (HbA$_{1c}$) of 8.5%. Although the patient never sustained a myocardial infarction, he has a complex and longstanding history of multivessel coronary artery disease (CAD), requiring two-vessel coronary artery bypass surgery (CABG) 7 years ago, and several subsequent percutaneous interventions (PCIs). Despite multiple interventions, patient continues to have chronic Canadian Cardiovascular Society (CCS) class 2–3 angina, with typical midsternal chest pressure upon mild-to-moderate physical activity—the pattern of angina has been stable for the past 5 years, but it interferes significantly with his quality of life.

One of the most enduring "medical myths" in cardiology is that patients with diabetes and CAD are less likely to experience typical angina than their nondiabetic counterparts. In large part, this originates from the assumption that because of diabetes-related autonomic neuropathy, patients with CAD and diabetes are much more likely to have "silent ischemia" than those without diabetes. This belief is based predominantly on several small and older studies and has not been confirmed in larger clinical trials. Specifically, one of the most rigorously conducted clinical studies to evaluate silent ischemia (the Asymptomatic Cardiac Ischemia Pilot) showed no difference in the prevalence of silent ischemia between patients with and without diabetes.[1] In fact, because patients with diabetes have more severe and diffuse CAD than those without diabetes, one would expect them to have more, not less, angina. Recent data have confirmed the higher prevalence of angina in patients with diabetes and CAD, as compared to those without diabetes. Analysis from a large, contemporary U.S.-based prospective registry showed that during 12 months after acute coronary syndrome, patients with diabetes experienced greater burden of angina at every time point—the magnitude of this difference was amplified over time, despite more aggressive angina management in patients with diabetes (Fig. 52.1).[2]

[1]Professor of Medicine, Saint Luke's Mid America Heart Institute, University of Missouri-Kansas City, Kansas City, MO.

DOI: 10.2337/9781580405713.52

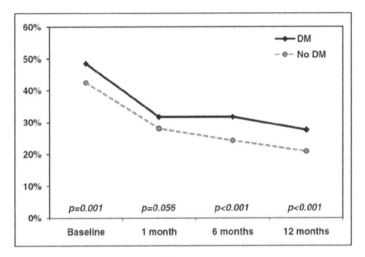

Figure 52.1—Patients reporting angina before and after myocardial infarction according to the presence or absence of diabetes.
As assessed with the Seattle Angina Questionnaire angina frequency domain: angina frequency score <100.

Source: Reprinted with permission from Arnold.[2]

Patient's cardiovascular medications include aspirin, high-dose atorvastatin, ACE-I, as well as a combination of metoprolol 25 mg daily, amlodipine 10 mg daily, and a long-acting nitrate (isosorbide mononitrate 60 mg daily) for angina management. His heart rate is in the mid-50s, and blood pressure is 125/70 mmHg on this regimen. He is inquiring whether any additional options are available to improve his angina symptoms and quality of life.

Unfortunately, the most recent coronary angiography showed no additional acceptable targets for PCI or surgery. Therefore, optimization of medical therapy remains the only additional option. β-Blockers and calcium channel blockers have both been demonstrated to be effective anti-anginal agents in patients with chronic stable CAD, while the data for long-acting nitrates (the oldest anti-anginal medication) are much more limited. Further uptitration of β-blockers is likely to be problematic in this patient, because of baseline bradycardia. Because of this patient's suboptimal glucose control, however, one could consider changing his metoprolol, a nonvasodilating β-blocker, to carvedilol, a vasodilating β-blocker.

Previous studies, including a dedicated randomized clinical trial, showed that carvedilol has a neutral effect on markers of chronic glycemia (such as HbA_{1c}) and fasting glucose, whereas metoprolol modestly worsens glycemic control over time. These differential effects of various β-blockers on glucose control are not widely known in the clinical community, and the vast majority of patients with diabetes are prescribed nonvasodilating β-blockers (i.e., metoprolol and atenolol) rather than carvedilol. Recent data also suggest that patients with diabetes discharged home on metoprolol and atenolol (vs. carvedilol) after acute myocardial infarction may experience worse glucose control during follow-up.[3]

One additional option to consider for this patient's angina management could be the addition of ranolazine, which is approved for angina treatment in the U.S., and has been shown to be effective in reducing angina frequency in patients with type 2 diabetes and stable CAD.[4] Post hoc analyses from clinical trials also suggest that ranolazine may lower fasting glucose and HbA_{1c} without causing hypoglycemia,[5] and its efficacy as a glucose-lowering agent currently is being tested in several ongoing prospective randomized trials.

Reevaluation of patient's glucose lowering medications may be of importance. Although SU are commonly used for type 2 diabetes management, they have been associated with increased risk of cardiovascular complications, including myocardial infarction. Early data also suggest that there is an association between SU use and greater angina frequency patients with type 2 diabetes, CAD, and stable angina. These data are preliminary, and in need of confirmation, but it is reasonable to consider using an alternative agent, on top of metformin, for glucose control in this patient.

Several medication adjustments were made over the course of the subsequent 6 weeks. Metoprolol was changed to carvedilol, and the patient was initiated on ranolazine and referred to an endocrinologist who increased the metformin dose, discontinued SU, and started the patient on an alternative glucose-lowering agent. Three months later, patient's angina symptoms were significantly improved, even though they did not completely resolve. In addition, his glucose control also improved, with HbA_{1c} decreasing from 8.5 to 7.7%.

REFERENCES

1. Caracciolo EA, Chaitman BR, Forman SA, et al. Diabetics with coronary disease have a prevalence of asymptomatic ischemia during exercise treadmill testing and ambulatory ischemia monitoring similar to that of nondiabetic patients. An ACIP database study. ACIP Investigators. Asymptomatic Cardiac Ischemia Pilot Investigators. *Circulation* 1996;93:2097–2105

2. Arnold SV, Spertus JA, Lipska KJ, et al. Association between diabetes mellitus and angina after acute myocardial infarction: analysis of the TRIUMPH prospective cohort study. *Eur J Prev Cardiol*. 2014 Apr 16. [Epub ahead of print] PubMed PMID: 24740679

3. Arnold SV, Spertus JA, Lipska KJ, et al. Type of beta-blocker use among patients with versus without diabetes after myocardial infarction. *Am Heart J* 2014 Sep;168(3):273–279.e1

4. Kosiborod M, Arnold SV, Spertus JA, et al. Evaluation of ranolazine in patients with type 2 diabetes mellitus and chronic stable angina: results from the TERISA randomized clinical trial (Type 2 Diabetes Evaluation of Ranolazine in Subjects with Chronic Stable Angina). *J Am Coll Cardiol* 2013;61:2038–2045

5. Chisholm JW, Goldfine AB, Dhalla AK, et al. Effect of ranolazine on A1C and glucose levels in hyperglycemic patients with non-ST elevation acute coronary syndrome. *Diabetes Care* 2010;33:1163–1168

Case 53

Glycemic Control in a Patient with Type 2 Diabetes Undergoing Cardiac Surgery

M. Kathleen Figaro, MD, MS[1]

A 55-year-old woman with a past medical history of type 2 diabetes, tobacco abuse, dyslipidemia, and hypertension presents for cardiac surgery after initial presentation with a slow-healing right heel ulcer. As a part of the evaluation of her right heel ulceration, she underwent vascular testing that revealed decreased perfusion to the right lower extremity. The patient was referred to an endovascular specialist who attempted an endovascular revascularization. The patient was found to have a chronic total occlusion of the right superficial femoral artery with collateral reconstitution of the popliteal artery and tibial runoff. Attempts at bridging the superficial femoral artery occlusion were not successful.

During the attempted dilation of this vessel, the vessel had a dissection that was resolved with a stent. The patient was referred for operative revascularization. After referral to the cardiac surgeon, evaluation by cardiac catheterization found depressed ejection fraction down to 35%, with three-vessel disease. The patient was scheduled for cardiac bypass (CABG). The patient was a heavy tobacco user and before admission was attempting to decrease the amount of her smoking. She stopped smoking ~1 week before admission for CABG. She was maintained on metformin 1,000 mg b.i.d. and insulin glargine 30 units nightly.

The patient was admitted at 7 A.M. for the CABG procedure. She had been told to decrease her glargine from 30 units to 15 units on the night before surgery and to stop metformin 2 days before surgery. Her blood glucose was >400 mg/dL (22.2 mmol/L). Surgery was canceled and the patient was transferred to the intensive care unit (ICU).

Hyperglycemia and insulin resistance frequently are seen in patients with diabetes and vascular disease. In addition, a relationship exists between preoperative A1C level and surgical outcomes. In patients undergoing CABG surgery, there is an association between high A1C values and surgical complications, including mortality, cerebrovascular accidents, and deep sternal wound infections.[1] Hypoglycemia intraoperatively puts extra cardiovascular stress on patients. Patients are often told to decrease insulin before surgery to avoid hypoglycemia. Actual treatment for a given patient should be individualized

---

[1]Medical Director, Diabetes Care Center, Endocrinology, Genesis Health Care, Bettendorf, IA.

DOI: 10.2337/9781580405713.53

and should be based on diabetes type, type of regimen, glycemic control, type of surgical procedure, and available expertise preoperatively.

Although hyperglycemia can delay surgery, as it did in this patient for 24 h, intravenous (i.v.) insulin infusion with potassium and glucose has been found to be an effective method for controlling hyperglycemia in intraoperative patients. Although it neither reduces myocardial damage nor improves intraoperative cardiac performance in patients without contractile dysfunction, it efficiently controlled glucose intraoperatively.[2] This gives an alternative course of action to simply cutting the basal insulin in half or, worse, holding all insulin before the surgical date and responding to the ensuing hyperglycemia.

Because of the patient's hyperglycemia before surgery, endocrinology was consulted. A glucostabilizer i.v. insulin protocol already exists in the hospital, and this was recommended to the referring provider. The patient's glucose levels were controlled after 4 h on the i.v. insulin protocol to <150 mg/dL (8.3 mmol/L). When the patient was converted from i.v. insulin to subcutaneous insulin therapy, the patient's glargine was not started for >8 h after the i.v. insulin was stopped. The patient had begun to eat and had no standing prandial insulin orders, only a correction dose to be used for glucose levels >150 mg/dL (8.3 mmol/L). The patient had elevations in glucose levels that prompted reconsultation of endocrinology to help with glycemic control.

Virtually every hospital has developed and refined protocols for i.v. insulin infusion; however, fewer hospitals use i.v. insulin during surgical procedures. Many hospitals use i.v. insulin postoperatively in the ICU, and protocols consider both blood glucose levels and sequential, usually hourly, changes in glycemic values. Although i.v. insulin protocols are frequently used in the postoperative period, the conversion between i.v. insulin and subcutaneous insulin is often poorly administered and patients develop hyperglycemia.

At the time of consultation, her workup revealed the following:

Weight	**110 kg**
Blood pressure	**142/85 mmHg**
Temperature	**37.3°C**
Pulse	**72 (regular)**
Respirations	**20/min**

The patient was alert, had 1+ pedal pulses, and post-CABG dressings. The rest of her physical exam was unremarkable:

Sodium	**136 mEq/L**
Potassium	**5.4 mEq/L**
Chloride	**106 mEq/L**
Carbon dioxide	**29 mEq/L**
Blood urea nitrogen	**27 mg/dL**
Creatinine	**1.45 mg/dL**
Glucose	**175 mg/dL (9.7 mmol/L)**

Her complete blood count showed the following:

White blood cell count	12.8
Hemoglobin	8.2 g/dL
Hematocrit	26.1%
Platelet count	299
Preoperative HbA$_{1c}$	8.9%
Thyroid-stimulating hormone	1.9 mIU/L
T4	1.0 ng/dL
T3	2.6 pg/dL
Cholesterol	308 mg/dL
Triglycerides	586 mg/dL
HDL	40 mg/dL

Her glucose had varied between 147 and 234 mg/dL (8.2 and 13 mmol/L) over the past 12 h. She was started back on glargine and lispro meal insulin with a correction scale, and within 24 h, her glucose levels were controlled and all <150 mg/dL (8.3 mmol/L).

The first task was to estimate her total daily dose of insulin (TDDI). We knew the patient administered 30 units of glargine daily at home and that her HbA$_{1c}$ was elevated. Assuming mealtime boluses are approximately equal to basal insulin, her TDDI needs were estimated to be about 60 units. This was divided in half and she was restarted on glargine 30 units and 10 units of lispro per meal. This was adjusted downward over the next 48 h to 28 units of glargine and 8 units of lispro as the stress of surgery dissipated.

Some surgeons consider it important to lower HbA$_{1c}$ levels to the goals recommended by the American Diabetes Association (<7% for most patients) before elective surgery, whereas others consider it less important because most evidence exists for acute hyperglycemia before surgery or directly after surgery.[3,4] The standard practice of lowering insulin before the operative day to avoid hypoglycemia should be reconsidered, especially in patients with high A1C levels both because HbA$_{1c}$ independently predicts poorer postsurgical outcomes[5] and because iatrogenically induced hyperglycemia can delay surgery and be a costly mistake for patients who already have uncontrolled diabetes.

REFERENCES

1. O'Sullivan CJ, Hynes N, Mahendran B, Andrews EJ, Avalos G, Tawfik S, Lowery A, Sultan S. Haemoglobin A1C (HbA1C) in non-diabetic and diabetic vascular patients. Is HbA1C an independent risk factor and predictor of adverse outcome? *Eur J Vasc Endovasc Surg* 2006;32(2):188–197

2. Shim YH, Kweon TD, Lee JH, Nam SB, Kwak YL. Intravenous glucose-insulin-potassium during off-pump coronary artery bypass surgery does not reduce myocardial injury. *Acta Anaesthesiol Scand* 2006;50(8):954–961

3. Halkos ME, Puskas JD, Lattouf OM, Kilgo P, Kerendi F, Song HK, Guyton RA, Thourani VH. Elevated preoperative hemoglobin A1C level is predictive of adverse events after coronary artery bypass surgery. *Thorac Cardiovasc Surg* 2008;136(3):631–640

4. Halkos ME, Lattouf OM, Puskas JD, Kilgo P, Cooper WA, Morris CD, Guyton RA, Thourani VH. Elevated preoperative hemoglobin A1C level is associated with reduced long-term survival after coronary artery bypass surgery. *Ann Thorac Surg* 2008;86(5):1431–1437

5. Kinoshita T, Asai T, Suzuki T, Kambara A, Matsubayashi K. Preoperative hemoglobin A1C predicts atrial fibrillation after off-pump coronary bypass surgery. *Eur J Cardiothorac Surg* 2012;41(1):102–107

Case 54

Inpatient Insulin Management for Complex Enteral Feedings

ANNA BETH BARTON, MD;[1] KATHRYN J. EVANS, DNP, FNP-BC;[2]
AND LILLIAN F. LIEN, MD[3]

C ritically ill medical or surgical patients often require enteral nutrition during hospitalization. A variety of formulas are available, each providing essential daily nutrients that can be more easily administered and tolerated during times of physiologic stress.[1] Inpatient registered dietitians (RD) develop enteral nutrition plans for individual patients based on such factors as weight-based caloric needs, nutrient requirements for wound healing, and underlying comorbidities that guide electrolyte restrictions.[1] For patients who also have diabetes, enteral nutrition can make glycemic control a challenge. This case illustrates the methods that endocrinologists in our institution often use to tailor insulin administration to cover complicated enteral feeding regimens.

A 65-year-old male patient with type 2 diabetes and longstanding achalasia refractory to myotomy was admitted for esophagectomy with cervical pharyngogastrostomy. Postoperatively, enteral tube feedings (TF) were initiated and administered on a continuous (24 h) basis. The primary team initially maintained the patient on a "sliding scale" of regular insulin alone, despite his known history of diabetes. As an outpatient, his diabetes regimen consisted of Januvia 100 mg/day, with the most recent A1C documented at 6.4% 2 months before his admission. On sliding-scale insulin alone, he was persistently hyperglycemic with blood glucose values ranging from 169 to 280 mg/dL (9.4–15.6 mmol/L). Thus, the inpatient Diabetes Management Service (DMS) was consulted for assistance with glycemic control. Of note, his postoperative course was complicated by an empyema thought to be related to aspiration resulting in sepsis requiring intravenous antibiotics, inotropic support, and chest tube placement. This led to intermittent initiation and discontinuation of tube feeds. At the time of consultation, he was afebrile with a blood pressure of 124/60 mmHg, heart rate of 100 bpm, and weight of 84 kg. He was sedated on mechanical ventilation. Physical exam was notable for a nasogastric tube in his naris and a chest tube draining purulent material. He was mildly tachycardic but without murmurs and

[1]Endocrinology Fellow, Department of Medicine Division of Endocrinology, Metabolism, and Nutrition, Duke University Medical Center, Durham, NC. [2]Division of Endocrinology, Metabolism and Nutrition, Duke University Medical Center, Durham, NC. [3]Medical Director, Duke Inpatient Diabetes Management Associate Professor, Department of Medicine Division of Endocrinology, Metabolism, and Nutrition, Duke University Medical Center, Durham, NC.

DOI: 10.2337/9781580405713.54

had decreased breath sounds on bilateral lung exam. There was no upper extremity edema but he did have trace edema in his lower extremities.

After an assessment of the medication administration record of insulin requirements to date, the DMS team estimated the patient would benefit from a regimen of subcutaneous (SQ) regular insulin 15 units every 6 h, as long as the patient remained on continuous TF, specifically, Isosource 1.5 kcal/ml (a 44% carbohydrate formula) at 65 mL/h providing a total of 2,340 kcal/day. Doses were gradually uptitrated to regular insulin 18 units every 6 h, and blood glucose was stable on this regimen, ranging from 136 to 159 mg/dL (7.6–8.8 mmol/L) (Table 54.1).

Many types of insulin regimens have been utilized to facilitate glycemic control on continuous TF. Although some clinicians believe that glargine insulin is safe and effective for use with enteral feedings,[2,3] our institution believes that the use of basal (long-acting) insulin is not ideal with TF because of common cessation or interruption of the feedings (resulting from a clogged tube or emergent NPO preprocedure), which, when unexpected, can cause profound hypoglycemia. Thus, our institution often prefers the use of shorter-acting regular insulin and intermediate acting NPH insulin. For this patient receiving continuous enteral TF, the DMS team initiated SQ regular insulin every 6 h, so that the insulin could match the effect of the TF regimen. Regular insulin peaks in 2–4 h and lasts 6–8 h making it an effective therapy for continuous (or q 3 h bolus) TF.[4]

On postoperative day 17, the primary surgical team decided to transition the patient to a cycled nocturnal TF regimen to allow for planned introduction of daytime oral intake. Thus, continuous TF was discontinued, and the new nutrition plan ordered was Nutren 2.0 kcal/ml (a 39% carbohydrate formula) cycled at 70 mL/h overnight from 4:00 p.m. to 10:00 a.m., providing 2,520 kcal/day. The DMS team accounted for these nocturnal feedings

Table 54.1—BG Values with Continuous Tube Feedings (24 h)

Dates: 7/24/13–7/25/13

Time	0600		1200		1800		0000		0600
Blood glucose (mg/dL)	136		138		159		145		
Insulin administered	18 units R		18 units R		18 units R		18 units R		
Enteral feeding (Isosource 1.5) in mL/h	65	65	65	65	65	65	65	65	65

BG, blood glucose; R, regular insulin; TDD, 72 units.

Table 54.2— BG Values with Cycled (Nocturnal) Tube Feedings from 4:00 p.m. to 10:00 a.m.

Date: 7/28/13 to 7/29/13

Time	0600	1000	1200	1600	1800	2200	0000	0600	1000	1200	1600	1800
Blood glucose (mg/dL)	121		148		149	177	188			132		147
Insulin administered	12 units R			20 units R		36 units N		12 units R			20 units R	
Enteral feeding (Nutren 2.0) in mL/h	70	off	off	Resume at 70	70	70	70	70	off	off	Resumed at 70	70

Time	2200	0300	0600	1000	1200	1600	1800	2200
Blood glucose (mg/dL)	168	127	127	131	139		166	177
Insulin administered	36 units N		12 units R			20 units R		36 units N
Enteral feeding (Nutren 2.0) in mL/h	70	70	70	off	off	Resumed at 70	70	70

BG, blood glucose; R, regular insulin; NPH, neutral protamine Hagedorn; TDD, 68 units.

with a carefully tailored SQ regimen of regular insulin three times daily with NPH insulin at bedtime. The doses were calculated to coordinate with the timing of the nutrition. The patient was started on 12 units of regular insulin given at 6:00 a.m., correction dose only at noon (as the patient was off TF and had minimal p.o. intake), 20 units regular given at 4:00 p.m., and 36 units NPH given at 9:00 p.m. (Table 54.2).

The DMS team considered many key factors in determining this new regimen. The team acknowledged that the patient had exhibited good glycemic control on the previous total daily dose (TDD) of 72 units while on continuous TF. The new nutrition formula was less carbohydrate-rich but contained more calories. The timing of the new regimen also required shifting of the insulin doses to match the nocturnal caloric burden.

To cover the 18 h of TF feeds with minimal sleep interruptions, the team estimated that one-half of the TDD (i.e., 36 units) could be given as NPH at bedtime. The remaining portion of the TDD was slightly reduced for safety, from 36 to 32 units, which could be divided easily into two separate regular insulin doses: 20 units (roughly two-thirds) given when tube feeds started at 4:00 P.M., and 12 units (roughly one-third) at 6:00 A.M. to account for the fact that the TF would continue running until 10:00 A.M. Because the patient was not on insulin as an outpatient without evidence of type 1 physiology, with minimal oral intake at lunchtime, and no TF on-board at noon, only correction dose insulin was given when needed at noon. With this regimen, adequate glycemic control was achieved (Table 54.2). Patients with diabetes usually require a short-acting insulin (regular) administered 30 min before the start of TF, along with a longer acting insulin, such as NPH, administered between 9:00 and 11:00 P.M. to cover carbohydrates overnight.[4]

This case illustrates an example of how to alter the insulin regimen, with regard to dosing, timing, and type of insulin, when enteral nutrition is adjusted from continuous to an atypical cycled schedule.

REFERENCES

1. McClave SA, et al. Guidelines for the provision and assessment of nutrition support therapy in the adult critically ill patient: Society of Critical Care Medicine and the Society for Parenteral and Enteral Nutrition. *J Parent Ent Nutr* 2009;33(3):277–316

2. Korytkowski MT, et al. Insulin therapy and glycemic control in hospitalized patients with diabetes during enteral nutrition therapy: a randomized controlled clinical trial. *Diabetes Care* 2009;32:594–596

3. Fatiti G, et al. Use of insulin glargine in patients with hyperglycemia receiving artificial nutrition. *Acta Diabetologica* 2009;42(4):182–186

4. Lien LF, Cox M, Feinglos MN, Corsino L. *Diabetes Control in the Hospitalized Patient: A Comprehensive Clinical Guide.* Springer: New York, 2010

Case 55

Glycemic Control in a Patient with Type 1 Diabetes and Severe Burns

R. Matthew Hawkins, PA-C,[1] and Boris Draznin, MD, PhD[1]

A 52-year-old man was brought to the emergency department after being found in a burning warehouse, a victim of a gas explosion that caused multiple fractures and severe burns to his upper body, face, neck, and upper and lower extremities. Presenting diagnoses included epidural and subdural hemorrhages; depressed skull fracture with pneumocephalus; pelvic and acetabular fractures; multiple facial fractures; transverse process fractures at the cervical, thoracic, and lumbar levels; and 14% body surface area burns. Past medical history obtained from the paramedics revealed type 1 diabetes. Patient was intubated and taken to the operating room. His blood glucose level was 476 mg/dL (26.6 mmol/L) with normal anion gap. Intravenous (i.v.) insulin infusion was initiated.

Hyperglycemia and insulin resistance are frequently seen in patients with severe trauma and especially in those with severe burns.[1] There are at least three different mechanisms working in concert to induce a hypermetabolic state and to elevate blood glucose levels in patients with severe burns: release of catecholamines, glucocorticoids, and cytokines.[2]

Catecholamines increase glycogenolysis, lipolysis, and proteolysis with release of glucose, glycerol, free fatty acids, and amino acids. Stress-induced elevations in glucocorticoids lead to enhanced gluconeogenesis and peripheral insulin resistance. Cytokines, such as tumor necrosis factor-α (TNFα), interleukin-6 (IL-6), and IL-18, cause severe insulin resistance by increasing serine phosphorylation of insulin receptor substrate-1 (IRS-1),[3] thus reducing intracellular signal transduction to phosphatidylinositol 3-kinase and downstream mediators of insulin action. Although release of catecholamines and glucocorticoid is increased 2- to 10-fold, the levels of cytokines and inflammatory mediators rise up to 100-fold and remain elevated for long periods of time. There are suggestions in the pediatric literature that insulin resistance remains prominent for months or even years post burn.[2,4]

The best method of controlling hyperglycemia in patients in intensive care and in the operating room is i.v. insulin infusion. Practically every hospital has developed and refined protocols for i.v. insulin infusion. Most protocols are run by the nursing staff and take into consideration both the actual blood glucose levels and changes in glycemic values.

[1]Division of Endocrinology, Diabetes and Metabolism, Department of Medicine, University of Colorado Anschutz Medical Center, Aurora CO.

DOI: 10.2337/9781580405713.55

Between April 7, 2011, and April 15, 2011, the patient underwent numerous surgical procedures for his fractures, hemorrhages, and burns. Enteral nutrition was initiated and i.v. insulin infusion continued. The Glucose Management Team (GMT) was consulted on April 18, 2011, to help with glycemic control.

At the time of consultation, his workup revealed the following:

Weight	92 kg
Blood pressure	140/55 mmHg
Temperature	37.2°C
Pulse	95 bpm (regular)
Respirations	28 (on mechanical ventilation via tracheostomy)

Patient was sedated, had 2+ pedal edema, and multiple dressings. The rest of his physical exam was unremarkable. Table 55.1 shows his i.v. insulin infusion rates.

The first task of the GMT was to estimate his total daily dose of insulin (TDDI). Without the benefit of knowing how much insulin the patient administered at home, one approach to estimating the TDDI is based on the patient's weight. For a patient with type 1 diabetes and increased BMI we approximate a need of 0.25 units of insulin per kilogram of body weight (BW) for basal needs. At 92 kg of BW and BMI of 29 kg/m^2, this would result in 23 units of basal insulin. Assuming meal-time boluses are approximately equal to basal insulin, one estimates his TDDI needs as 46 units.

The alternate calculations can be based on the amount of carbohydrate the patient received via continuous tube feeding (TF). Our patient received Nutren 2.0 at 55 ml/h, delivering 258.7 g/24 h of carbohydrates. Assuming the starting carbohydrate to insulin ratio (C:I) of 10:1 (1 unit of insulin for every 10 g of carbohydrates), we estimated his nutritional needs to be 25.8 units of insulin for 24 h. Adding has basal insulin requirements (0.25 units/kg BW × 92 kg = 23 units), his TDDI was calculated to be 49 units.

Patient's i.v. insulin requirement, however, was much higher (Table 55.1), on average at 9.6 units/h, a TDDI of 230 units, reflecting his severe insulin resistance. The decision was made to continue i.v. insulin for another day in anticipation of improvement in his insulin sensitivity. On the next day, his TDDI came down to 180 units (Table 55.2). His i.v. insulin infusion was discontinued and subcutaneous insulin started.

Because the patient was still on continuous enteral nutrition, we used premixed biphasic 70/30 insulin three times daily. A number of insulin regimens are used successfully in patients on continuous TF, including the use of basal-bolus regimen with long-acting and fast-acting insulins, intermediate-action NPH insulin three or four times daily, and 70/30 insulin twice or three times daily. In a small study, we compared the efficacy and safety of a basal-bolus regimen with 70/30 insulin administered either twice or three times daily in patients receiving continuous enteral feeding.[5] Administration of 70/30 insulin three times daily produced more even glycemic control and

Table 55.1—Glucose Control April 18, 2011

Time	0000	0200	0400	0600	0700	0800	0915	1030	1130	1300	1400	1600	1700
BG	224	197	180	141	114	132	144	113	115	120	118	97	101
GTT rate	9	10	12	11	9	10	11	9	9	9	9	7	7
TF rate	55					55						55	

Average GTT rate of 9.6 units/h; 24 h × 9.6 units/h = 230.4 total daily dose.
BG, blood glucose in mg/dL; GTT, i.v. insulin infusion rate in units per hour; TF, tube feeding in mL/h.

Table 55.2—Glucose Control April 19, 2011

Time	0100	0200	0300	0400	0500	0600	0700	0800	0900	1000	1100
BG	160	153	139	131	117	129	140	141	152	119	126
GTT rate	7	8			7		8		9	7	
TF rate	55				55				55		

Average GTT rate of 7.6 units/h over the last 24 h; 24 h × 9.6 units/h = 182.4 total daily dose.
BG, blood glucose in mg/dL; GTT, i.v. insulin infusion rate in units per hour; TF, tube feeding in mL/h.

fewer hypoglycemic events than comparators. Because of interruptions in enteral feeding caused by either medical decisions, mechanical malfunctions (the tube can be occluded or dislodged), or by patients themselves (pulling the tube out), the presence of long-acting insulin on board may result in hypoglycemia. Most institutions have standing orders to initiate D-10% i.v. infusion when the TF is interrupted. Nevertheless, insulin of a shorter duration appears to be a safer option. We also prefer using 70/30 insulin over NPH because of its faster onset of action, although both insulins provide the same length of glucose lowering effect.

The patient was started on 60 units of 70/30 insulin three times daily with corrections with fast-acting insulin every 6 h, using 1 unit of insulin for every 25 mg/dL (1.4 mmol/L) of blood glucose >125 mg/dL (6.9 mmol/L). The doses of insulin were adjusted daily and by May 18, 2011, the patient was on 30 units of 70/30 three times daily. The TF continued at 55 mL/h.

By this time, he was breathing on his own and able to communicate. Diabetes history revealed that he had type 1 diabetes from the age of 14 years. His latest HbA$_{1c}$ 6 months before admission was 7.8%, and he had no chronic complications of diabetes. Before admission, he controlled his diabetes with 28 units of glargine nightly and lispro with C:I ratio of 10:1 and a correction factor (CF) of 1 unit for every 25 mg/dL (1.4 mmol/L) of blood glucose >100 mg/dL (5.6 mmol/L); and a TDDI of 55 units, very close to our initial estimate.

When TF was discontinued and oral intake resumed, he was started on his home insulin regimen. He was discharged to a rehabilitation unit and then sent home 2 months later on 22 units of long-acting insulin and fast-acting insulin at C:I ratio of 10:1 with a CF of 1 unit for every 25 mg/dL (1.4 mmol/L) of blood glucose >100 mg/dL (5.6 mmol/L).

REFERENCES

1. Jeschke MG, Finnerty CC, Herndon DN, Song J, Boehning D, Tompkins RG, Baker HV, Gauglitz GG. Severe injury is associated with insulin resistance, endoplasmic retirulum stress response, and unfolded protein response. *Ann Surg* 2012;255:370–378

2. Gauglitz GG, Herndon DN, Kulp GA, Meyer WJ 3rd, Jeschke MG. Abnormal insulin sensitivity persists up to three years in pediatric patients post-burn. *J Clin Endocrinol Metab* 2009;94:1656–1664

3. Morino K, Petersen KF, Shulman GI. Molecular mechanisms of insulin resistance in humans and their potential links with mitochondrial dysfunction. *Diabetes* 2006;55(Suppl. 2):S9–S15

4. Cree MG, Fram RY, Barr D, Chinkes D, Wolfe RR, Herndon DN. Insulin resistance, secretion and breakdown are increased 9 months following severe burn injury. *Burns* 2009;35:63–69

5. Hsia E, Seggelke SA, Gibbs J, Rasouli N, Draznin B. Comparison of 70/30 biphasic insulin with glargine/lispro regimen in non-critically ill diabetic patients on continuous enteral nutrition therapy. *J Clin Nutr* 2011;26:714–717

Case 56

Combined Effect of Intravenous Insulin Infusion and Subcutaneous Rapid-Acting Insulin for Glycemic Control in Severe Insulin Resistance

Magdalena Szkudlinska, MD,[1] and Irl B. Hirsch, MD[1]

A 60-year-old morbidly obese (BMI >40 kg/m^2) Caucasian man with a 24-year history of type 2 diabetes and recent diagnosis of acute lymphocytic leukemia was admitted to the hematology/oncology service. The patient's home diabetes regimen consisted of insulin pump therapy with U-500 regular insulin.[1-3] Home insulin pump settings are shown in Table 56.1.

Table 56.1 — Because U-500 Insulin Is Used in the Pump, Actual Doses of Insulin Are Fivefold Higher

Time	Units/h
0:00	0.600
7:30	1.45
12:30	0.750
22:00	0.500
22:00	0.500
24-Hour Total	19.875 units

Time	Carbohydrate Ratio (g/unit)
0:00	3.5
11:00	8.0

Time	Insulin Sensitivity (mg/dL per unit)
0:00	20

[1]University of Washington School of Medicine, Division of Metabolism, Endocrinology, & Nutrition, Seattle, WA.

   DOI: 10.2337/9781580405713.56

Upon admission, given the anticipated increase in insulin requirements in the setting of high-dose steroids, the patient was started on an intravenous insulin infusion. Initially, the patient's blood glucose values were well controlled in the 140–180 mg/dL range (7.8–10.0 mmol/L), requiring 14 units/h with 5% dextrose in normal saline at 75 mL/h. Of note, over 24 h, this amount, equivalent to 67.2 units of U-500 insulin (336 units of U-100 regular insulin), was already significantly more than his home insulin requirement of 19.875 units (99 units of U-100 regular insulin). After receiving two doses of daily dexamethasone of 40 mg and being transitioned from not eating (NPO status) to carbohydrate-controlled diet, postprandial blood glucose values increased, as would be expected. Despite requiring a maximal insulin infusion rate of 40 units/h (per hospital protocol), glucose levels remained uncontrolled (Fig. 56.1).

Next, the decision was made to add a subcutaneous rapid-acting insulin analog with meals. Insulin lispro was provided with an insulin-to-carbohydrate ratio of 1 unit/2 g, along with continuation of the intravenous insulin infusion for basal and correction dosing per hospital protocol. Over 24 h, improvement in blood glucose control was seen (Fig. 56.2).

The challenge of using high-dose steroids in the setting of high insulin resistance is compounded in this case because of oral intake while receiving intravenous insulin infusion. The continuation of intravenous insulin infusion while the patient transitions to oral intake is an all-too-common practice, resulting in retrospective, frequent insulin infusion titrations that only become more difficult as oral intake increases. This case demonstrates a novel approach by combining intravenous insulin infusion along with rapid-acting analog for mealtime and steroid-induced postprandial hyperglycemia coverage.

The use of two different portals of insulin delivery appears to be effective in managing severely insulin-resistant patients in the hospital who are eating. Use of intravenous insulin alone cannot keep up with food intake. Major changes in basal insulin resistance are difficult to manage with subcutaneous basal insulin,

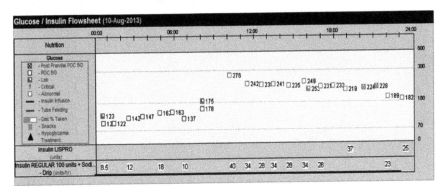

Figure 56.1—Uncontrolled glucose levels.

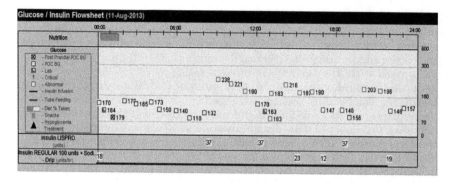

Figure 56.2—Improvement in blood glucose control.

where traditionally adjustments are initiated after consistent patterns of fasting glycemia are noted, usually after several days. For severely insulin-resistant patients who subsequently require steroid therapy, this is not possible. This combination of using two portals of insulin delivery deserves formal study.

REFERENCES

1. Cochran E, et al. The use of U-500 in patients with extreme insulin resistance. *Diabetes Care* 2005;28(5):1240–1244

2. Davidson MB, et al. U-500 regular insulin: clinical experience and pharmacokinetics in obese, severely insulin-resistant type 2 diabetic patients. *Diabetes Care* 2010;33(2):281–283

3. Lane WS, et al. High dose insulin therapy: is it time for U-500 insulin? *Endocr Pract* 2009;15(1):71–79

Case 57

Therapeutic Hypothermia and Severe Insulin Resistance in Patients with Diabetes and Cardiac Arrest

STACEY SEGGELKE, RD, MS, CDE,[1] AND BORIS DRAZNIN, MD, PhD[1]

J.M., a 45-year-old man had a witnessed cardiac arrest at the airport on December 30 at 10:30 P.M. Emergency medical services (EMS) arrived at the scene and found him in pulseless electrical activity. He was intubated, and epinephrine and bicarbonate were administered en route to the hospital. Upon arrival to the emergency room, the patient had pulses and cardiac activity. He was in severe acidosis with blood glucose levels >1,400 mg/dL (77.8 mmol/L). Patient was found to wear an insulin pump with the following settings:

Basal insulin total	21.1 units
Carbohydrate-to-insulin ratio	14:1
Sensitivity (correction factor)	40
Blood glucose levels before admission	209–289 mg/dL (11.6–16.1 mmol/L)

Cooling protocol was initiated and intravenous insulin infusion started.

Therapeutic hypothermia (also called targeted temperature management) is used widely in patients with out-of-hospital cardiac arrest. Therapeutic hypothermia significantly improves neurological deficit and survival in these patients.[1] Duration of cooling varies considerably, ranging from 2–3 days to up to 10 days. Body temperature can be lowered to 34–35.9°C (93.2–96.6°F), 32–33.9°C (89.6–93.0°F), or 30–31.9°C (86–89.4°F) for mild, moderate, or moderate-deep hypothermia, respectively.[2] Deep hypothermia (<30°C [86°F]) is rarely used as it is associated with a much greater risk for severe side effects.[3] In fact, a recent international, multicenter, randomized trial suggested that a temperature <36°C (96.8°F) (targeted at 33°C [91.4°F]) did not confer any additional benefit.[4]

When the core temperature drops to 32°C (89.6°F), the metabolic rate decreases to 50–65% of normal, oxygen consumption and CO_2 production decrease by the same percentage. At the same time, there is an increase in the levels of free fatty acids, ketones, and lactate.[5]

[1]Division of Endocrinology, Diabetes and Metabolism, Department of Medicine, University of Colorado Anschutz Medical Campus, Aurora, CO.

DOI: 10.2337/9781580405713.57

Table 57.1—Blood Glucose Levels and Intravenous Insulin Infusion (Gtt) Rates during the First 12 h of Admission

	Insulin Gtt (12/31)						
Time	0000	0130	0300	0400	0600	0930	1200
Glucose (mg/dL)	1019			883	749	673	626
Gtt Rate (units/h)		16	16	18	18	25	25
IV Bolus (units)		10	10	10	10		

Another important consequence of hypothermia is decreased insulin secretion and moderate to severe insulin resistance leading to hyperglycemia, particularly in patients with diabetes.

Despite repeated intravenous (i.v.) boluses of insulin and a high rate of i.v. insulin infusion, patient's glycemia remained significantly elevated (Table 57.1) and the glucose management team was consulted. Even though his insulin pump settings suggested that he was reasonably sensitive to insulin, his current insulin requirement clearly indicated severe insulin resistance.

The mechanism of severe insulin resistance in hypothermia is not well understood, but it certainly diminished insulin binding to its receptor as well as diminished signal transduction, and GLUT-4 function (recruitment of glucose transporters to the plasma membrane and their subsequent internalization) played a significant role.[4] All steps involved in mediating insulin action on glucose transport and intracellular metabolism are diminished by lower temperature. Impaired insulin release could contribute to hyperglycemia. The mechanism of this impairment is said to include diminished intracellular metabolism of glucose and slower rates of fusion and fission of insulin-containing secretory vesicles in the pancreatic β-cells under hypothermic conditions.

As a result, in some patients, hyperglycemia can be extreme approaching or exceeding 1,000 mg/dL (55.6 mmol/L). Insulin requirement is greatly increased and, frequently, insulin infusion even at the very high rate is unable to control hyperglycemia.

J. M. required an insulin infusion rate of 30 units/h to bring his glycemia to 300 mg/dL (22 mmol/L) 24 h after admission. At that point, a gradual rewarming phase was initiated, and his insulin sensitivity increased rapidly with a rapid decrease in insulin requirement (Table 57.2).

Temperature-dependence of insulin action is particularly important in the rewarming phase. With the core temperature rising, insulin action improves dramatically, and with large quantities of insulin on board, hypoglycemia may ensue precipitously. Insulin infusion rate must be decreased aggressively in the rewarming phase to avoid hypoglycemia. In practical terms, the danger of

Table 57.2 — Blood Glucose Levels and Intravenous Insulin Infusion (Gtt) Rates 24–32 h Postadmission

	Insulin Gtt (1/1)								
Time	0000	0100	0200	0300	0400	0500	0600	0700	0800
Glucose (mg/dL)	306	261	234	194	139	114	89	71	97
Gtt Rate (units/h)	30	27			20	14	0	0	0

hypoglycemia during the rewarming phase is the most important point to remember during the management of glycemia in patients with therapeutic hypothermia. Infusion of D-10% may be needed to stabilize glycemia in the rewarming phase.

REFERENCES

1. The Hypothermia after Cardiac Arrest Study Group. Mild therapeutic hypothermia to improve the neurologic outcome after cardiac arrest. *N Eng J Med* 2002;346:549–556

2. Polderman KH, Herold I. Therapeutic hypothermia in the intensive care unit: practical considerations, side effects, and cooling methods. *Crit Care Med* 2009;37:1101–1120

3. Polderman KH. Mechanisms of action, physiological effects, and complications of hypothermia. *Crit Care Med* 2009;37(Suppl.):S186–S202

4. Nielsen N, Wetterslev J, Cronberg T, Erlinge D, Gasche Y, Hassager C, et al. Targeted temperature management at 33°C versus 36°C after cardiac arrest. *New Eng J Med* 2013;369:2197–2206

5. Aoki M, Nomura F, Stromski ME, Tsuji MK, Fackler JC, Hickey PR, Holtzman DH, Jonas RA. Effects of pH on brain energetics and hypothermic circulatory arrest. *Ann Thorac Surg* 1993;55:1093–1103

Case 58

Extreme Insulin Resistance Following Heart Transplant

Suruchi Gupta, MBBS, MPH;[1] Diana Johnson Oakes, APRN-BC;[1] Ashley Therasse, MD;[1] Amisha Wallia, MD, MS;[1] and Mark E. Molitch, MD[1]

A 60-year-old Caucasian woman presented with 2 weeks of worsening fatigue and shortness of breath. Past medical history revealed adriamycin-induced cardiomyopathy, for which she required a left ventricular assist device (LVAD) and a subsequent heart transplant. She did not have a history of diabetes. Her blood glucose (BG) average 3 months before the transplant was 112 ± 30 mg/dL (6.2 ± 1.7 mmol/L). Her preoperative glucose was 80 mg/dL (4.4 mmol/L) and her intraoperative BG levels ranged from 95 to 342 mg/dL (5.2–19 mmol/L). There were no complications during surgery. She received a single dose of 500 mg of intravenous (i.v.) methylprednisone intraoperatively.

Hyperglycemia is a well-known phenomenon in critically ill patients during the postoperative period. It is associated with increased risks of infection, inpatient mortality, and other adverse events in both diabetic and nondiabetic patients.[1] Intensive insulin therapy in the intensive care unit (ICU) has been shown to reduce morbidity and mortality in such patients with current recommendations that BG targets be in the 140–180 mg/dL (7.8–10 mmol/L) range.[2] Heart transplant patients are some of the most challenging to treat; they receive high-dose steroids, have several comorbidities, are treated by multiple providers, and often have prolonged hospital stays.[3] Hypoglycemia can be a limiting factor, and safe and effective implementation of insulin protocols can be difficult in these patients.[4] Here, we present an example of a particularly challenging subset of these patients who are very insulin resistant, require very high doses of insulin, and are particularly prone to hypoglycemia.[4]

At Northwestern Memorial Hospital (NMH) all hyperglycemic heart transplant patients are placed on an i.v. insulin drip protocol postoperatively.[5] This protocol has effectively achieved good glycemic control with an acceptable amount of hypoglycemia in such patients.[4,5] When transferred to the floor, glycemic control continues with subcutaneous insulin. Both ICU and floor protocols are overseen by a glucose management service (GMS) (nurse practitioners working with an attending endocrinologist).

[1]Division of Endocrinology, Metabolism and Molecular Medicine, Northwestern University Feinberg School of Medicine, Chicago, IL.

DOI: 10.2337/9781580405713.58

Postoperatively, the patient was admitted to the ICU. Her vital signs were stable, her BMI was 23.1 kg/m², and her BG was 447 mg/dL (24.8 mmol/L). She was started on an initial insulin drip at a rate of 8 units/h and received a bolus of 8 units by the ICU nurse as per protocol. While she was on the insulin drip, she was also being treated with several pressors (dobutamine, epinephrine, isoproterenol, and vasopressin). Her i.v. insulin infusion rates and BG levels are shown in Fig. 58.1.

This protocol was developed by the GMS team specifically for transplant patients and was modified over the years based on data obtained from several hundred patients. Cardiac transplant patients at NMH receive i.v. methylpred-nisone in the following doses: 500 mg intraoperatively once, 125 mg every 8 h for 24 h followed by 16 mg daily with subsequent conversion to prednisone 20 mg orally with diet advancement. The drip rate is based on the initial BG upon arrival in the ICU and adjusted according to the hourly rate of change of BG (whether the BG increases or decreases and whether the rate of change of BG is > or <60 mg/dL [3.3 mmol/L]). At high BG levels (>200 mg/dL [11.1 mmol/L]), the drip rate always goes up at the time of the next BG level if the BG is higher or if the BG is still >200 mg/dL and the BG decrease is <60 mg/dL. The drip rate goes down for BG decreases >60 mg/dL or for smaller decreases if the BG is <200 mg/dL.

This patient had severe insulin resistance on admission to the ICU. During the first 10–12 h in the ICU, her BG levels were still in the 400s (22.2 mmol/L) and drip rates were increased from 8 to 64 units/h according to the protocol under supervision of the GMS. Over the next few hours, her insulin resistance "broke" and BG levels fell. To prevent hypoglycemia, the GMS nurse practitioner decided to decrease the insulin dose more than outlined in the protocol. The dose was reduced by 50% every hour for the next 5 h until the drip was stopped. Even with appropriate dose

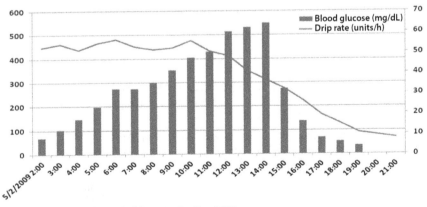

Figure 58.1—BG and drip rate in the ICU.

reduction and discontinuation of the drip, her BG level fell to 69 mg/dL (3.8 mmol/L).

Several questions are raised in the management of a patient like this: *1)* How do we predict the severe insulin resistance? Some potential risk factors, such as BMI, use of pressors, age, and BG at the beginning of surgery were not found to be significant when analyzed (unpublished data). With a small number of patients, we have not been able to develop a profile to predict insulin resistance for such patients. *2)* Should insulin doses continue to increase until glucose levels fall significantly or should the dose be capped at a certain point while we wait for the BG to come down? Are we saturating all the insulin receptors at high insulin doses? Whether the insulin receptors are saturated at such high insulin doses still remains unclear. *3)* How do we determine why and when the insulin resistance breaks and how do we avoid hypoglycemia in such patients? Frequent monitoring, peak drip alerts, and endocrine and pharmacy consultation for those above certain parameters may be necessary. Certain institutions have already developed maximum drip rates allowed and have these parameters in place.

Her drip was restarted at 3 units/h 8 h later and was stable during the remainder of her ICU stay of 5 days. Upon transfer to the floor, she was started on a clear liquid diet, 20 units of insulin glargine, and 2 units of insulin aspart according to the conversion formulas used by the GMS team. She continued to recover well on the floor. Her liver enzymes trended down. She was in the hospital for a total of 11 days after her transplant surgery. She did not require any diabetes medications during the last 3 days of hospitalization or at discharge.

This patient illustrates problems that may arise for a particular subset of patients with extreme insulin resistance. Such patients are important to recognize to avoid periods of prolonged hyperglycemia and to avoid hypoglycemia when the resistance suddenly "breaks."

REFERENCES

1. Umpierrez GE, Isaacs SD, Bazargan N, et al. Hyperglycemia: an independent marker of inhospital mortality in patients with undiagnosed diabetes. *J Clin Endocrinol Metab* 2002;87:978–982

2. Moghissi, ES, Hirsch IB, Kortykowski MT, et al. American Association of Clinical Endocrinologists and American Diabetes Association consensus statement on inpatient glycemic control. *Diabetes Care* 2009;32(6):1119–1131

3. Lang CC, Beniaminovitz A, Edwards N, Mancini DM. Morbidity and mortality in diabetic patients following cardiac transplantation. *J Heart Lung Transplant* 2003;22(3):244–249

4. Garcia C, Wallia A, Gupta S, et al. Intensive glycemic control after heart transplantation is safe and effective for diabetic and non-diabetic patients. *Clinical Transplantation* 2013;27:444–454

5. DeSantis AJ, Schmeltz LR, Schmidt K, et al. Inpatient management of hyperglycemia: the Northwestern experience. *Endocr Pract* 2006;12(5):491–505

Case 59

Glycemic Control after Left Ventricular Assist Device Placement in a Patient with Type 2 Diabetes

Gitana Staskus, MD[1]

A 63-year-old man with severe coronary artery disease, ischemic cardiomyopathy, underwent a repeat coronary artery bypass grafting (CABG) with aortic valve replacement and mitral valve repair on November 1, 2012, in a regional hospital. He had difficulty weaning off of cardiopulmonary bypass despite an intraaortic balloon pump placement and inotropic support. He was transferred to the cardiothoracic surgery (CT) service at the University of Utah Hospital on November 2, 2012, in critical condition with an open chest and on extracorporeal membrane oxygenation (ECMO).

His past medical history revealed poorly controlled type 2 diabetes for 13 years and CABG in 1996. His home insulin regimen was glargine 85 units once daily and glulisine 6 units with meals 3 times a day.

The patient's admission glucose level was 219 mg/dL (12.2 mmol/L). His serum creatinine was 2.35 mg/dL. Intravenous (i.v.) insulin infusion with regular insulin was initiated in the surgical intensive care unit (ICU). His initial total daily insulin requirements were 100–170 units and his daily blood glucose average was 130–160 mg/dL (7.2–8.9 mmol/L).

Severe heart failure (HF) independently of its etiology has been associated with increased insulin resistance (IR). High insulin requirements are common in patients with type 2 diabetes and advanced chronic heart failure. The mechanisms of increased insulin resistance are thought to be multifactorial because of numerous positive and negative hormonal and hemodynamic effects on various proinflammatory and anti-inflammatory cytokines, leading to a worsening of insulin resistance:

1. Retinol binding protein 4 (RBP4). Increased levels of an adipocytokine RBP4 in patients with diabetes and severe HF may be contributing to increased insulin resistance by increasing hepatic gluconeogenesis via the enhanced expression of phosphenolpyruvate carboxykinase and impaired insulin signaling in skeletal muscle.[1]

2. Tumor necrosis factor-α (TNFα). High levels of tumor necrosis factor-α are found in patients with severe HF. TNFα is a proinflammatory cytokine capable of producing dilated cardiomyopathy, pulmonary edema, and

[1]Assistant Professor of Medicine, Division of Endocrinology, Metabolism and Diabetes, University of Utah, School of Medicine.

DOI: 10.2337/9781580405713.59

death. Its increased levels have been associated with peripheral insulin resistance and decreased insulin-mediated glucose disposal.[2]

3. Adiponectin. Adiponectin is an insulin sensitizing and antiatherogenic adipocytokine. There are suggestions in the literature that downregulation of adiponectin receptors may result in its functional resistance with a loss of its protective "insulin sensitizing" role.[3]

4. Resistin. Because resistin is found in higher concentrations in patients with heart failure, this association may contribute to increased insulin resistance in heart failure.[4]

After the initial reexploration of the chest for mediastinal hemorrhage, the patient underwent removal of ECMO, placement of intracorporeal left ventricular assist device (LVAD), extracorporeal right ventricular assist device (RVAD), and mitral valve repair on November 5, 2012. Between November 5, 2012, and November 14, 2012, he underwent another reexploration of the chest for bleeding, RVAD removal, and sternotomy closure.

Enteral nutrition (tube feeding [TF]) was initiated on November 2, 2012, with the rate increased to 90 mL/h over the period of 15 days. The total daily dose of insulin (TDDI) increased to 240 units before sternotomy closure and RVAD removal. The subcutaneous NPH insulin (30 units every 12 h) was added to i.v. insulin infusion.

The patient remained in the surgery ICU in critical condition. As his NPH insulin dose was titrated up to 80 units every 12 h, the i.v. insulin infusion rate was decreased. His TDDI remained 150–200 units. The Inpatient Glucose Management Service was consulted on November 30, 2012, to help with glycemic control after the patient was transferred to a cardiovascular medical unit (CVMU). The NPH insulin was stopped 1 day earlier because of an episode of hypoglycemia (blood glucose <60 mg/dL [<3.3 mmol/L]) and blood glucose levels were on a rise.

At the time of consultation, his workup showed the following:

Weight	**108 kg**
Blood pressure	**110/76 mmHg**
Temperature	**36.7°C (98.1°F)**
Pulse	**77 bpm**

The patient had trace bilateral pedal edema and multiple dressings. His 6:00 P.M. blood glucose was 231 mg/dL (12.8 mmol/L). He remained on continuous tube feeding at 90 mL/h.

Several insulin regimens can be used for patients during continuous enteral nutrition. We used a basal-bolus regimen with long-acting glargine insulin and scheduled doses of regular insulin in addition to correction of blood glucose levels >180 mg/dL (10 mmol/L) every 6 h. Patients on enteral nutrition often experience unexpected interruptions in TF, and with rapid decrease in carbohydrate intake, the danger of hypoglycemia arises. To avoid hypoglycemia should TF interruption occur, we prefer using only ~30% of a total daily insulin dose in a form of long-acting insulin. The remaining 70% of a TDDI we divide into four equal doses of regular insulin every 6 h to be administered only if tube feeding is running.

"Stop" insulin orders in place for nursing staff instruct them not to administer the next dose of regular insulin if TF is interrupted unexpectedly. A lower dose of long-acting insulin and administration of regular insulin every 6 h allowed us to avoid institution of standing orders of D-10% i.v. infusion, which often is not desirable in a cardiovascular patient on fluid restriction and risk of fluid overload.

The patient was transferred to an acute inpatient rehabilitation unit on December 19, 2012. His insulin requirements continued to decrease despite stable weight. His daily average blood glucose remained 130–150 mg/dL (7.2–8.3 mmol/L) with glargine 12 units once daily and lispro 4 units three times a day after the TF was stopped and the patient was eating on his own. Because of small insulin requirements and stable kidney function, a decision was made to transition the patient to oral hypoglycemic agents. Mealtime lispro was replaced with sitagliptin 100 mg once daily and glargine was discontinued a few days later.

The patient was sent home on January 10, 2013, on monotherapy with sitagliptin 100 mg once daily.

LVADs are increasingly used to treat severe congestive heart failure as destination therapy or as a bridge to heart transplantation. Published studies in the literature support evidence of improved glycemic control in diabetic patients with severe heart failure treated with LVADs.[5] The mechanisms responsible for improved insulin sensitivity are yet to be completely understood and may include recovery of cardiac output and circulation with improved peripheral tissue oxygenation and improved systemic inflammation and decreased various inflammatory cytokines, including interleukin-8, leading to reduction of diabetogenic RBP4.

Our patient demonstrated a dramatic improvement in his insulin resistance and glycemic control after the LVAD placement; his insulin requirements decreased from >200 units/day when critically ill to becoming insulin free at the time of discharge to home (Table 59.1).

Table 59.1 — Total Daily Dose of Insulin and Glucose Control during Hospital Stay

Hospitalization day	2	3	10	20	26	37	46	53	59	69
Blood glucose average (mg/dL)	153	135	147	140	75	130	136	107	133	117
Blood glucose average (mmol/L)	8.5	7.5	8.2	7.8	4.2	7.2	7.5	5.9	7.4	6.5
Total daily dose of insulin (units)	97	166	240	188	0	59	54	30	20	0

REFERENCES

1. Chavarria N, Kato R, Khan, R, Chokshi A, Akashi H, Takayama H, Naka Y, Farr M, Mancini D, Schulze PC. Increased levels of retinol binding protein 4 in patients with advanced heart failure correct after hemodynamic improvement through ventricular assist device placement. *Circulation J* 2012;76:2148–2152

2. McGaffin KR, Moravec CS, McTiernan CF. Tumor necrosis factor α and insulin resistance in obese type 2 diabetic patients. *Int J Obes* 2003;27(1):88–94

3. Van Berendoncks AM, Garnier A, Beckers P, Hoymans VY, Possemiers N, Fortin D, Martinet W, Van Hoof V, Vrints CJ, Ventura-Clapier R, Conraads VM. Functional adiponectin resistance at the level of the skeletal muscle in mild to moderate chronic heart failure. *Circ Heart Fail* 2010;3(2):185–194

4. Butler J, Kalogeropoulos A, Georgiopoulou V, de Rekeneire N, Rodondi N, Smith AL, Hoffmann U, Kanaya A, Newman AB, Kritchevsky SB, Vasan RS, Wilson PWF, Harris TB. Serum resistin concentrations and risk of new onset heart failure in older persons: the Health, Aging, and Body Composition (Health ABC) Study. *Arterioscler Thromb Vasc Biol* 2009;29(7):1144–1149

5. Uriel N, Naka Y, Colombo PC, Farr M, Pak S, Cotarlan V, Albu JB, Gallagher D, Mancini D, Ginsberg HN, Jorde UP. Improved diabetic control in advanced heart failure patients treated with left ventricular assist devices. *Eur J Heart Fail* 2011;13:195–199

Case 60

Management of Diabetic Ketoacidosis in a Patient on Hemodialysis

ROOPASHREE PRABHUSHANKAR, MD;[1] SOFIA SYED, MD;[1] AND JAMES R. SOWERS, MD, FACE, FACP, FAHA[1-3]

A 47-year-old woman with type 1 diabetes (T1D) on hemodialysis (HD) presented with altered mental status, vomiting, and abdominal pain. She had frequent admissions for similar episodes in the past because of nonadherence to insulin. Past medical history is significant for uncontrolled T1D (A1C 10.7%), diabetic retinopathy with blindness, and end-stage renal disease (ESRD); she was producing urine of ~100 mL/day. On admission, pulse rate was 110/min and blood pressure 110/60 mmHg. Her dry weight was documented at 68 kg, and her admission weight was 67 kg. She appeared dehydrated with dry mouth and eyes. Otherwise the physical examination was unremarkable. Labs showed the following:

Sodium	133 mmol/L
Potassium	3.4 mmol/L
Chloride	85 mmol/L
Bicarbonate	12 mmol/L
Blood urea nitrogen	32 mg/L
Creatinine	4.61 mg/L
Serum glucose	576 mg/dL (32 mmol/L)
Anion gap	36 mmol/L

She was diagnosed with diabetic ketoacidosis (DKA) with dehydration.

ESRD increases morbidity and mortality in diabetic patients.[1] Annually, DKA occurs in 4.6–8.0 per 1,000 people with T1D. Data on the incidence and management of DKA in hemodialysis patients is lacking, likely related to a low incidence that could be due to factors such as prolonged insulin half-life in the setting of ESRD and frequent monitoring of such patients during HD. However, these patients are prone to infections,[2] which can trigger DKA. Our patient had blindness, which limited her ability to use the prescribed doses of insulin, and frequent titration of her insulin regimen secondary to rapidly fluctuating blood glucose led to medication nonadherence, resulting in multiple DKA episodes.

[1]Division of Endocrinology, Diabetes and Metabolism, Department of Medicine, University of Missouri, Harry S. Truman Memorial Veterans' Hospital, Columbia, MO. [2]Department of Medical Pharmacology and Physiology, University of Missouri, Harry S. Truman Memorial Veterans' Hospital, Columbia, MO. [3]Diabetes and Cardiovascular Center, University of Missouri, Harry S. Truman Memorial Veterans' Hospital, Columbia, MO.

DOI: 10.2337/9781580405713.60

Furthermore, the patient was started on an insulin drip and was given serial intravenous normal saline (NS) boluses. Labs to assess recovery of metabolic acidosis and hypokalemia were followed regularly. She required a 6-h insulin drip to attain a normal anion gap and bicarbonate level.

DKA is a complex metabolic disorder resulting from absolute or relative insulin deficiency, which leads to hyperglycemia, ketonemia, and anion gap metabolic acidosis.

In patients with preserved renal function, hyperglycemia leads to osmotic diuresis and increases serum osmolality resulting in dehydration. The consortium of the metabolic derangements often results in electrolyte disturbances like hyperkalemia, hyponatremia, and hyperchloremia. Osmotic diuresis also depletes phosphates, ketones, glucose, and free water. Free water loss in DKA is ~3–6 L or nearly 100 mL/kg of body weight. Thus, the cornerstone in DKA management for patients with preserved renal function is vigorous intravenous fluid replacement and correction of ketosis via insulin infusion followed by electrolyte replacement.

Our patient was dehydrated due to vomiting in addition to a small component of osmotic diuresis as she was still producing urine. Her weight on admission was less than her dry weight. She was given NS boluses of 500 mL to a total of 1,500 mL over the initial 12 h and serially monitored for signs of volume overload with parameters like jugular venous distention, auscultation of lungs for pulmonary edema, and blood pressure. On follow-up examination, there was normalization of vital signs and hydration status with no evidence of volume overload.

In patients requiring HD, there are preexisting metabolic derangements resulting from the renal disease and, hence, DKA can present in a different manner. Various factors are to be considered when managing such patients.

FLUID RESUSCITATION

Patients requiring HD are commonly anuric and osmotic diuresis is absent. Hence, they generally are not fluid depleted and do not require rapid intravenous fluid resuscitation. Correction of ketosis and hyperglycemia by insulin infusion alone can be sufficient in restoring the fluid balance. In a subset of HD patients who still have sufficient urine output, however, osmotic diuresis can cause hyperosmolarity and dehydration. Coexistent vomiting, diarrhea, fever, or sepsis can contribute to intravascular volume contraction, and fluid replacement is warranted in such instances. These patients are unable to excrete the free water and can easily become volume overloaded, resulting in hypertension and pulmonary edema. A thorough history and physical examination can give us a good estimate of the volume status, especially with the knowledge of their dry weight. In patients who develop hypovolemia because of extra renal causes, modest saline boluses can be given cautiously with close monitoring of volume status.

ANION GAP METABOLIC ACIDOSIS

Patients on HD, when not in DKA, may already have low bicarbonate and anion gap metabolic acidosis secondary to renal failure. Diagnosing DKA in such patients can be misleading if based exclusively on anion gap and low bicarbonate levels. The β-hydroxybutyrate levels can help distinguish DKA from hyperglycemia in such instances. In addition, DKA can present as a mixed acid base disorder. Arterial blood gas analysis and the awareness of the baseline bicarbonate, PCO_2, and anion gap can be resourceful.

ELECTROLYTE IMBALANCES

Mild hyperkalemia is often present at baseline in HD patients. With development of DKA, it can worsen, which is directly related to the mean glucose levels and hyperosmolarity. Insulin therapy often brings the potassium levels back to baseline by promoting potassium shift from extracellular fluid to intracellular fluid. Hence, serial monitoring of potassium while on insulin infusion is absolutely required. If the patient develops hypokalemia, potassium should be replaced cautiously only after acidosis is corrected and with telemetry monitoring. Serum sodium concentration can also provide a clue to the volume status after the ketosis and hyperglycemia has resolved. If sodium levels are high, then free water deficit can be calculated and replaced. If the sodium levels are low when compared to their baseline, HD will likely be needed to remove the excess fluid. This emphasizes the serial monitoring of electrolytes during and after insulin therapy.

EMERGENCY DIALYSIS

Emergency HD for DKA is indicated for severe hyperkalemia with electrocardiogram changes[3] and if pulmonary edema develops,[4] both of which are life threatening. HD, however, carries the risk of rapid decline in tonicity, which can be detrimental and can cause seizures.[5] Benefits of HD in the treatment of DKA have not been established.

REFERENCES

1. Port FK. Morbidity and mortality in dialysis patients. *Kidney Int* 1994;46(6):1728–1737

2. Sarnak MJ, Jaber BL. Mortality caused by sepsis in patients with end-stage renal disease compared with the general population. *Kidney Int* 2000;58:1758–1764

3. Montoliu J, Revert L. Lethal hyperkalemia associated with severe hyperglycemia in diabetic patients with renal failure. *Am J Kidney Dis* 1985;5:47–48

4. Tzamalokas AH, Rohrscheib M, Ing TS, Siamopoulos KC, Elisaf MF, Spalding CT. Serum tonicity, extracellular volume and clinical manifestations in symptomatic dialysis-associated hyperglycemia treated only with insulin. *Int J Artif Organs* 2005;27:751–758

5. Gupta A, Rohrscheib M, Tzamaloukas AH. Extreme hyperglycemia with ketoacidosis and hyperkalemia in a patient on chronic hemodialysis. *Hemodial Int* 2008;12(Suppl. 2):S43–S47

New Diabetes Emergency: Acute Rhabdomyolysis Complicating Hyperglycemic Hyperosmolar Coma

CHERIE VAZ, MD,[1] AND AJAY CHAUDHURI, MD, MRCP[2]

A 57-year-old man with a history of hypertension and recently diagnosed diabetes, presented with polyuria, polydipsia, generalized weakness, and confusion. He was drowsy on arrival and Glasgow Coma Scale (GCS) deteriorated to eye (E), motor (M), and verbal (V) responses E2M4V1 in a few hours. He was fully functional at baseline. He was brought in when his mental status deteriorated over just a few hours. He was started on metformin 500 mg twice daily for diabetes and was apparently taking it inconsistently since diabetes was diagnosed 1 week earlier. Initial laboratory workup showed the following:

White blood cell count	8.7
Hemoglobin	16
Platelets	291,000
Sodium (Na)	137 mEq/L
Potassium	4.8 mEq/L
Bicarbonate	22
Blood urea nitrogen (BUN)	116 mg/dL
Creatinine	3.22
Anion gap	22
Glucose	1,710 mg/dL
Corrected Na	162 mEq/L
Calculated osmolality	370 mOsm/kg
Arterial pH	7.22
Serum ketones	positive (small)
Urine ketones	trace positive
Magnesium	5.2 ng/mL (elevated)
Phosphate	3.3 mg/dL (normal)

In the emergency department, the patient was treated with 15 units of subcutaneous regular insulin and 10 units intravenous regular insulin. He was started on an insulin drip at 3.5 units/h. He received 2 L of normal saline. HbA$_{1c}$ checked during hospitalization was 12.4%.

[1]Section of Endocrinology, Department of Medicine, Temple University School of Medicine, Philadelphia, PA. [2]Department of Endocrinology, State University of New York, University at Buffalo and Kaleida Health, Buffalo, NY.

DOI: 10.2337/9781580405713.61

Table 61.1 – Laboratory Data

	Arrival	6h	12h	24h	36h	Day 2	Day 3	Day 4	Day 5
Na (mEq/L)	137	153	158	166	161	158	151	141	141
K (mEq/L)	4.8	3.1	4	4.6	3.9	3.5	3.6	3.8	3.6
Cl (mEq/L)	93	117	124	136	130	132	124	115	112
HCO_3 (mEq/L)	22	24	26	26	24	20	25	24	23
BUN (mg/dL)	116	93	75	48	34	21	21	22	16
Cr (mg/dL)	3.22	2.7	1.6	1.41	1.19	0.85	0.9	0.96	0.87
Corrected Na	162.7	165	164.5	167.7	163.8	158.3	152	143.5	142
Ca (mg/dL)	9.6	8.7	9	9.2	8.6	6.7	7.8	8.1	8.1
Glucose (mg/dL)	1,710	883	512	211	278	122	172	256	166
Mg (1.7–2.7) (mg/dL)	5.2	4.5	4.1	3.1	2.7	2	2.4	2.5	2.1
P (2.6–4.9) (mg/dL)	3.3	3.3	2.7	–	3	–	2.5	–	–
Alkp (30–125) (units/L)	128	113	101	–	79	–	75	113	136
AST (5–50) (units/L)	35	42	72	–	584	–	346	299	311
ALT (5–50) (units/L)	42	38	42	–	160	–	140	169	228
Troponin I (0–0.06) (ng/mL)	0.03	0.05	0.01	–	0.12	0.1	0.09	–	–
CK (0–180) (units/L)	2,379	5,730	21,767	–	48,897	41,748	29,289	12,180	2,872
CK MB (≤5) (ng/dl)	7	15	42	–	85	61	34	15	<5

Endocrinology was consulted for management of hyperglycemic hyperosmolar coma. At the time of consultation the patient was very lethargic. His height was 179 cm, weight 74.8 kg, temperature 36°C, pulse 88, blood pressure 128/84 mmHg, respiratory rate 18, O$_2$ saturation 96%. Physical exam was otherwise unremarkable. Urine in the Foley bag was noted to be of pink color. He was on folic acid, thiamine, metoprolol, amlodipine, pantoprazole, heparin, 5% dextrose in half normal saline at 100 mL/h. He had received several boluses of normal saline. A comprehensive workup for altered mental status was negative. He had negative imaging of chest and normal head computerized tomography. As flexeril was listed as his medication, we checked serum and urine quantitative and qualitative levels for cyclobenzaprine (by high-performance liquid chromatography), which were negative. Workup for infection was negative.

Blood glucose trended down on the insulin drip. It was titrated to 7 units/h overnight during the first few hours following presentation, then titrated to 2 units/h the next morning when glucose was 219 mg/dL (12.2 mmol/L). The anion gap had closed, and BUN/creatinine was trending down. Six hours later, Na was 158 mEql/L. As he had pink urine and we were looking for precipitating factors for the hyperglycemic crisis, we checked a creatine kinase (CK). Initial CK was 2,379 units/L and it increased to 21,767 units/L in 24 h with CKMB 42 ng/dL (<4). TSH was 1.47 mcU/mL (normal 0.4–5). Serum and urine toxicology and alcohol screen were negative. Troponin 0.03 ng/mL was negative on admission and peaked at 0.12 ng/mL 28 h later. Urine was positive for hemoglobin, and initially negative for protein; however, 24 h later, protein was 2+. Phosphate was 3.3 mg/dL (normal 2.6–4.9) on presentation and remained within normal. Calcium was 9.6 ng/dL (normal 8.5–10.5) and remained within normal. Urine myoglobin was >10,000 ng/mL (normal <1). CK isoenzyme analysis on successive samples was 100% MM and 0% MB (<4) and 0% BB fractions (not detected). Renal ultrasound was normal. These findings were suggestive of rhabdomyolysis, which we speculated was a complication of the hyperglycemic hyperosmolar state.

The patient remained on the insulin drip at a continuous rate of 1–2 units/h with D5 in half normal saline at 150 mL/h with 1 ampule of bicarbonate. Na continued to trend up over the next day and peaked at 168 mEq/L 24 h later. Measured serum osmolality was 364 mOsm/kg (275–295). CK trended up over the next day and peaked at 48,897 units/L 28 h later with peak CKMB of 85 ng/mL. Aspartate aminotransferase (AST)/ alanine aminotransferase (ALT), which were initially normal, and were elevated on day 3 at 584 units/mL and 160 units/mL, respectively, consistent with rhabdomyolysis.

The pathogenesis of this nontraumatic rhabdomyolysis is multifactorial and includes inhibition of the sodium pump by hyperosmolar states, acidosis, hypernatremia, potassium deficiency, hypophosphatemia, and a

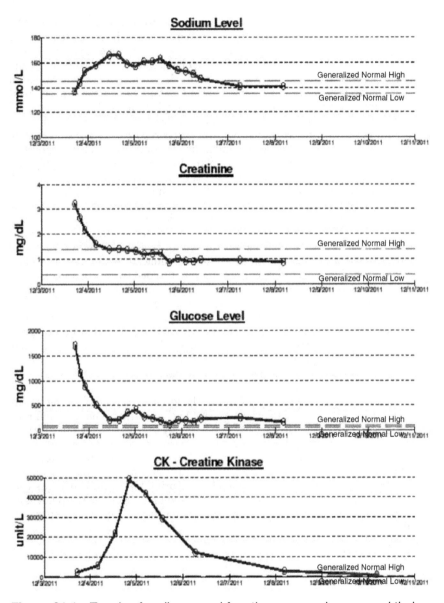

Figure 61.1 — Trends of sodium, renal function, serum glucose, and their temporal relation to CK levels.

decrease in intramuscular energy supply due to insulin deficiency.[1] The resultant fall in the transmembrane potential, and elevated intracellular calcium, activates proteases with subsequent leakage of muscle enzymes, contributing to the development of rhabdomyolysis.[2] Serum osmolality levels and blood glucose are thought to be the major determinants for occurrence of rhabdomyolysis in the hyperglycemic state.[1] We hypothesize that the prothrombotic state that is induced by severe hyperglycemia could result in muscle tissue infarction with subsequent elevated CK levels, further confirmed in our patient as 100% from MM fraction. A previous report of hyperosmolar state complicated with rhabdomyolysis and ischemic colitis would also support our hypothesis.[3] Another important risk factor for developing rhabdomyolysis is the severity of insulin deficiency. This is demonstrated in our patient with hemoglobin A1C 12.4% while not receiving insulin.

We were able to successfully treat this patient with severe nontraumatic rhabdomyolysis and massive myoglobinuria, despite his poor prognosis from very low GCS at presentation. Treatment includes aggressive intravenous hydration with normal saline, a bicarbonate drip, and an insulin drip. Blood glucose control was achieved within 12 h. Creatinine normalized in 28 h. Magnesium, which was elevated on presentation, trended to normal as creatinine improved. Sodium peaked in 24 h and gradually corrected over the next 3 days. Rhabdomyolysis became pronounced once acute renal failure and hyperglycemia had, in fact, resolved. Insulin drip was continued at a continuous rate of 2 units/h following correction of blood glucose and normalization of anion gap to correct the state of insulin deficiency, which is thought to precipitate rhabdomyolysis. CK peaked at 28 h and trended down to 881 units/L on day 7. The patient's mental status gradually improved from day 3, and he was back to baseline on day 4.

Without early recognition of severe rhabdomyolysis complicating hyperglycemic emergencies, patients could have fatal outcomes. The temporal relationship of hyperosmolar state and rhabdomyolysis is depicted in our case with peak sodium occurring just before peak CK (Fig. 61.1). Rhabdomyolysis can aggravate acute renal failure in these patients if not diagnosed and treated early. Current guidelines do not dictate routine measurement of CK in hyperosmolar hyperglycemic states. We recommend monitoring CK in these patients with particular attention to cases with very high sodium. Given the temporal association demonstrated in this case, we suggest CK be rechecked daily after peak glucose and serum osmolality.

REFERENCES

1. Singhal PC, Abramovici M, Ayer S, Desroches L. Determinants of rhabdomyolysis in the diabetic state. *Am J Nephrol* 1991;11:447–450

2. Singhal PC, Schlondorff D. Hyperosmolal state associated with rhabdomyolysis. *Nephron* 1987;47:202–204

3. Izumi T, Shimizu E, Imakiire T, Kikuchi Y, Oshima S, Kubota T, Hakozaki Y. Successfully treated case of hyperosmolar hyperglycemic state complicated with rhabdomyolysis, acute kidney injury, and ischemic colitis. *Intern Med* 2010;49(21):2321–2326

4. Sani MA, Campana-Salort E, Begu-LeCorroller A, Baccou M, Valéro R, Vialettes B. Non-traumatic rhabdomyolysis and diabetes. *Diabetes Metab* 2011;37(3):262–264

Case 62

Transitioning from Intravenous to Subcutaneous Insulin in a Complicated Patient

Kathryn J. Evans, DNP, FNP-BC,[1] and Lillian F. Lien, MD[2]

A 60-year-old man with uncontrolled type 2 diabetes (A1C 8.2%) pre-sented after 3 weeks of fevers and chills associated with chronic left foot ulcers that had progressed to wet gangrene. The patient reported poor compliance with his home diabetes medications: lispro 75–25 (30 units every morning and 36 units every evening), metformin, and Januvia. On admission he had a blood glucose (BG) of 400 mg/dL (22.2 mmol/L) and an anion gap of 11. He was admitted for a planned below-the-knee amputation (BKA) by the general surgical service and started on an intravenous (i.v.) insulin drip, i.v. fluids, and antibiotics. Between December 1, 2013, and December 6, 2013, the patient under-went several surgical procedures, ending with a left completion BKA on December 6, 2013.

On December 7, 2013, the patient was still requiring i.v. insulin. He weighed 90.7 kg. Vital signs included

Temperature	37.4°C (99.3°F)
Heart rate	94 bpm
Respirations	16
Blood pressure	125/60 mmHg

The inpatient Diabetes Management Service (DMS) was consulted to assist with postoperative glycemic management in the setting of uncon-trolled diabetes, variable food intake, and transitioning from i.v. to subcuta-neous (SQ) insulin.

When BG is uncontrolled, i.v. insulin is initiated in the inpatient setting to allow safe and rapid attainment of glycemic control.[1] Complex patients may also benefit from i.v. insulin to determine changing insulin requirements.[1,2] In our institution, we routinely prescribe i.v. insulin for patients with type 1 or

[1]Division of Endocrinology, Metabolism and Nutrition, Duke University Medical Center, Durham, NC. [2]Duke Inpatient Diabetes Management, Department of Medicine, Division of Endocrinology, Metabolism, and Nutrition, Duke University Medical Center, Durham, NC.

DOI: 10.2337/9781580405713.62

Table 62.1 — Blood Glucose Value, December 7, 2013

	1200	1300	1400	1500	1600	1700	1800	1900	2000	2100	2200	2300
BG	159	151	151	139	195	181		155	161		173	169
GTT rate	0.78	0.78	0.78	0.70	0.70	0.84	1.01	1.22	0.84	0.92	1	1.1
SQ Lantus										12		
SQ Lispro	4						4					

BG, blood glucose; GTT rate, i.v. insulin drip rate; SQ, subcutaneous.

type 2 diabetes who present with diabetic ketoacidosis (DKA), hyperglycemic hyperosmolar nonketotic syndrome (HHNK), infection, myocardial infarction, surgical complications, and trauma, among other conditions. Intravenous insulin allows a safe dose of insulin to be administered on an hourly basis, is easily adjusted in the face of complex comorbidities, and provides a smooth transition to appropriate SQ dosing.

The patient tolerated the surgical procedure well and on postoperative day 1 (December 7, 2013) was ordered a no-concentrated-sweets diet. The patient had erratic eating patterns with substantial intake by mouth and the DMS team initiated a four-shot basal-bolus SQ insulin regimen while continuing the i.v. insulin drip. Because i.v. insulin is not intended to cover prandial intake (without significant variability in drip rates), orders were placed for 4 units lispro SQ t.i.d. with meals and 12 units glargine SQ every night (qHS). The nurses were instructed to continue titrating the i.v. insulin drip on an hourly basis, according to our institutional policy (Table 62.1).

Ideally, i.v. insulin is used to correct basal insulin requirements. If the patient is allowed to eat, prandial SQ insulin should also be given to prevent the i.v. drip rate from increasing dramatically and to prevent loss of optimal glucose control after food intake. Although some literature suggests that SQ insulin can be given at least 1–2 h before complete discontinuation of the insulin drip (in favor of SQ insulin use alone),[3,5] our institution commonly uses basal and prandial SQ insulin concurrently with i.v. insulin to facilitate glucose control in complicated patients. The i.v. insulin is titrated on an hourly basis as usual, and the rapid-acting SQ insulin covers food intake, while the SQ 24-h basal insulin gradually brings down the drip rates. Furthermore, continued titration of the i.v. insulin allows the provider to assess how much insulin the patient is still requiring over and above the SQ amount, so that subsequent SQ doses can be adjusted before discontinuing the i.v. insulin. Our institution typically recommends stopping the i.v. insulin when drip rates are <0.5 units/h. The use of SQ insulin in addition to i.v. insulin has been supported by other researchers.[3–5]

Table 62.2—Blood Glucose Values, December 8, 2013

	1200	1300	1400	1500	1600	1700	1800	1900	2000	2100	2200	2300
BG	141	120	118	113	104	121	156	137		122		105
GTT rate	2.6	1.6	1.4	1.3	1.1		1.2			1.11	1.11	1.11	0.77
SQ Lantus										20		
SQ Lispro	4					4						

BG, blood glucose; GTT rate, i.v. insulin drip rate; SQ, subcutaneous.

In this case, the SQ dose selections (glargine 12 units qHS and lispro 4 units t.i.d. with meals) were weight-based: 90 kg using a cautious 0.3 units/kg = 27 units total daily dose (TDD). This was split into 50% basal (13.5 units) and 50% bolus (3.3 units per meal). The final basal dose was conservative because the patient remained on i.v. insulin. Another method of verifying appropriate SQ dosing is to use the overnight insulin drip rate (presumably the basal requirement). For this patient, the overnight drip rate on postoperative day 1 was an average of 0.7 units/h (0.7 × 24 h = 16.8 units; 75% of this dose is 12 units basal). This calculation is based on studies that have suggested that using 70–80% of the 24-h i.v. insulin requirement for SQ transition produces optimum results.[5]

On December 8, 2013, the patient was postoperative day 2 and recovering favorably, although his i.v. drip rates remained at 1–2 units/h. These residual elevated i.v. drip rates were believed to be due to use of a conservative initial weight-based SQ estimate (0.3 units/kg as opposed to ≥0.5 units/kg) as well as residual infection, stress, and intermittent postoperative pain. His orders were altered to reflect continuation of i.v. insulin, including the continuation of 4 units lispro SQ t.i.d. with meals, but an increase to 20 units glargine SQ qHS (Table 62.2).

By December 9, 2013, the i.v. drip rates dropped substantially, the i.v. insulin was discontinued, and the patient continued on 4 units of lispro SQ t.i.d. and 20 units glargine SQ qHS. The insulin drip remained off with continued stabilization of the blood glucose on only the SQ regimen. From December 10 to 11, the patient continued to have improved food intake with some variability in the amount of meal consumption. His lispro doses were adjusted to 4 units (breakfast), 5 units (lunch), and 7 units (dinner). His glargine dose was ultimately increased to 24 units qHS. With these doses, the patient's blood glucose ranged from 143 to 170 mg/dL (7.9–9.4 mmol/L), which is within goal according to the inpatient American Diabetes Association guidelines recommending blood glucose values ranging from 140 to 180 mg/dL (7.8–10 mmol/L) (Table 62.3).[2]

Table 62.3—Blood Glucose Values, December 9, 2013

	0000	0100	0200	0300	0400	0500	0600	0700	0800	0900	1000	1100	1200	1300	1400	1500	1600	1700
BG		118	101	121	110	129	114	116	125	141	125		154					149
GTT rate	0.69	0.62	0.62	0.62	0.43	0.43	0.3	0.27	0	0	0	0	0					
SQ Lantus																		
SQ Lispro									4				4					4

BG, blood glucose; GTT rate, i.v. insulin drip rate; SQ, subcutaneous.

This patient had many factors that contributed to his hyperglycemic state. Postoperative stress, pain, variable oral intake, infection, and underlying insulin resistance are all complicating factors in his glycemic management.[2] Patients require close monitoring and daily titration to match the amount of insulin to changing requirements. The use of SQ insulin, specifically glargine, along with i.v. insulin has been shown to significantly reduce rebound hyperglycemia (>180 mg/dL or 10 mmol/L) after discontinuing the insulin drip.[4]

REFERENCES

1. Bode B, Braithwaite S, Steed R, Davidson P. Intravenous insulin infusion therapy: Indications, methods, and transition to subcutaneous insulin therapy. *Crit Care Med* 2012;40(12):3251–3276

2. Lien LF, Cox M, Feinglos MN, Corsino L. *Diabetes Control in the Hospitalized Patient: A Comprehensive Clinical Guide*. Springer, New York, 2010

3. Furnary A, Braithwaite S. Effects of outcome on in-hospital transition from intravenous insulin to subcutaneous therapy. *Am J Cardiology* 2006;98(14):557–564

4. Braithwaite S. The transition from intravenous insulin to long-term diabetes therapies: the argument for insulin analogs. *Semin Thorac Cardiovasc Surg* 2006;18(4):366–378

5. Hsia E, Seggelke S, Gibbs J, Hawkins M, Cohlmia E, Draznin B. Subcutaneous administration of glargine to diabetic patients receiving insulin infusion prevents rebound hyperglycemia. *J Clin Endocrinol Metab* 2012;97:3132–3137

Case 63

Failure to Coordinate Diabetes Care between Hospital and Ambulatory Settings: A Threat to Safe and Quality Patient Care

Shawn Peavie, DO,[1] and Mercedes Falciglia, MD[1,2]

A 61-year-old man with a history of type 2 diabetes, chronic kidney disease, stroke, vascular dementia, hypertension, coronary artery disease, and depression presented to the hospital from a nursing home with altered mental status and weakness. The patient had been residing in a nursing home due mainly to dementia. On admission, he and his wife reported he had been experiencing altered mental status with increasing confusion over the past few months. On admission to the hospital, his ambulatory insulin regimen from the nursing home was continued. This regimen consisted of glargine 15 units subcutaneous every night and lispro 4 units subcutaneous with each meal, as well as a correction scale of 1 unit for every 50 mg/dL (2.8 mmol/L) >150 mg/dL (8.3 mmol/L).

On night 2 of hospital admission, his blood glucose decreased to 64 mg/dL (93.6 mmol/L), and the primary medical team decreased his glargine dose to 10 units nightly. On day 6 of hospital admission, his blood glucose dropped further to 49 mg/dL (2.7 mmol/L) in the evening prompting the primary team to discontinue the glargine dosing with continuation of only prandial dosing with lispro. On day 7 of hospital admission, his blood glucose was 41 mg/dL (2.3 mmol/L) at noon. The primary team consequently decreased lispro to 3 units before meals. He was then discharged back to the nursing home on day 8. His discharge summary that was sent to the nursing home facility did not include any record of the hypoglycemic events that he experienced while hospitalized or that the insulin doses had been significantly decreased. The medication reconciliation record at discharge listed the same ambulatory insulin regimen and doses from before his admission. This regimen was resumed upon admission instead of the modified regimen from the time of discharge, which had substantially reduced dosing.

During the patient's hospitalization, several factors were proposed by the primary and consulting teams as contributing to the altered mental status for which he was admitted. These included worsening fronto-temporal dementia and possible bacteremia. However, hypoglycemia in the months preceding

[1] University of Cincinnati College of Medicine; Division of Endocrinology, Diabetes, and Metabolism, Cincinnati, OH. [2] Cincinnati Veterans Affairs Medical Center, Cincinnati, OH.

DOI: 10.2337/9781580405713.63

hospitalization was not invoked as a cause and hypoglycemia was not mentioned in the medical record of the patient's glycemic status before admission. Our review of the medical record revealed that the patient's HbA_{1c} 3 months before admission was 8.8%, while at the time of admission it was 5.3%. According to the medical record during hospitalization, the patient had similar dietary intake while in the hospital as he did at the nursing home facility.

This case raises important points for consideration, the most important of which is the lack of coordination between hospital and ambulatory care, thereby posing a serious safety threat to the patient both in the hospital and after discharge to the nursing home. The patient's discharge summary did not mention the numerous occurrences of hypoglycemia and subsequent reductions in doses of insulin taking place during hospitalization. Furthermore, the medication reconciliation record that was sent to the nursing home incorrectly noted the same insulin regimen continued from the nursing home on admission. Continuing an insulin regimen that substantially exceeded his current requirement at discharge predisposed the patient to severe hypoglycemia after discharge.

Safe and effective transitions for hospitalized patients with hyperglycemia and diabetes are hampered by well-established inadequacies in the coordination of care between inpatient and outpatient settings.[1] Diabetes-specific care coordination for hospitalized patients is further challenged because although diabetes is a common comorbidity in hospitalized patients, diabetes is the principal reason for admission in only 1–2% cases.[2] Although individuals hospitalized with diabetes often have poor control, the postdischarge period lacks appropriate outpatient medication regimen adjustment or scheduled follow-up visits.[1] Hospitalized individuals with diabetes are more likely to suffer adverse events after hospital discharge and have more frequent hospitalizations and readmissions.[1]

In this case, the lack of awareness among hospital providers about the significant decline in HbA_{1c} in the months before admission represents another lapse in diabetes care coordination that obscures an important potential contributor to the patient's worsening mental function—recurrent and severe hypoglycemia. The risk of hypoglycemia appears to be increased in older adults who may have more neuroglycopenic manifestations of hypoglycemia (dizziness, weakness, delirium, confusion) compared with adrenergic manifestations (tremors, sweating).[3] Severe hypoglycemia requiring hospitalization has been associated with an increased risk of dementia, and older adults with diabetes who develop dementia have a higher risk of hypoglycemia.[4] Recurrent and severe hypoglycemia has been associated with cognitive impairment in elderly persons with diabetes.[5]

This case illustrates the need for effective and reproducible methods to coordinate diabetes-specific care between hospital and primary care settings for people with diabetes or hyperglycemia. Such mechanisms, together with diabetes care that is individualized for an individual's life expectancy and comorbidities, could improve the health of a population at high-risk for morbidity, mortality, and cost to the health care system.[5]

REFERENCES

1. Wheeler K, Crawford R, McAdams D, Benel S, Dunbar VG, Caudle JM, et al. Inpatient to outpatient transfer of care in urban patients with diabetes: patterns and determinants of immediate postdischarge follow-up. *Arch Intern Med* 2004;164(4):447–453

2. Fraze T, Jiang HJ, Burgess J. Hospital stays for patients with diabetes, 2008. HCUP Statistical Brief No. 93 [Internet], August 2010. Rockville, MD, Agency for Healthcare Research and Quality. Available from http://www.hcup-us.ahrq.gov/reports/statbriefs/sb93.pdf

3. Cryer PE. The barrier of hypoglycemia in diabetes. *Diabetes* 2008;57(12):3169–3176

4. Yaffe K, Falvey CM, Hamilton N, Harris TB, Simonsick EM, Strotmeyer ES, et al. Association between hypoglycemia and dementia in a biracial cohort of older adults with diabetes mellitus. *JAMA Intern Med* 2013;173(14):1300–1306

5. Kirkman MS, Briscoe VJ, Clark N, Florez H, Haas LB, Halter JB, et al. Diabetes in older adults: a consensus report. *J Am Geriatr Soc* 2012;60(12):2342–2356

Case 64

Preventing Readmission: Translating the Hospital Diabetes Regimen into a Home Regimen that Is Safe, Effective, and Easy to Follow

JANE JEFFRIE SELEY, DNP, MPH, MSN, BC-ADM, CDE, CDTC[1]

A 71-year-old woman of Caribbean descent with a 15-year history of type 2 diabetes, hypertension, and hyperlipidemia is sent to the emergency room of a large academic medical center by her podiatrist. The podiatrist correctly suspects that a draining ulcer at the base of her left third toe indicates underlying osteomyelitis. Under the care of a primary care physician, the patient's home diabetes regimen has been the same since diagnosis 15 years earlier: glyburide 10 mg twice daily and metformin 850 mg twice daily. The patient is admitted to a general medicine floor with a blood glucose (BG) level of 201 mg/dL (11.2 mmol/L) and is started on basal/bolus insulin therapy, intravenous (i.v.) antibiotics, and wound care. Her HbA_{1c} is 12.2%.

A comprehensive insulin order set was used to place orders for BG monitoring, a consistent carbohydrate meal plan, treatment for hypoglycemia, and both basal and bolus insulin therapy (see Fig. 64.1). A medium dose insulin order set autocalculated the basal insulin dose (75.2 kg weight × 0.2 units/kg for medium dose = 15 units) and a prandial aspart scale:

0 units for BG 70–100 mg/dL

3 units for BG 101–150 mg/dL

4 units for BG 151–200 mg/dL

6 units for BG 201–250 mg/dL

7 units for BG 251–300 mg/dL

8 units for BG 301–350 mg/dL

9 units for BG 351–400 mg/dL

10 units for BG 401–999 mg/dL

A bedtime aspart correction scale was also ordered:

3 units if BG 301–350 mg/dL

4 units if BG 351–400 md/dL

5 units if BG 401–999 mg/dL

[1]New York Presbyterian/Weill Cornell Medical Center, New York, NY.

DOI: 10.2337/9781580405713.64

Over the course of the 7-day hospital stay, the glargine was titrated up to 20 units at 9:00 P.M. based on fasting BG levels in the 200–300 mg/dL (11.1–16.7 mmol/L) range, while the aspart scale was maintained at a medium dose. Three days before discharge, the medicine team ordered diabetes education for insulin instruction as well as a nutrition consult. The registered nurse caring for the patient that day documented insulin teaching with the aspart pen.

On the day of discharge, the diabetes nurse practitioner was consulted to teach the patient how to calculate an insulin dose based on the current BG level. Up until this time, the patient had not been involved in determining the insulin dose despite being given a calculated dose 3–4 times a day. She could not state her current glargine dose and did not understand carbohydrate counting. A dietitian saw her 2 days earlier, but the patient did not have any recollection of the visit. When asked what she planned to eat for breakfast after she takes her mealtime insulin postdischarge, she replied "cheese." She understands that she has a high HbA_{1c} and that the diabetes pills she was taking are no longer effective. She is interested and willing to learn intensive therapy to control her hyperglycemia and to prevent further foot problems.

Ordinarily in a case like this, given that this patient is older, lives alone, and has no experience with insulin administration or dose calculation, I would gravitate toward basal insulin and a fixed dose of mealtime insulin or a premixed insulin at the time of discharge and hope that the regimen could be advanced in the outpatient setting. Unfortunately, I was meeting the patient for the first time on the day of discharge.

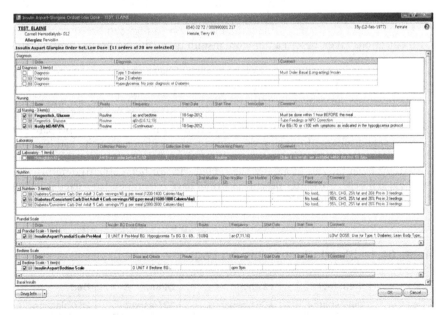

Figure 64.1 — Partial view of aspart-glargine order set.

INPATIENT DIABETES SELF-MANAGEMENT EDUCATION

Inpatient diabetes self-management education has been associated with shorter lengths of stay and improved outcomes postdischarge.[1] Clinicians caring for patients with diabetes in the acute care setting may not feel they have sufficient knowledge and experience to provide education in "survival skills," such as insulin administration and home BG monitoring. To make matters worse, they often have competing priorities and limited time to devote to patient education.[2,3] Diabetes self-management education can be incorporated into usual nursing care, coaching the patient to participate in BG monitoring and insulin administration throughout hospitalization instead of on the day of discharge, leaving the patient with little opportunity to practice new skills and build confidence. If diabetes education is offered whenever a patient is due for glucose monitoring or insulin, it will take a great deal less staff time.

DETERMINING A SAFE AND EFFECTIVE DISCHARGE REGIMEN

Determining the best home regimen is more art than science. Similar to the American Diabetes Association and the European Association for the Study of Diabetes position statement on the management of hyperglycemia in type 2 diabetes, a patient-centered approach that tailors the regimen to each patient is key. Factors to consider include diabetes duration, HbA_{1c}, weight, age, comorbidities, cost, and complexity of the regimen. The art is in matching the "right" regimen to each individual patient. Table 64.1 is the patient's recent BG levels and insulin usage.[4,5] Table 64.2 is an adaptation of a helpful guide by Umpierrez et al.[1] to transition patients home on a regimen based on diabetes medications taken before admission, insulin usage during hospitalization, and current HbA_{1c}.

Since this patient's HbA_{1c} was *double digits*, it is clear that basal-bolus insulin therapy would be the best choice. Although she was older, lived alone, and had not practiced survival skills until the afternoon of her discharge, she was highly motivated to learn. It took two 1-h sessions with the diabetes nurse practitioner and one 0.5-h session with the dietitian in one afternoon to prepare her for a safe discharge following the same insulin regimen that she had been on in the hospital. This high concentration of staff time was avoidable had the patient been taught on a daily basis. Had she not been able to demonstrate these skills correctly after practice, I would have recommended a fixed regimen of glargine 20 units at 9:00 P.M. and four units of aspart before each meal. As a

Table 64.1—Blood Glucose/Insulin Log

	Breakfast	Lunch	Dinner	Bed
Day 1	158/aspart 4	361/aspart 9	197/aspart 4	267/glargine 20
Day 2	273/aspart 7	184/aspart 4	Discharged	

Table 64.2—Transition Guide for Diabetes Medications from Inpatient to Outpatient

A1C <7%	A1C 7–9%	A1C >9%
Return to the same regimen as prior to admission.	Restart preadmission medications, keep on basal insulin at half the inpatient dose.	Basal-bolus at the inpatient dose. Consider premixed insulin or basal insulin + glinide.

Source: Adapted from Umpierrez.[1]

precautionary measure, a follow-up phone call was planned for the next day, a primary care appointment in 1 week, and an appointment with an endocrinologist in 2 weeks. The patient declined a one-time safety visit by a visiting nurse as she wanted to return to work as soon as possible.

REFERENCES

1. Umpierrez GE, Hellman R, Korytkowski M, Kosiborod M, Maynard G, Montori VM, Seley JJ, Van den Berghe G. Management of hyperglycemia in hospitalized patients in non-critical care setting: an Endocrine Society Clinical Practice Guideline. *J Clin Endocrinol Metab* 2012;97:16–38

2. Seley JJ, Wallace M. Meeting the challenge of inpatient diabetes education: an interdisciplinary approach. In *Educating Your Patient with Diabetes*. Weinger K, Carver CA, Eds. New York, Humana Press, 2008, 81–96

3. American Association of Diabetes Educators. AADE position statement: diabetes inpatient management. *Diabetes Educator* 2012;38(1):142–146

4. American Diabetes Association. Clinical practice recommendations. *Diabetes Care* 2014;37:S14–S80

5. Inzucchi SE, Bergenstal RM, Buse JB, Diamant M, Ferrannini E, Nauck M, Peters AL, Tsapas A, Wender R, Matthews DR. Management of hyperglycemia in type 2 diabetes: a patient centered approach. *Diabetes Care* 2012;35(6):1364–1379

Case 65

Novel Combination Therapy for Type 2 Diabetes

Donna White, RPh, CDE, BCACP,[1] and Svetlana Goldman, PharmD[1]

A 59-year-old woman presented to the endocrinology clinic with elevated blood glucose (HbA$_{1c}$ 8.9%) following a recent hospitalization requiring high-dose steroids for an allergic reaction to an anesthesia induction agent. This patient had diabetes for the past 7 years and was previously well controlled on metformin 1,000 mg twice daily (all prior HbA$_{1c}$ <7%). She had previously tried a sulfonylurea, but this was discontinued because of one severe hypoglycemic event. Her past medical history included hypertension, hyperlipidemia, atrial fibrillation, and obesity. During hospitalization, glucose control was maintained by insulin infusion, and she was discharged on insulin glargine 20 units daily. Metformin was continued and blood glucose levels remained as high as 300 mg/dL (16.7 mmol/L). She was instructed to titrate insulin until fasting blood glucose were <150 mg/dL (8.3 mmol/L). The patient titrated to 85 units of insulin daily with blood glucose averages remaining >190 mg/dL (10.5 mmol/L). Her steroid taper was completed 2 months before her initial endocrine visit. The patient expressed frustration with poor blood glucose control and weight gain. A plan to address her glucose control and her weight gain included discontinuation of her insulin, continuation of her metformin, and the addition of canagliflozin 100 mg daily, titrated to 300 mg daily initially with subsequent addition of a glucagon-like peptide-1 (GLP-1) inhibitor, liraglutide, 0.6 mg titrated to 1.8 mg daily.

Recent updates to diabetes treatment guidelines (American Diabetes Association and American Association of Clinical Endocrinologist [AACE]) have focused on more patient-centered approaches to glycemic control.[1,2] Treatment choices focus more on minimizing potential medication side effects, including hypoglycemia and weight gain, and maximizing the benefits of HbA$_{1c}$ lowering and cardioprotective effects. Insulin is often the best therapy for hospitalized patients and is the most effective agent for lowering HbA$_{1c}$, but it is limited by the potential for weight gain and an increased risk of hypoglycemia as goals are realized. Obesity is an independent risk factor for hypertension and cardiovascular disease. Other options to consider for obese patients with type 2 diabetes include dual or triple therapy with less potential for weight gain and hypoglycemia.

Twenty percent of glucose homeostasis is contributed by the kidneys. Recent U.S. Food and Drug Administration (FDA) approval of several oral sodium glucose cotransporter 2 (SGLT2) inhibitors adds an additional

[1]University of Virginia Health System, Department of Pharmacy, Charlottesville, VA.

DOI: 10.2337/9781580405713.65

Table 65.1—Changes in Weight and HbA$_{1c}$

Date	Weight (kg)	HbA$_{1c}$ (%)
8/23/13 started canagliflozin	118.6	8.9
9/20/13 started liraglutide	114.5	—
1/09/14	102.3	6.6

target for lowering blood glucose. SGLT2 inhibitors work by increasing glucose excretion in the urine by reducing reabsorption of filtered glucose and decreasing the renal glucose threshold. SGLT2 inhibitors are effective in all stages of diabetes, as they act independently of pancreatic β-cell function.

One phase 3 clinical study demonstrated an HbA$_{1c}$ lowering for canagliflozin of –0.77% to –1.03% (100 mg vs. 300 mg dose, respectively) and weight loss of –2.5 kg to –3.4 kg (100 mg vs. 300 mg dose, respectively).[3] Although these agents have beneficial HbA$_{1c}$ lowering and weight loss (wasting 240–320 calories per day as long as energy is not increased), they also are associated with an increased risk of mycotic infections, urinary tract infections, hypotension, and hyperkalemia because of osmotic diuresis and reduced intravascular volume.[4]

This patient previously discontinued sulfonylurea therapy because of hypoglycemia; therefore, an agent with a lower risk of hypoglycemia would be preferred. Also, with an initial BMI of 42.2 kg/m^2 (height 5′ 6″; weight 261 lb), this patient would benefit from an agent that has the potential for weight loss rather than weight gain. Although an SGLT2 inhibitor is not a first-line agent, in utilizing a more patient-centered approach to clinical decision making, this medication has the potential benefits of weight loss and low risk of hypoglycemia, a favorable profile for this particular patient.

Follow-up appointment in 1 month showed an improvement in blood glucose with most readings 150–200 mg/dL (8.3–11.1 mmol/L). Recorded weight was 252 lb (9 lb loss). Patient did report one vaginal yeast infection treated with fluconazole, but denied any other side effects. Because blood glucose remained above goal, a GLP-1 receptor agonist was initiated. Patient was instructed to start liraglutide 0.6 mg daily and titrate to a therapeutic dose of 1.8 mg daily.

Incretins are hormones secreted at low levels during the fasting state and stimulate insulin secretion in a glucose-dependent manner following an oral glucose load.[5] GLP-1 is one of the endogenous incretins that also suppresses glucagon secretion. Because these incretins are released in response to a meal, insulin stimulation occurs in proportion to the actual glucose amount ingested. Thus, GLP-1 receptor agonists (GLP-1 RA) have much lower potential for hypoglycemia than insulin secretagogues, such as sulfonylureas.

Liraglutide is a GLP-1 RA that is given as a once-daily subcutaneous injection, improving compliance over the twice-daily injection of exenatide. These agents typically lower HbA$_{1c}$ by 0.4 to 1.6%.[5,6] They also have added benefits of weight loss, reduction in triglycerides, and decrease in blood pressure.

Weight loss and HbA$_{1c}$ lowering has been greater for GLP-1 RAs versus dipeptidyl peptidase 4 (DPP-4) inhibitors in head-to-head trials, placing them higher in the treatment hierarchy developed by the AACE and ACE (American College of Endocrinology).[2]

For our patient, liraglutide was an appropriate next-line treatment option because our patient remained above goal on dual hypoglycemic therapy and could benefit from further weight loss.

Patient presented 3 months later to the endocrinologist with significant reductions in blood glucose values and improvement in HbA$_{1c}$ (6.6%) (Table 65.1). She lost an additional 27 lb since last visit and a total of 36 lb since starting canagliflozin.

REFERENCES

1. American Diabetes Association. Standards of medical care in diabetes, 2015. *Diabetes Care* 2015;38(Suppl. 1):S1–S93

2. Handelsman Y, Mechanick JI, Blonde L, et al. American Association of Clinical Endocrinologists medical guidelines for clinical practice for developing a diabetes mellitus comprehensive care plan. *Endocr Pract* 2011;17(Suppl. 2):1–53

3. Stenlof K, Cefalu WT, Kim KA, et al. Efficacy and safety of canagliflozin monotherapy in subjects with type 2 diabetes mellitus inadequately controlled with diet and exercise. *Diabetes Obes Metab* 2013;15:378–382

4. *Invokana (canagliflozin), prescribing information.* Titusville, NJ, Janssen, 2013

5. Nauck MA. Incretin-based therapies for type 2 diabetes mellitus: properties, functions, and clinical implications. *Am J Med* 2011;124(1 Suppl.):S3–S18

6. Inzucchi SE, Bergenstal RM, Buse JB, et al. Management of hyperglycemia in type 2 diabetes, 2015: a patient-centered approach: update to a position statement of the American Diabetes Association and the European Association for the Study of Diabetes. *Diabetes Care* 2015;38:140–149

Case 66

Do Many People with Type 2 Diabetes *Really* Need Insulin?

Stanley S. Schwartz, MD[1,2]

A 74-year-old woman was seen for endocrine consultation, after admission for bronchitis, type 2 diabetes, and hypertension. She had been treated for 35 years for her diabetes, with noninsulin therapy for her initial 15 years and with insulin for the past 20 years. She was taking 15 units U-500 insulin q.i.d. (= 300 units regular insulin), and eating concentrated sweets. Careful questioning revealed that she was having nocturnal hypoglycemia and awakening in the morning with sweats. She had gained 58 lb since starting insulin therapy, 30 of which she gained over the past 5 years that she was on U-500.

Her pre-admission HbA_{1c} was 9.3% on November 20, 2012. No weight was documented in the hospital.

She had been started on insulin at a time during which she was not following a diet, eating both the "wrong stuff," simple sugars, and too much of the "right stuff," everything else. Typically, such patients have quick weight gain, and then, at a time when food intake is decreased for a few days, develop hypoglycemia—adrenergic or neuroglycopenic symptoms—as well as clues of hypoglycemic unawareness, such as awaking with a headache they did not go to sleep with; awaking with nightmares, vivid, or eerie dreams; or awaking with bed sheets or pajamas soaked with sweat; and experiencing undue hunger during the day. Some physicians do not recognize or do not know these symptoms. It is believed that 42% of patients with type 2 diabetes have hypoglycemic unawareness episodes.[1]

In the hospital, we started a no-concentrated sweet (NCS) diet and sitagliptin 100 mg. As she was starting a diet, insulin dose was reduced by 50%. She eventually was discharged home on 7 units U-500 q.i.d. (140 units regular insulin daily).

As one starts a hypocaloric or a low simple carbohydrate (CHO) diet, it is critical to reduce insulin doses proportionately for estimated reduction in CHO calories. We reduce insulin doses by ~25%, a rule of thumb that works well, for an estimate of excess insulin causing hypoglycemia, and by an additional 25% for the estimated reduction in simple CHO caloric intake; also, a modest reduction is employed on starting a dipeptidyl peptidase 4 (DPP-4)

[1]Main Line Health System, Wynnewood, PA. [2]University of Pennsylvania, Philadelphia, PA.

DOI: 10.2337/9781580405713.66

inhibitor (we usually decrease boluses 30% and basal insulin 10% for DPP-4 initiation).[2]

The patient was seen in the office ~2 weeks later, weight 219 lb, BMI 36.44 kg/m², blood glucose levels in the low 100 mg/dL (5.6 mmol/L) range; liraglutide was started, 1.2 mg daily (sitagliptin was discontinued), and U-500 insulin reduced to 6 units q.i.d. (120 units regular insulin daily; this combination is used off-label).

It is well known that GLP-1 receptor agonists have greater effectiveness than DPP-4 inhibitor in lowering HbA$_{1c}$ and promoting weight loss.[3] Thus, we further reduced insulin 15%, for the switch from DPP-4 to GLP-1.

On December 27, 2012 (2 weeks later), her weight was 213 lb (BMI 35.44 kg/m²), a loss of an additional 6 lb. Liraglutide was increased to 1.8 mg daily, insulin decreased to 4 units of U-500 q.i.d. (as she was having some hypoglycemic reactions) (80 units of regular insulin daily).
On February, 21, 2013, her weight was 203 lb (BMI 33.78 kg/m²), a loss of 10 lb more. Her next HbA$_{1c}$ was 6.8%.
In July 2013, she deviated from her diet and increased U-500 insulin to 5 units q.i.d. (100 units of regular insulin daily). At this point, the importance of diet was readdressed, canagliflozin 100 mg was added to her regime, and she was switched to 40 units of glargine.

The combination of SGLT-2 inhibitor and GLP-1 induced ~3.5% additional body weight loss and an additional drop of 1% in HbA$_{1c}$.[4]

She was seen 4 weeks later and demonstrated a 6 lb weight loss, down to 198 lb (BMI 32.95 kg/m²). Her glargine was reduced to 30 units once daily. Metformin was added for additional glycemic benefit. On October 19, 2013, insulin was stopped and pioglitazone started.
On November 25, 2013, essentially 1 year after starting diet and alternative antidiabetic agents, she required no *insulin*, she maintained her 36-lb weight loss, and her HbA$_{1c}$ was now 6.9%.

This is an exaggerated example (weaning off 300 units of insulin), but with the common result in our office of stopping insulin in patients with type 2 diabetes by following general principles of diabetes management.[2] Patients on <40 units/day total insulin and eating sweets, having hypoglycemia (with careful questioning for hypoglycemic unawareness), are advised to decrease doses of insulin by 25% at the start of a hypocaloric diet, with an additional 25% decrease to account for hypoglycemia. We also advise to decrease insulin dose by 20% when initiating GLP-1 receptor agonists, and by 25% when initiating SGLT-2 inhibitors. The cumulative result is to stop insulin and provide careful follow-up.
We use the same percentage reductions of doses in patients on >40 units of total daily insulin as in this case. In the process, we recommend stopping bolus insulin (when calculated dose per meal is >5 units), and we keep basal insulin until, as patients lose weight, we may add metformin and/or pioglitazone (all of which decrease insulin resistance), or until blood glucose levels decrease

further, with a possibility of discontinuing insulin altogether, as outlined by this case.

The key points of this case are that patients with type 2 diabetes can lose weight and be taken off insulin by compliance with a diet and addition of non-hypoglycemia agents. This will facilitate weight loss, eliminate hypoglycemia, and may reduce cardiovascular risk factors. This case also emphasizes the value of combining GLP-1 receptor agonists with SGLT-2 inhibitors, which improve β-cell dysfunction and use agents that decrease insulin resistance.[5]

REFERENCES

1. Chico A, Vidal–Rios P, Subira M, Novials A. The CGMS is useful for detecting unrecognized hypoglycemias in patients with type 1 and type 2 diabetes but is not better than frequent capillary glucose measurements for improving metabolic control. *Diabetes Care* 2003;26:1153–1157

2. Schwarz SS. Optimizing glycemic control and minimizing the risk of hypoglycemia in patients with type 2 diabetes. *Drugs in Context* 2013;212–255. doi:10.7573/dic.212255

3. DeFronzo RA, Okerson T, Viswanathan P, Guan X, Holcombe JH, MacConell L. Exenatide vs sitagliptin MOA study. *Curr Med Res Opin* 2008;24(10):2943–2952

4. Wysham CH, Woo VC, Mathieu C, Desai M, Alba M, Capuno G, Meinenger G. Canagliflozin (CANA) added on to dipeptidyl peptidase-4 inhibitors (DPP-4i) or glucagon-like peptide-1 (GLP-1) agonists with or without other antihyperglycemic agents (AHAs) in type 2 diabetes mellitus (T2DM) [abstract]. 1080-P, ADA Meeting, Chicago, IL, June 21–25, 2013

5. Defronzo R, Eldor R, Abdul-Ghani A. Pathophysiologic approach to therapy in patients with newly diagnosed type 2 diabetes. *Diabetes Care* 2013;36:S127–S138

Case 67

Glycemic Control in a Patient with Type 1 Diabetes and Peritoneal Dialysis

Nadir Khir, MD;[1] Stephen Brietzke, MD;[1] and James R. Sowers, MD[1]

A 51-year-old Caucasian woman with longstanding type 1 diabetes (T1D), with end-stage renal disease on maintenance peritoneal dialysis (PD), developed increasingly labile glycemia and frequent, severe hypoglycemia and hypoglycemia unawareness. Diabetes Service was consulted during hospitalization for severe hyperglycemia and hypoglycemia, which persisted on a basal-bolus insulin regimen of glargine and lispro.

Review of her records identified a temporal association between increasing glycemic variability and the introduction of icodextrin to her dialysis protocol. Hypoglycemic episodes occurred nocturnally, before breakfast in the fasting state, or in the late morning, after breakfast. Her insulin regimen, which had been tailored toward nocturnal dialysate exchanges, consisted of glargine 10 units each morning and NPH insulin, 8 units at the start of PD exchanges each night. Mealtime aspart boluses, were administered at 2 units/15 g of carbohydrate, plus a correction dose of 1 unit per increment of 25 mg/dL (1.4 mmol/L) >150 mg/dL (8.3 mmol/L) by point-of-care testing. At home, she used a OneTouch UltraMini meter, performing at least four tests daily, and glycemia ranged from 30 to >600 mg/dL (1.7 to >33.3 mmol/L) despite frequent insulin correction dosing.

Hypoglycemia unawareness is an important limitation in insulin therapy for diabetes and is defined by the absence of warning "adrenergic" symptoms before neurocognitive dysfunction. Defective glucose counter-regulation, with impaired response of glucagon and epinephrine secretion in response to hypoglycemia, as well as nonsuppressible, exogenous insulin in excess of requirement, contributes to the problem. Management consists of a shift in priority from control of hyperglycemia to avoidance of hypoglycemia. A number of acute and chronic conditions potentially can contribute to recurrent hypoglycemia, and include cortisol and growth hormone deficiency, inborn errors of metabolism, alcohol, and medication intoxications (notably, sulfonylureas, salicylates, propranolol, and of course, exogenous insulin). Other contributors include longstanding type 1 diabetes with autonomic neuropathy, gastroparesis, and total loss of C-peptide reserve. Renal disease can contribute because of failure of renal gluconeogenesis, reduced degradation and elimination of exogenous insulin, and medications that promote hypoglycemia.

---

[1]Division of Endocrinology, Diabetes and Metabolism, Department of Medicine, University of Missouri, Columbia, MO.

                    DOI: 10.2337/9781580405713.67

Patients receiving PD using icodextrin are prone to home monitor device error that falsely reads high blood glucose following peritoneal dialysis with icodextrin. Correction of falsely elevated blood glucose on blood glucose meter checks can lead to catastrophic hypoglycemia.[1] Icodextrin (7.5% wt/vol; Extraneal; Baxter Healthcare, Chicago, IL), a peritoneal dialysate used in patients with concomitant diabetes, consists of a glucose polymer derived from cornstarch that is hydrolyzed in the systemic circulation to maltose metabolites. These metabolites may affect the enzymatic glucose determinations used in many bedside blood glucose meters and lead to erroneously elevated glucose measurements. Meters using the enzyme glucose dehydrogenase pyrroloquinoline quinone (GDH-PQQ) tend to return falsely elevated blood glucose values in patients receiving infusions of other glucose, such as maltose dialysis fluids.[2] This effect can persist for 2 weeks after stopping icodextrin. New test strips have been designed to minimize interference with nonglucose sugars. Blood glucose meters using glucose oxidase as the test reagent do not detect maltose and are recommended for use in patients treated with icodextrin dialysate.

The patient was found by a nutritionist to have excellent carbohydrate-counting skills. HbA$_{1c}$ averaged 8.5% over a 4-year period, ranging from 7.5 to 9.3%. Her most recent HbA$_{1c}$ was her personal lowest, 7.5%, and she had not had a blood transfusion for >1 year.

The HbA$_{1c}$ target that is associated with the best outcome in dialysis patients has not been established. Among dialysis patients, HbA$_{1c}$ goal of 7 to 8%, with the specific goal in individual patients based on the risk of hypoglycemia and presence of comorbid conditions.[3] The patient's recent HbA$_{1c}$ 7.5%—was felt to reflect her trend toward more frequent and more severe hypoglycemia—and hence, rather than being "good," was a call to action. Her longstanding diabetes and end-stage renal disease were felt to confer additional risk for hypoglycemic unawareness. Gastroparesis, previously documented by an abnormal gastric-emptying study, was felt causative of her breakfast postprandial hypoglycemia and contributory to the wide swings in glycemia. Overcorrection of hyperglycemia was suspected as likely, based on the patient's concurrent use of a GDH-PQQ-dependent meter, in the presence of icodextrin dialysate solution.

The patient's PD routine used six cycles of 2.5% dextrose in 2,000 ml fill volumes for 9 h overnight, and 1,000 ml of icodextrin (equivalent to a 4.25% dextrose solution) during the day. Point-of-care blood glucose testing using a glucose oxidase-dependent capillary blood glucose meter, confirmed by venous blood glucose measurements, established significant fasting hyperglycemia, even as daytime hypoglycemia was corrected. This finding led to the conclusion that the patient was absorbing a significant amount of both hypertonic dextrose and icodextrin, as the cause of the fasting hyperglycemia. Her insulin regimen was gradually titrated to glargine 14 units each morning plus insulin NPH 6 units and regular insulin 10 units, subcutaneously at the start of each night's PD exchanges, and insulin lispro 2 units/15 g carbohydrate and correction of 1 unit per increment of 50 mg/dL (2.8 mmol/L) in capillary blood glucose >175 mg/dL (9.7 mmol/L). On an ongoing basis, the

regimen resulted in narrower glycemic excursions and far fewer episodes of hypoglycemia.

PD patients have different peritoneal membrane transport characteristics. These differences are best classified and determined by use of the peritoneal equilibration test.[4] Patients with diabetes on continuous ambulatory PD who have uncontrolled hyperglycemia should undergo a peritoneal equilibration test. High transporters, who can have enormous glucose loads from rapid peritoneal glucose absorption, usually will benefit from transfer to multiple short-dwell exchange sessions of nocturnal PD.[5] Absorption of dialysate would cause a loss of osmotic gradient and the potential for suboptimal ultrafiltration volumes and inadequate solute clearance.

A glucose oxidase–based blood glucose meter should be used in the setting of icodextrin-based PD. True hyperglycemia following PD exchanges can represent a rapid transporter state of the peritoneal membrane, and patients should undergo a peritoneal equilibration test. Choice of insulin during PD is important to avoid potential hyperglycemia. A combination of short-acting and intermediate-acting insulin seems to be a better option for some patients.

REFERENCES

1. Kroll HR, Maher TR. Significant hypoglycemia secondary to icodextrin peritoneal dialysate in a diabetic patient. *Anesth Analg* 2007;104:1473–1474

2. Sloand JA. Dialysis patient safety: safeguards to prevent iatrogenic hypoglycemia in patients receiving icodextrin. *Am J Kidney Dis* 2012;60:514–516

3. KDIGO. Chapter 1: Definition and classification of CKD [article online]. *Kidney Int Suppl* 2013;3:19. Available from http://www.kdigo.org/clinical_practice_guidelines/pdf/CKD/KDIGO_2012_CKD_GL.pdf Accessed 4 March 2013

4. Twardowski ZJ. Clinical value of standardized equilibration tests in CAPD patients. *Blood Purif* 1989;7:95–108

5. Diaz-Buxo JA. Blood glucose control in diabetics: I. *Semin Dial* 1993;6:392–393

Case 68

Insulin Allergy in an Insulin-Requiring Patient

Nestoras Mathioudakis, MD[1]

A 60-year-old woman with a 6-year history of type 2 diabetes was referred for a second opinion regarding management of uncontrolled diabetes in the context of "an allergy to all types of insulin." One year before her initial visit, the patient had been started on detemir injections at bedtime because of unsatisfactory glycemic control on multiple oral agents. Immediately after injecting insulin, the patient developed urticaria at the injection site, surrounded by an erythematous and pruritic rash. There was no generalized urticaria or angioedema. Neither changing needles nor taking antihistamines could prevent this reaction. Subsequently, she was given a trial of exenatide, which produced the same reaction. Glycemic control was not significantly improved by glargine or exenatide.

The clinical presentation in this case was suggestive of a type I immediate hypersensitivity reaction, the most common type of allergic reaction to human insulin. In mild cases, there is localized urticaria at the injection site, whereas moderate to severe cases can present with generalized urticaria, angioedema, and rarely anaphylaxis. The first step in the investigation of a suspected insulin allergy is to exclude a reaction to the needles and confirm a reaction to insulin.[1] Some insulin vials are enclosed with latex, which could lead to contamination of the needle when drawing up insulin; silicone or other lubricants contained in some needles also can be allergenic.[1] In mild cases, switching needles and ensuring a latex-free delivery method are reasonable first steps in the evaluation. Poor injection technique can also lead to localized skin reactions from repeated inflammation.[2]

Although insulin allergy is rarely encountered in clinical practice (0.1–3% of insulin-treated patients),[1] it can present diagnostic and management challenges. The allergen can be a component within the insulin preparation, including impurities and additives, or the insulin protein itself. Although recombinant DNA technology has circumvented the problem of immunogenicity of animal insulin, there continue to be reports of allergies to all types of synthetic insulin, presumably because of hypersensitivity to microbial components used during synthesis or alterations in protein folding.[1]

The reaction to both basal insulin and a glucagon-like peptide 1 (GLP-1) agonist raised suspicion that the allergen may not have been insulin but rather

---

[1]Assistant Professor of Medicine, Division of Endocrinology, Diabetes, & Metabolism, Johns Hopkins University School of Medicine, Baltimore, MD.

DOI: 10.2337/9781580405713.68

some other substance common to detemir insulin and extenatide preparations. The poor glycemic response to both injectable medications was consistent with decreased drug efficiency from local skin inflammation.

The past medical history was notable for extensive drug and food allergies, atopic dermatitis, and exercise- and cold-induced asthma. Since the age of 40 years, the patient had undergone multiple attempts at desensitization and required frequent courses of oral glucocorticoids. Six months before the initial visit, she underwent an umbilical hernia repair. Perioperatively, she had received stress doses of dexamethasone for concerns of secondary adrenal insufficiency from prolonged courses of glucocorticoids. She developed marked steroid-induced hyperglycemia but was able to tolerate aspart insulin injections without any allergic manifestations. The patient was discharged home on multiple daily injections of aspart insulin, but after resuming her baseline steroid dose of prednisone 40 mg daily, again she developed localized skin reactions to aspart injections.

As is commonly reported with insulin allergy, this patient had several risk factors, including her gender, multiple drug allergy syndrome, allergic asthma, and food allergies. Her ability to tolerate insulin injections while receiving systemic steroids further supported the idea of a hypersensitivity reaction. Indeed, steroids are reserved for the treatment of insulin allergy when there is no alternative to treatment (i.e., type 1 diabetes), but they obviously are not an ideal therapeutic option given the hyperglycemia and insulin resistance that they induce.[1]

After extensive allergy skin testing, it was determined that she had a glycerol allergy. The patient saw an outside endocrinologist who had no advice for her and suggested that she add cycloset to maximal doses of other oral agents; however, this approach was ineffective. At the time of her initial visit, the patient's hemoglobin A1c was 9.9%. Her diabetes regimen included: metformin 2.5 g/day, sitagliptin 100 mg/day, and glimepiride 8 mg/day.

Intradermal insulin skin testing is the gold standard to confirm the diagnosis of insulin allergy.[1] Once the allergen was identified, it was important to verify its presence in all of the available types of insulin. Review of the summary product characteristics of the most common commercially used types of insulin revealed the excipients shown in Table 68.1.

As shown in Table 68.1, there is significant variability in the noninsulin components, with insulin glulisine being the only available insulin that does not contain glycerol. Both types of insulin that the patient previously attempted were confirmed to contain glycerol. Exenatide does not contain glycerol, but it does contain other preservatives. She was advised to use injections of insulin glulisine before meals and at bedtime and to discontinue oral glucose–lowering medications, with the exception of metformin. She tolerated the glulisine injections well. Successful treatment of allergy to rapid-acting insulin analogues has been reported with glulisine, presumably because of its unique profile of additives compared with the other rapid-acting analogues.[3]

Table 68.1—Characteristics of the Most Common Commercially Used Types of Insulin

Component	Function	Regular	Lispro	Aspart	Glulisine	NPH	Detemir	Glargine
Metacresol	Preservative	+	+	+	+	+	+	+
Phenol	Preservative	-	-	+	-	+	+	-
Trometamol	Buffering agent	-	-	-	+	-	-	-
Disodium hydrogen phosphate	Buffering agent	-	+	+	-	+	+	-
Sodium chloride	Tonicity agent	-	-	+	+	-	+	-
Glycerol	Tonicity agent	+	+	+	-	+	+	+
Zinc	Complexing agent	+	+	+	-	+	+	+
Polysorbate	Emulsifier	-	-	-	+	-	-	+
Protamine sulfate	Protracting agent	-	-	-	-	+	-	-
Sodium hydroxide	Alkalizing agent	+	+	+	+	+	+	+
Hydrochloric acid	Acidifying agent	+	+	+	+	+	+	+
Water for injection	Solvent	+	+	+	+	+	+	+

With titration of glulisine, her HbA_{1c} gradually declined from 9.9% to 7.5% over a 6-month period; however, without basal insulin, the patient continued to experience fasting hyperglycemia, prompting a decision to transition to an insulin pump (OmniPod) containing glulisine. After 3 months on the insulin pump, her HbA_{1c} was 7.3%.

This patient's "insulin allergy" was due to an additive within the insulin preparation and the solution was straightforward: simply switching to an alternative insulin preparation free of this additive. In insulin-requiring patients who fail to respond to changing insulin preparations, however, the management can prove challenging. Treatment approaches include the addition of nonsedating antihistamines, topical corticosteroids, inhaled β-agonists for bronchospasm, sedating anthistamines, leukotriene receptor antagonists, systemic steroids, omalizumab (anti-IgE monoclonal antibodies), systemic immunosuppression, and desensitization.[1] Insulin pump therapy also has been reported to be a successful approach to insulin allergy under the notion that continuous exposure helps to maintain tolerance.[4]

REFERENCES

1. Jacquier J, Chik CL, Senior PA. A practical, clinical approach to the assessment and management of suspected insulin allergy. *Diabet Med* 2013;30:977–985

2. Sanyal T, Ghosh S, Chowdhury S, Mukherjee S. Can a faulty injection technique lead to a localized insulin allergy? *Indian J Endocrinol Metab* 2013;17:S358–S359

3. Mollar-Puchades MA, Villanueva IL. Insulin glulisine in the treatment of allergy to rapid acting insulin and its rapid acting analogs. *Diabetes Res Clin Pract* 2009;83:e21–e22

4. Radermecker RP, Scheen AJ. Allergy reactions to insulin: effects of continuous subcutaneous insulin infusion and insulin analogues. *Diabetes Metab Res Rev* 2007;23:348–355

Case 69

Use of 3-Day Continuous Glucose Monitoring to Investigate Persistent Fasting Hyperglycemia in Type 2 Diabetes

MICHELLE GRIFFITH, MD,[1] AND MARY KORYTKOWSKI, MD[1]

A 38-year-old woman with type 2 diabetes for 13 years, complicated by peripheral neuropathy, was seen in a university-based diabetes clinic. Additional medical history was significant for hypertension and hyperlipidemia. Her HbA$_{1c}$ varied from 8.1 to 8.9% over the past 2 years.

Her medications included metformin 1,000 mg twice per day in combination with a basal-bolus insulin (BBI) regimen of glargine 20 units in the morning and 60 units in the evening and lispro with meals: 16 units with breakfast, 30 units with lunch, and 36 units with dinner. She reported that glargine had been increased from 50 units nightly to the current split dosing over the past 6 months.

Review of her home capillary blood glucose (CBG) readings demonstrated persistent fasting hyperglycemia with values in the 200–300 mg/dL (11.1–16.7 mmol/L) range, despite the fact that she denied snacking overnight or after dinner. Her prelunch and predinner CBG ranged between 118 and 170 mg/dL (6.6–9.4 mmol/L), with occasional values >200 mg/dL (11.1 mmol/L). She infrequently tested at bedtime. CBG values at 2:00 A.M. performed to investigate for nocturnal hypoglycemia were "normal." She denied any symptoms of nocturnal hypoglycemia.

On physical examination, she was obese with a weight of 135 kg and BMI 47.9 kg/m². Pulse was 64 and blood pressure 128/86 mmHg. She had no lipohypertrophy at the injection sites. Monofilament sensation was diminished in both feet. Her remaining physical examination was normal.

In individuals without diabetes, fasting blood glucose normally is maintained by overnight hepatic glucose output, with a circadian variation that is matched by compensatory insulin secretion. In patients with diabetes, overnight surges of counter-regulatory hormones—including cortisol, catecholamines, and in particular growth hormone—without adequate insulin release, contribute to fasting hyperglycemia.[1] The differential diagnosis of fasting hyperglycemia includes insufficient dosing of basal insulin, carbohydrate intake at bedtime or during the night, and the dawn phenomenon. Dawn phenomenon is a transient increase in insulin resistance in the early morning hours, likely related to exaggerated response to counter-regulatory hormones, typically with an increase in hepatic glucose output after 4:00 A.M.[1]

[1]Division of Endocrinology and Metabolism, Department of Medicine, University of Pittsburgh School of Medicine, Pittsburgh, PA.

DOI: 10.2337/9781580405713.69

Additionally, obstructive sleep apnea (OSA) has been associated with insulin resistance and may cause worsening of nocturnal hyperglycemia in patients with diabetes independent of other factors such as BMI.[2]

With consideration of possible dawn phenomenon, the patient's basal insulin was changed from glargine to detemir at doses of 30 units in the morning and 50 units in the evening. She was referred for a sleep study. Moderate OSA was diagnosed and continuous positive airway pressure (CPAP) therapy was initiated. She was also referred to a nutritionist.

The pharmacokinetics of detemir vary by dose but can include a more pronounced peak at higher doses than what is observed with glargine.[3] Although it was anticipated that this change in basal insulin would improve her morning control, the evening dose was reduced compared with the previous evening dose of glargine to minimize the risk of hypoglycemia.

With some dietary changes and initiation of CPAP, the patient lost 15 lb. Improvements were observed in her diastolic blood pressure. Fasting hyperglycemia still predominated 3 months later: fasting CBG 175–313 mg/dL (9.7–17.4 mmol/L); before lunch and dinner 100–180 mg/dL (5.6–10 mmol/L). She tested a few overnight blood glucose values and reported them being in the 150–160 mg/dL range (8.3–8.9 mmol/L). HbA$_{1c}$ was 8.7%. The dose of detemir was increased to 30 units in the morning and 70 units in the evening. At this time, she underwent 3 days of blinded continuous glucose monitor (CGM) system (CGMS iPro system by Medtronic) evaluation to investigate potential causes of her fasting hyperglycemia.

With a blinded CGM, the patient does not see real-time information regarding interstitial glucose levels. CGM devices with real-time data transmission are meant to be used as a tool by both the patient and the provider and can prompt patient action. In contrast, the blinded 3-day system functions as a data recorder and is designed to help with therapeutic decision making by collecting continuous data for analysis by the provider. Data on the impact of short-term, blinded CGM devices on glycemic control do not always support benefit to HbA$_{1c}$ levels.[4]

While wearing the CGM, the patient kept a precise log of CBG testing, food intake, and insulin dosing. Her downloaded CGM tracings

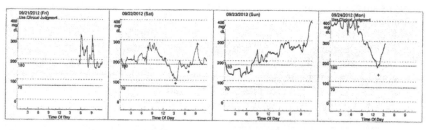

Figure 69.1 — Interstitial glucose in mg/dL vs. time of day for 72 h of monitoring (Medtronic iPro 2.2).

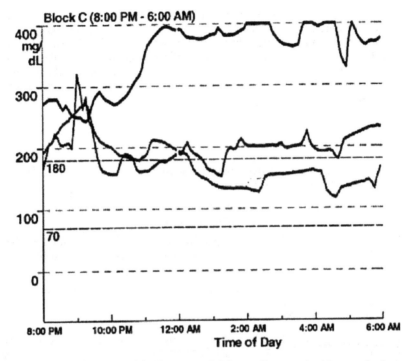

Figure 69.2—Overlay of 8:00 P.M. to 6:00 A.M. time period for each day; interstitial glucose in mg/dL vs. time of day.

demonstrated large increases in glucose levels approximately 3 h after dinner on all 3 days of the study. This information was not captured by her self-monitoring of CBG (Fig. 69.1). In one instance, without a bedtime snack, the postdinner glucose reading rose to 400 mg/dL on the CGM. The degree of morning hyperglycemia was related to the postprandial peak after dinner (Fig. 69.2). Her CBG improved during the daytime hours, likely the result of correctional insulin dosing and daytime activity.

Her insulin regimen was modified by increasing the dinnertime lispro from 36 to 42 units and the breakfast lispro from 16 to 26 units. A glucagon-like peptide 1 (GLP-1) agonist, liraglutide, was added at an initial dose of 0.6 mg daily for 1 week and then was increased to 1.2 mg daily. Over the next 2 months the predinner dose of lispro was gradually increased to 52 units and liraglutide to the maximal dose of 1.8 mg/day. At recent follow-up, she had achieved HbA$_{1c}$ of 6.9% and had lost 20 lb. Fasting CBG improved to the 120–160 mg/dL (6.7–8.9 mmol/L) range.

Although the short-term CGM data was helpful in this case, similar findings likely could have been deduced by scrupulous inclusion of bedtime blood glucose testing. Additionally, with obese insulin-resistant patients, improving the diet and exercise remain is important and additional pharmacological therapies contribute to improvements in glycemic control. Liraglutide is approved by the U.S. Food and Drug Administration for use with basal insulin but not with BBI. Its use in combination with insulin therapy for type 1 diabetes has been reported.[5] This patient's final regimen represents off-label use, but it has the potential benefit of weight neutrality and weight loss effects in some patients.

REFERENCES

1. Sheehan JP. Fasting hyperglycemia: etiology, diagnosis, and treatment. *Diabetes Technol Ther* 2004;6(4):525–533

2. Fendri S, et al. Nocturnal hyperglycaemia in type 2 diabetes with sleep apnoea syndrome. *Diabetes Res Clin Pract* 2011;91:e21–e23

3. Novo Nordisk. Insulin detemir product monograph [Internet]. Revised 10/2013. Available from http://www.novo-pi.com/levemir.pdf. Accessed 22 December 2013

4. Pepper GM, Steinsapir J, Reynolds K. Effect of short-term iPRO continuous glucose monitoring on hemoglobin A1C levels in clinical practice. *Diabetes Technol Ther* 2012;14(8):654–657

5. Kuhadiya ND, Malik R, Bellini NJ, et al. Liraglutide as additional treatment to insulin in obese patients with type 1 diabetes mellitus. *Endocr Pract* 2013;19(6):963–967

Case 70

Insulin Injections: What You "See" May Not Be What You Get

Robert J. Rushakoff, MD;[1] Mary M. Sullivan, DNP, RN, ANP-BC, CDE, FAAN;[2] Arti Shah, MD;[3] and Heidemarie Windham MacMaster, PharmD, CDE[4]

INSULIN VIAL, SYRINGE WITH AIR

A 78-year-old thin man was seen for high glucose levels. Despite follow-up with certified diabetes educators (CDEs) and physicians, glucose values were >300 mg/dL. He was prescribed 50 units of lispro before each meal and 100 units of glargine. His elderly wife was administering the shots. When asked, "How long does a bottle of insulin last?" she said at least a month (should have been about 6 days).

She was given a vial of insulin and syringe and asked to demonstrate how she gives insulin. She took the syringe, drew back to 50 units, pushed it into the vial sitting on the desk, pushed the air into the vial, and then promptly drew back 50 units of air back into the syringe.

Instructed on insulin pen use, glucose levels have been controlled with <20 units premixed insulin twice a day.

MISSING PEN NEEDLE

A 50-year-old woman was discharged from the hospital following total pancreatectomy. Prior to discharge, the CDE instructed her on insulin pen use and the patient demonstrated self-injection.

Postdischarge, the patient had two visits to her local emergency room where diabetic ketoacidosis (DKA) was diagnosed and treated. She was seen by her primary care physician who asked her to demonstrate her injection technique. She dialed the appropriate dose of insulin and then proceeded to try and inject the insulin without any attached needle. The patient had not received a prescription for pen needles and neither the pharmacy nor the patient questioned this.

[1]Division of Endocrinology and Metabolism, University of California, San Francisco, CA. [2]Department of Nursing, University of California, San Francisco, CA. [3]Division of Endocrinology and Metabolism, University of California, San Francisco, CA. [4]Department of Pharmaceutical Services, University of California, San Francisco, CA.

DOI: 10.2337/9781580405713.70

COVERED PEN NEEDLE

A 60-year-old woman was discharged from the hospital with a new requirement for insulin. Before discharge, she learned and successfully demonstrated her pen technique. At follow-up, glucose levels were 200–300 mg/
dL. When asked to demonstrate injection technique, she put a new needle
on the pen, dialed in the correct insulin dose, and then "injected" herself.
The patient, however, did not take the plastic cap off the pen needle.

INJECT INSULIN AND COUNT TO 10

A 78-year-old woman was referred for "brittle" diabetes. She was taking
4 units lispro premeal and nightly glargine. Using pens, she perfectly
described how she would dial in the dose, inject, and count to 10. When asked
to demonstrate, she dialed in the correct number, inserted the pen needle
under her skin, fully pushed the plunger, and immediately pulled the pen
needle out, holding the insulin pen at arm's length while she counted to 10.

DISCUSSION

When assessing insulin use, medical providers consider the dose and type of insulin, renal function, diet, and exercise. Despite diabetes self-care education and
frequent medical follow-up, poor insulin injection technique can lead to DKA,
hyperglycemia, and "brittle" diabetes.

INSULIN VIAL, SYRINGE WITH AIR

Even with multiple CDE and physician visits, and aggressive insulin titration,
glucose levels remained out of control. Asking, "How long does a bottle of insulin
last?" revealed the amount of insulin reportedly given was not what was ordered.

Using a syringe and vial for insulin administration can be difficult,[1] and dosing
errors occur, especially in the elderly. Patients with poor vision may believe they
have injected their insulin, with the insulin actually injected onto their skin. Experienced patients may have been taking their insulin appropriately, but with changes
in their health and vision, the technique that the patient and providers took for
granted became the unknown weak link in their management. Insulin pens generally are thought to be easier to use and to allow for more accurate dosing than
with insulin syringes, especially when low doses are used.[2,3] When the response to
changes in insulin do not make sense (as with a thin elderly patient needing
>200 units/day), consider basic technique problems.

MISSING PEN NEEDLE

This patient had demonstrated correct insulin pen technique. No insulin pen
needles were ordered at the time of discharge. Neither the patient, nor pharmacist, nor anyone in the emergency room realized that the pen needles were not

present. We previously have reported that problems with writing insulin prescriptions for discharge to home from the hospital can occur.[4]

COVERED PEN NEEDLE

Before being discharged to home, the patient demonstrated that she could use the insulin pen correctly. Once home, the patient had all of her diabetes supplies, but never actually injected her insulin dose as she left the plastic cap that covers the needle in place. For nurse safety, hospitals utilize single use safety-cap insulin pen needles. This safety cap covers the needle and the patient never actually sees the needle, before or after the injection. Thus, as far as the patient was concerned, having the cap on the needle was normal.

INJECT INSULIN AND COUNT TO 10

Although instructed in use of insulin pens, technique was never confirmed. She did not wait several seconds after the injection before withdrawing the pen, but dutifully counted those seconds off, tightly holding the pen while it was in the air. Some of the insulin was injected on the skin and some in the air, but little subcutaneously. Patients with diabetes, even longstanding diabetes and previous diabetes education, may have developed poor habits. Technique needs to be observed for errors, especially if diabetes control remains problematic.[5]

TAKE-HOME MESSAGES

1. Patients should be instructed and demonstrate using all components of the specific insulin delivery device that they will have at home.
2. Patients need printed educational material in their preferred language informing them of all of the components and steps necessary for a successful insulin injection.
3. Discharge prescriptions for insulin must include everything needed (i.e., the syringe if using a vial, the pen needles if using pens, lancets for fingersticks, and glucose test strips).
4. When ongoing glucose control remains difficult, having the patient demonstrate all aspects of insulin injection technique should be part of the evaluation. This is true even if the patient had mastered the technical aspects of insulin self-administration.
5. Elderly patients may need additional reinforcement of diabetes instruction despite years of diabetes experience.

REFERENCES

1. Bell DH, Clements RS Jr, Perentesis G, Roddam R, Wagenknecht L. Dosage accuracy of self-mixed vs premixed insulin. *Arch Intern Med* 1991;151(11): 2265–2269

2. Thurman JE. Insulin pen injection devices for management of patients with type 2 diabetes: considerations based on an endocrinologist's practical experience in the United States. *Endocr Pract* 2007;13(6):672–678

3. Molife C, Lee LJ, Shi L, Sawhney M, Lenox SM. Assessment of patient-reported outcomes of insulin pen devices versus conventional vial and syringe. *Diabetes Technol Ther* 2009;11(8):529–538

4. Kimmel B, Sullivan MM, Rushakoff RJ. Survey on transition from inpatient to outpatient for patients on insulin: what really goes on at home? *Endocr Pr Off J Am Coll Endocrinol Am Assoc Clin Endocrinol* 2010;16(5):785–791

5. Spray J. Type 1 diabetes: identifying and evaluating patient injection technique. *Br J Nurs Mark Allen Publ* 2009;18(18):1100–1105

Case 71

Prolonged Insulin-Free Management of Type 1 Diabetes

Danielle Castillo, MD,[1] and Joseph Aloi, MD, FACE[1]

A 32-year-old white man with no prior medical problems presented to the emergency room 7 years ago with a 2-week history of polyuria, polydipsia, weight loss, and blurry vision. He was found to have a blood glucose of 700 mg/dL (38.9 mmol/L), an anion gap of 17 mEq/l, and positive ketones in his urine. His A1C was 12.2%. He was treated for diabetic ketoacidosis (DKA). His discharge medications included an ACE inhibitor, basal insulin 30 units before breakfast and 35 units at bedtime, and analog insulin with meals.

On follow-up 1 week after discharge, his C-peptide level was 1.9 ng/mL with a blood glucose of 143 mg/dL (7.9 mmol/L). Four months later, his C-peptide level was 2.4 ng/mL and rose to 5.4 ng/mL following a can of Ensure. Glutamic acid decarboxylase antibodies (GADAb) were positive with a titer of 87.1 units/mL, insulin antibodies were 2.2 units/mL (normal 0–0.9), and islet cell antibodies were negative. A1C was 5.8%.

His C-peptide levels suggested that he retained some β-cell function. His insulin requirements pointed to a significant component of insulin resistance and therapies directed at improving insulin resistance and possibly preserving β-cell function were added.

Between the time of his initial presentation and subsequent follow-up, his weight improved from 258 lb (BMI 31.4 kg/m²) to 238 lb (BMI 29.0 kg/m²) as a result of exercise and dietary changes. Pioglitazone and metformin were added to his regimen and his mealtime insulin was able to be discontinued. Exenatide 10 mcg twice daily was added to his regimen later that year. He continued to lose weight by running several miles a day and 1 year after his initial presentation, his BMI was normal. Basal insulin was stopped 7 months after diagnosis, and he has remained on the pioglitazone, metformin, and exenatide with excellent glycemic control for the past 7 years.

The effects of lifestyle interventions greatly improved his "acquired" insulin resistance. Addition of pharmacological agents known to improve insulin sensitivity was successful in helping achieve an A1C in the prediabetic range for a long duration. It is tempting to ascribe some preservation of β-cell function to his pharmacologic regimen.

[1]Division of Endocrinology & Metabolism, Eastern Virginia Medical School, Norfolk, VA.

DOI: 10.2337/9781580405713.71

His A1C has remained well controlled, ranging from 6.0 to 6.8% over the past 7 years. His human insulin antibodies were undetectable 5 years after his initial presentation. Currently, 7 years after his initial presentation, his GADA remains elevated at 40.7 units/mL, C-peptide detectable at 1.8 units/mL, and he remains off of insulin.

GAD antibody often is used to guide clinicians in diagnosis of the type of diabetes. It is also used to predict an increased likelihood of insulin requirement. Data from several studies suggest that this is an acceptable practice.[1-3] On initial presentation, our patient did require insulin, as do many patients with type 2 diabetes, but he was able to discontinue insulin therapy after weight loss and dietary changes. Seven years after discontinuation of insulin, his C-peptide level remains stable and he does not require insulin. The factors that contribute to this extremely long "honeymoon" include his ability to adhere to a carbohydrate restricted diet and active exercise program. It is intriguing but unclear whether the use of GLP agonist has slowed β-cell loss through its effects on apoptosis or simply through antagonism of glucagon.

REFERENCES

1. Turner R, Stratton I, Horton V, et al. UKPDS 25: autoantibodies to islet-cell cytoplasm and glutamic acid decarboxylase for prediction of insulin requirement in type 2 diabetes. UK Prospective Diabetes Study Group. *Lancet* 1997;350:1288–1293

2. Davis TM, Wright AD, Mehta ZM, et al. Islet autoantibodies in clinically diagnosed type 2 diabetes: prevalence and relationship with metabolic control (UKPDS 70). *Diabetologia* 2005;48:695–702

3. Tuomildhto J, Zimmet P, Mackay IR, et al. Antibodies to glutamic acid decarboxylase as predictors of insulin-dependent diabetes mellitus before clinical onset of disease. *Lancet* 1994;343:1383–1385

Case 72
Delayed Response to NPH Insulin
Mayer B. Davidson, MD[1]

A 58-year-old lean woman with type 2 diabetes was referred to the diabetes clinic for control of her diabetes. Diabetes was diagnosed 12 years ago and she had been taking insulin for 1 year after failing oral medication. Her insulin regimen at the time of referral was 20 units of NPH insulin before breakfast and 12 units before supper. Her BMI was 25.1 kg/m² and her HbA$_{1c}$ level was 9.5%. She was motivated to improve her control. Table 72.1 summarizes our initial experience with her. Glucose values (mg/dL) are the range (median). The interval between visits was 3 weeks unless otherwise noted.

VISIT 1 (INITIAL)

Because the fasting glucose levels were at target but the before-supper values were high, the morning NPH insulin dose was increased and the before-supper dose remained the same.

VISIT 2

As is done routinely for referred patients taking only NPH insulin, we added a short-acting insulin after the initial visit. Because the before-supper glucose levels remained high and some fasting levels were low, the before-breakfast NPH dose was increased and the before-supper NPH dose was decreased.

VISIT 3

Because her before-supper glucose levels remained high and her fasting levels continued to contain some hypoglycemic values, the before-breakfast NPH dose was increased and the before-supper NPH dose was decreased. Furthermore, both doses of regular insulin were increased because the before-lunch and before-bedtime snack values were high.

[1]Department of Internal Medicine, Charles R. Drew University, Los Angeles, CA.
DOI: 10.2337/9781580405713.72

Table 72.1 — Insulin Doses and Self-Monitored Blood Glucose Values over Time

Visit	Current insulin doses (units)	Before breakfast (mg/dL)	Before lunch (mg/dL)	Before supper (mg/dL)	Before bedtime snack (mg/dL)	New insulin doses (units)
1	20 Nᵃ 12 Nᶜ	68–141 (110)	ND	192–243 (212)	ND	22 Nᵃ 12 Nᶜ
2	22 Nᵃ 12 Nᶜ	52–128 (82)	168–218 (180)	187–228 (202)	222–302 (250)	24 N/4 Rᵃ 10 N/4 Rᶜ
3	24 N/4Rᵃ 10 N/4 Rᶜ	67–118 (75)	143–191 (162)	175–213 (190)	183–254 (220)	26 N/6 Rᵃ 8 N/6 Rᶜ
4	26 N/6 Rᵃ 8 N/6 Rᶜ	45–78 (62)	123–162 (140)	169–223 (185)	176–233 (195)	26 N/8 Rᵃ 4 N/6 Rᶜ
5	26 N/8 Rᵃ 4 N/6 Rᶜ	47–82 (65)	113–154 (128)	172–234 (195)	163–222 (187)	26 N/8 Rᵃ 6 Rᶜ
6	26 N/8 Rᵃ 6 Rᶜ	53–90 (72)	97–138 (122)	168–214 (183)	158–201 (173)	24 N/8 Rᵃ 4 Rᵇ 6 Rᶜ
7	24 N/8 Rᵃ 4 Rᵇ 6 Rᶜ	74–105 (90)	86–140 (128)	136–185 (159)	138–177 (155)	4 N/8 Rᵃ 6 Rᵇ 6 Rᶜ
8	24 N/8 Rᵃ 6 Rᵇ 6 Rᶜ	76–119 (105)	92–143 (119)	114–152 (133)	127–172 (151)	24 N/8 Rᵃ 6 Rᵇ 8 Rᶜ
9	24 N/8 Rᵃ 6 Rᵇ 8 Rᶜ	67–133 (110)	88–123 (108)	116–158 (127)	121–161 (143)	24 N/8 Rᵃ 6 Rᵇ 10 Rᶜ

ND, not done; N, NPH insulin; R, regular insulin.
[a]before breakfast; [b]before lunch; [c]before supper.

VISIT 4

At this visit, delayed peaking of NPH insulin was suspected and the before-supper dose was halved. Although the before-supper glucose levels remained high, the morning dose of NPH was not changed for two reasons: If, indeed, NPH insulin had a delayed peak of action, changing the before-breakfast dose would not affect the before-supper glucose values. Second, if both doses were changed, it would be more difficult to determine which dose change was responsible for the subsequent fasting glucose levels. The morning dose of regular insulin was increased because the before-lunch glucose values were high. The before-supper dose of regular insulin was not changed because the change in glucose values between supper and bedtime was close to zero. In addition, there was a concern that if the before-supper glucose levels were lowered to target, then an increased dose of regular insulin might cause hypoglycemia.

VISIT 5

The before-breakfast glucose levels remained low. To confirm delayed peak action of NPH insulin, it was discontinued before supper. No other changes were made. The HbA$_{1c}$ level measured at this visit was 8.2%.

VISIT 6

With delayed peaking of NPH insulin documented and hypoglycemic values before breakfast, the morning dose of NPH insulin was decreased. Because NPH insulin taken before breakfast would not have much effect on before-supper glucose levels, a before-lunch injection of regular insulin was introduced. The before-supper dose of regular insulin was not changed.

VISIT 7

Because the fasting glucose values were now at target without hypoglycemia, the morning dose of NPH insulin was maintained. Because the before-supper glucose levels were still too high, the before-lunch dose of regular insulin was increased. The before-supper dose of regular insulin was not changed.

VISIT 8

Because the before-supper glucose levels were nearly at target but the before-bedtime values were high, the before-supper dose of regular insulin was increased. No other changes were made. Because the insulin doses were relatively stable, the patient was next seen in 6 weeks.

VISIT 9

Because the before-bedtime snack glucose values were still slightly above target, the before-supper dose of regular insulin was again increased with no other changes made. The HbA$_{1c}$ level measured at this visit was 7.3%. The patient was subsequently followed at 6-week intervals.

The approach of our diabetes program with insulin-requiring patients taking two or more injections per day is to see them every 3 weeks when out of control and substantial dose adjustments may be necessary. Our dose adjustments are also relatively conservative to avoid hypoglycemia. We routinely ask patients to test preprandially because the most important determinant of postprandial glucose levels are the preprandial ones. That is, the increment over the preprandial level is similar regardless of the preprandial value.[1-3] Therefore, postprandial hyperglycemia is best treated by lowering preprandial glycemia. We use the preprandial American Diabetes Association (ADA) glucose target of 80–130 mg/dL.[4] Although we (like most providers) prefer that patients taking more than one injection of insulin test four times a day, realistically most will not test that often. Our goal is to have them test at least twice a day.

The response to regular insulin in this patient was appropriate. This response to lispro insulin also tends to be appropriate. This strongly suggests that the delay in the peak action must be due to a delay in the dissociation of insulin from the protamine in the NPH insulin preparation. The defining pattern is normal or low fasting glucose levels in spite of decreasing, and finally no, evening NPH insulin[5] and the lack of response of the before-supper glucose tests (and often more fasting hypoglycemia) as the morning NPH insulin dose is increased. Because the afternoon glucose levels are not affected much by the morning NPH insulin, short- or rapid-acting insulin is necessary before lunch.

Thus, the eventual insulin regimen that effectively controls these patients is a basal-bolus regimen with the morning NPH insulin as the basal insulin.

These patients are described as "delayed peakers" and they are rare. In my 50 years of caring for people with diabetes, I would estimate seeing ~20 cases. For those of us who follow challenging patients, it is important to recognize them. If not, adjusting their insulin doses can be very frustrating, and they are at increased risk of overnight hypoglycemia as well as daytime hyperglycemia.

REFERENCES

1. Cusi K, Cunningham GR, Comstock JP. Safety and efficacy of normalizing fasting glucose with bedtime insulin alone in NIDDM. *Diabetes Care* 1995;18:843–851

2. Monnier L, Colette C, Dunseath GJ, Owens DR. The loss of postprandial glycemic control precedes stepwise deterioration of fasting with worsening diabetes. *Diabetes Care* 2007;30:263–269

3. Bonomo K, DeSalve A, Fiova E, et al. Evaluation of a simple policy for pre- and post-prandial blood glucose self-monitoring in people with type 2 diabetes not on insulin. *Diabetes Res Clin Pract* 2010;87:246–251

4. American Diabetes Association. Standards of medical care in diabetes, 2015. *Diabetes Care* 2015;38(Suppl. 1):S1–S93

5. Davidson MB. Delayed response to NPH insulin. *Diab Res Clin Pract* 2004;64:229

Case 73

Reversal of Type 2 Diabetes by Weight Loss Despite Presence of Macro- and Microvascular Complications

CARL PETERS, MB, CHB;[1] SARAH STEVEN, MB, CHB;[1] AND ROY TAYLOR, MD[1]

A 48-year-old man was diagnosed with type 2 diabetes in July 2008, presenting with marked hyperglycemia (blood glucose >500 mg/dL) and HbA$_{1c}$ of 12.9%. He was morbidly obese at 265 lb. Peripheral neuropathy was present at diagnosis, with pain sufficient to interrupt sleep becoming severe within 3 months. Over the following 2 years, metformin and glipizide were ineffective at maintaining glycemic control and not well tolerated because of gastrointestinal adverse effects. In July 2010, insulin was commenced (insulin glargine once daily with insulin lispro before meals). Glycemic control remained suboptimal, however, with HbA$_{1c}$ ~12.5%. Access to medical services was limited for the patient, who had no medical insurance.

Diagnosis of type 2 diabetes is often significantly delayed and presentation can be years after hyperglycemia has already developed. The initial presentation can be with hyperglycemic emergencies, including hyperglycemic hyperosmolar state or ketoacidosis. The presence of neuropathy at diagnosis supports the likelihood of a prolonged period of unrecognized hyperglycemia. Difficult access to health care providers because of financial constraints often contributes to delayed diagnosis and limits treatment options for patients based on affordability. Metformin and sulphonylureas are cheap and usually effective agents for improving glycemic control. Metformin is recommended as a first-line therapy for chronic management of type 2 diabetes by the American Diabetes Association,[1] although gastrointestinal side effects may be dose limiting. Newer hypoglycemic therapies are typically more expensive and unaffordable for some patients. Insulin is an effective strategy for those unable to achieve glycemic control with alternative agents. Recombinant human insulin (regular or NPH) is usually the least expensive. Analog insulin would incur greater cost and may contribute to nonadherence as affordability is limited.

Diabetes complications progressed in 2010, including ischemic ulceration affecting the right foot and recurrent bouts of fungal otitis externa requiring multiple courses of therapy. In February 2011, he suffered a myocardial infarction. By May 2011, a left foot ulcer developed and rapidly spread over the dorsum of the foot, eventually becoming necrotic.

[1]Newcastle Magnetic Resonance Centre, Campus for Ageing and Vitality, Newcastle upon Tyne, England.

DOI: 10.2337/9781580405713.73

The association between diabetes and cardiovascular disease is profound, although its mechanisms are not completely understood. Cardiovascular disease is the leading cause of death among patients with diabetes, and there has been growing interest in primary prevention. Although trials of aspirin for primary prevention have been disappointing, statin therapy and blood pressure lowering are clearly effective and are now recommended for selected patients according to clinical guidelines and cardiovascular risk algorithms. The effect of improvement of glycemic control on cardiovascular outcomes is modest,[2] and the microvascular benefits are well proven.

Following development of the left foot ulcer, he felt his life was over, with threatened amputation and heart disease both resulting from uncontrolled diabetes. In July 2011, he came across media coverage citing evidence of reversal of type 2 diabetes with a very-low-calorie diet. Calorie intake of ordinary foodstuffs was self-reduced to 1,000 kcal/day and 2 weeks later reduced further to 600 kcal/day. Body weight at commencement of the very-low-calorie diet was 265 lb and HbA$_{1c}$ 12.8%. All hypoglycemic therapy, including insulin, was discontinued by the patient at the commencement of the very-low-calorie diet. Within 2 weeks, morning fasting blood glucose had fallen from 372 mg/dL (20.7 mmol/L) to 127 mg/dL (7.0 mmol/L) and weight by 10 lb. The very-low-calorie diet was well tolerated and continued over the following 9 weeks. No angina occurred, and there were no gastrointestinal symptoms, other than occasional hunger, which was managed with portions of salad and nonstarchy vegetables. Weight continued to fall throughout the dietary period and blood glucose levels normalized (Fig. 73.1). There were no hypoglycemic episodes.

In 2011, Lim et al. published a study testing the hypothesis that hypocaloric diet alone could achieve normalization of glucose control in type 2 diabetes. Eleven subjects with type 2 diabetes (duration <4 years) were shown to normalize fasting blood glucose within 7 days by reducing dietary calorie intake to 600–800 kcal/day.[3] This occurred at the same time as normalization of both hepatic glucose sensitivity and intrahepatic triglyceride content seen on MRI. Pancreatic β-cell function was slower to respond, with first phase and maximal insulin responses normalizing over the 8-week intervention period, again in step with normalization of pancreas triglyceride content. Peripheral insulin sensitivity remained unchanged throughout the study period. This study demonstrated that hypocaloric diet can reverse the twin pathophysiologic mechanisms of type 2 diabetes and normalize blood glucose levels, similar to the effect of bariatric surgery. Type 2 diabetes was therefore not an inexorably progressive condition as had previously been thought. The paper received widespread attention including media coverage and, consequently, many health-motivated individuals underwent the same dietary restriction by reducing consumption of ordinary foodstuffs with the goal of reversing their diabetes. The diet was undertaken at home with some suggested advice on dietary modification and patients were advised to discuss discontinuing hypoglycemic therapy with their doctor. Extensive email feedback was received and among those who communicated their efforts to the research center, 61% achieved reversal of diabetes with a mean weight loss of 14.8 kg.[4]

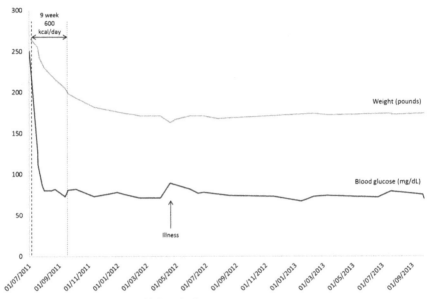

Figure 73.1—Weight and blood glucose.

At the end of the subject's 9-week very-low-calorie diet, calorie intake gradually was increased to 1,500 kcal/day and then maintained at that level for 4 months before returning to normal eating at around two-thirds of previous calorie intake. Weight loss continued for 3 months following the very-low-calorie diet and had plateaued at around 174 lb (total weight loss 91 lb) by January 2012, remaining steady over the subsequent 18 months (Fig. 73.1). No further episodes of otitis externa occurred and the foot ulceration healed completely. There was also a subjective resolution of pain in the feet from diabetic peripheral neuropathy.

It is commonly believed that very-low-calorie diets offer little success for obesity management beyond an initial rapid weight loss, as patients regain to above the baseline value, and it is poorly performed in routine practice. In 2013, Lean et al. published on a program of approximately 800 kcal/day low-calorie liquid diet performed within routine primary care supported by specialist dietitians who provided a sympathetic but firm directed approach to weight regain.[5] At 12 months, weight was recorded for 75% of patients with a mean weight loss of 12.5 kg. One-third of patients achieved >15 kg weight loss and the program was well accepted within primary care. Importantly, weight regain was avoided in this large population based group over the 12-month period.

Following the very-low-calorie diet, blood glucose remained normal over 30 months and HbA$_{1c}$ in February 2012 was 5.3% with no hypoglycemic medications and 1 year later 5.4%, again without therapy. From contemplating amputation, he now enjoys a high quality of life.

REFERENCES

1. American Diabetes Association. Standards of medical care in diabetes, 2015. *Diabetes Care* 2015;38(Suppl. 1):S1–S93

2. Holman RR, Paul SK, Bethel MA, Matthews DR, Neil HAW. 10-year follow-up of intensive glucose control in type 2 diabetes. *N Engl J Med* 2008;359:1577–1589

3. Lim EL, Hollingsworth KG, Chen MJ, Mathers JC, Taylor R. Reversal of type 2 diabetes: normalisation of beta cell function in association with decreased pancreas and liver triacylglycerol. *Diabetologia* 2011;54:2506–2514

4. Steven S, Lim EL, Taylor R. Population response to information on reversibility of type 2 diabetes. *Diabet Med* 2013;30:e135–e138

5. Lean M, Brosnahan N, McLoone P, McCombie L, Higgs AB, Ross H, Mackenzie M, Grieve E, Finer N, Reckless J, Haslam D, Sloan B, Morrison D. Feasibility and indicative results from a 12-month low-energy liquid diet treatment and maintenance programme for severe obesity. *Br J Gen Pract* 2013;63:e115–e124

Case 74

Glycemic Control in Older Adults with Diabetes and Use of New SGLT2 Inhibitors

Carolyn Horney, MD,[1] and Jeffrey Wallace, MD, MPH[1]

An 81-year-old man is seen in a seniors clinic for care of his type 2 diabetes (T2D), stage III chronic kidney disease (CrCl 55 mL/min), hypertension, and benign prostatic hypertrophy. His current medications are liraglutide 1.2 mg subcutaneous daily, metformin 1,000 mg every evening, aspirin, atorvastatin, and tamsulosin.

This patient is one of many older adults living with diabetes. The prevalence of T2D among adults ≥65 years is between 22 and 33%.[1,2] Although much of the increasing rate of T2D in older adults is tied to increasing rates of obesity and longer lifespans, several changes associated with aging, including increased adiposity, sarcopenia, physical inactivity, and impaired pancreatic islet function also are implicated. People ≥75 years have the highest rates of diabetes complications (amputation, visual impairment, and end-stage renal disease) and also have higher risks from diabetes treatment as evidenced by a twofold increase in rates of emergency department visits for hypoglycemia compared with the general population.[1]

The patient's blood pressure is 141/63 mmHg. His last glycosylated hemoglobin (HbA_{1c}) 4 months ago was 6.5%. He is up to date on his eye and foot exams, has no evidence of retinopathy, and has normal urine microalbumin levels.

In 2013, the American Geriatrics Society (AGS) released updated guidelines for improving the care of older adults with diabetes. They recommend monitoring HbA_{1c} levels at least every 6 months when individual targets are not met, while every 12 months may be appropriate when HbA_{1c} levels have been stable. Self-monitoring of blood glucose levels should be considered but adjusted depending on functional and cognitive abilities.

AGS guidelines suggest a target blood pressure of <140/90 mmHg but emphasize the potential harm of lowering systolic blood pressure <120 mmHg. Solid evidence supports the use of statin therapy up to age 75 years, and although data are lacking for patients >80 years, age alone should not be used to determine lipid management. In general, statin therapy should be prescribed unless contraindicated, not tolerated, or felt to be inappropriate because of overall health status and limited life expectancy.

[1]University of Colorado Health Sciences Center, Division of Geriatric Medicine, Aurora, CO.
DOI: 10.2337/9781580405713.74

After an initial evaluation, patients at higher risk for eye disease should have a dilated eye exam at least annually. Those at lower risk may extend their screening interval to every 2 years. Albumin levels should be checked annually unless life expectancy is limited or if the patient is already taking an ACE inhibitor or angiotensin receptor blocker. Older adults with diabetes are at increased risk of falls, major depression, and cognitive impairment and should be screened for these conditions.

Patient desires tight control and is concerned about fasting blood glucose levels in the 120–130 mg/dL (6.7–7.2 mmol/L) range. He denies any symptoms of hypoglycemia or blood glucose readings <70 mg/dL.

This patient demonstrates some of the challenges of managing diabetes in older adults, particularly balancing individual patient goals and the benefits and risks of tight glycemic control. The foundation of diabetes management among older adults remains lifestyle and diet modification.[3] In fact, intensive lifestyle modification may be disproportionately successful among older participants. The AGS guideline for glycemic control recommends a target HbA_{1c} of 7.5–8%. The guidelines, however, support an individualized approach to glycemic control in older adults based on burden of comorbid disease, functional status life expectancy, and patient preferences rather than a one-size fits all approach to HbA_{1c} goals.[3] A goal of 7–7.5% may be considered in healthy older adults if it can safely be achieved. Higher HbA_{1c} targets of 8–9% may be appropriate for older adults with multiple comorbid illnesses or limited life expectancy. Metformin is the preferred first-line agent, although dosing must be reduced for estimated glomerular filtration rate (~eGFR) 30–60 mL/min and use avoided with eGFR <30 mL/min. Sulfonylureas are associated with increasing risk of hypoglycemia with advancing age and should be used with great caution. Insulin can be used safely in healthy older adults with careful monitoring, education, and ongoing cognitive assessment.[3]

The AGS guidelines highlight the potential harms of tight glycemic control and that there is no evidence that using medications to achieve tight glycemic control in older adults is beneficial.[3] Trials of improved glycemic control in younger adults indicate that it takes roughly 10 years to achieve reductions in microvascular complications.[2–4] On the basis of this evidence, this 81-year-old patient with several major comorbid conditions actually may benefit from a slightly higher HbA_{1c}.

At his next visit, metformin is discontinued because of gastrointestinal symptoms. At his request, the patient was started on canagliflozin 100 mg p.o. daily. Two months later he complains of increased fatigue, mild orthostatic dizziness, and occasional dysuria.

Canagliflozin, a sodium-glucose cotransporter 2 (SGLT2) inhibitor, is a new therapy for treating T2D. The SGLT2 is overexpressed and overactivated in patients with T2D. This transporter is responsible for 80–90% of renal glucose reabsorption and SGLT2 inhibitors work by reducing renal glucose reabsorption, thus resulting in increased urinary glucose excretion.[5]

As a class, SGLT2 inhibitors reduce HbA_{1c} levels by roughly half to 1%, both as monotherapy and as add-on therapy.[5] These improvements in glycemic control are similar to those seen with other oral diabetes medications. SGLT2 inhibitors also have a positive effect on decreasing body weight and lowering blood pressure. SGLT2 inhibitors have a lower incidence of hypoglycemia than insulin or sulfonylureas, but they have been associated with a higher risk of both urinary (5% incidence) and genital tract infections (10% incidence), as well as with an increased risk of hypotension and hyperkalemia. They should not be used in patients with reduced renal function (eGFR <45 mL/min).

Because of his symptoms, his canagliflozin was stopped. His orthostasis and dysuria resolved. Four months later his HbA_{1c} had risen to 7.1%, and he was feeling much better.

This case demonstrates the need to balance patient preferences, individualized therapy decisions, guidelines, and evidence when managing diabetes in older adults. Having achieved an HbA_{1c} of 7.0–7.5% while avoiding hypoglycemia is an excellent outcome for this patient who preferred tight control and according to AGS guidelines that recommend less aggressive management in older adults with multiple comorbid conditions.

REFERENCES

1. Kirkman S, et al. Diabetes in older adults: a consensus report. *J Am Geriatr Soc* 2012;60:2342–2356

2. Kirkman S, et al. Diabetes in older adults. *Diabetes Care* 2012; 35:2650–2664

3. AGS Expert Panel on the Care of Older Adults with Diabetes Mellitus. Guidelines abstracted from the AGS Guidelines for Improving the Care of Older Adults with Diabetes Mellitus: 2013 update. *J Am Geriatr Soc* 2013;61:2020–2026

4. Moreno G, Mangione CM. Management of cardiovascular disease risk factors in older adults with type 2 diabetes mellitus: 2002–2012 literature review. *J Am Geriatr Soc* 2013;61:2027–2037

5. Vasilakou D, et al. Sodium-glucose cotransporter 2 inhibitors for type 2 diabetes: a systematic review and meta-analysis. *Ann Intern Med* 2013;159:262–274

Case 75

Blood Glucose Control of Patients with Hypertriglyceridemia

Henning Beck-Nielsen, DMSc[1]

O ur patient was 48 years old when she was hospitalized the first time with acute abdominal pain. Until then she had been well and had not received any medication. She had never before been hospitalized except for the birth of her two children: a daughter and a son. Her abdominal pain started in the evening after a heavy meal. The pain was located in the middle of the abdomen and extended to her back. It had continued for 2 h when she was hospitalized with the diagnosis of appendicitis. A computed tomography scan of the abdomen showed an enlarged and echogenic pancreas, whereas the appendix and gallbladder appeared normal. An elevated amylase concentration was consistent with the diagnosis of acute pancreatitis. The patient also said that she had lost 4–5 kg during the last 6 months and also had developed a tendency to fall asleep when sitting in a chair. She denied drinking alcohol regularly. A blood glucose (BG) level was elevated at 12 mmol/l (216 mg/dL) and confirmed the diagnosis of diabetes.

The patient was treated with saline infusion supplemented with potassium based on repetitive measurements of serum potassium, analgesics, and placement of a gastric tube. Rapid-acting insulin treatment was started with subcutaneous injections every 3 h based on an algorithm (Table 75.1), aiming for a BG level of approximately 6–9 mmol/L (108–162 mg/dL). BG was measured every 3 h at the bedside. After 2 days the patient had recovered, the gastric tube was removed, and she started to eat. Amylase values dropped dramatically.

Pancreatitis often develops secondary to gallbladder stones, alcoholism, or specific genetic defects. Our patient did not suffer from the two first diseases, but she told us that her father died at the age of 48 years from myocardial infarction. Whether or not he had suffered from diabetes was unknown. On the basis of that information, her pancreatitis could be hereditary.

Her plasma triglyceride (TG) concentration was measured together with plasma cholesterol, both low-density lipoprotein (LDL) and high-density lipoprotein (HDL). Total cholesterol was 6.5 mmol/L (250 mg/dL), LDL 30 mmol/L (116 mg/dL), HDL 1.0 mmol/L (39 mg/dL), but plasma TG was 52 mmol/L (4,602 mg/dl) (normal is <2 mmol/L).

[1]Department of Endocrinology, Odense University Hospital, Odense, Denmark.

 DOI: 10.2337/9781580405713.75

Table 75.1—Insulin Algorithm

Blood glucose (BG) levels are measured every 3 h and subcutaneous rapid-acting insulin injections are given based on BG values.	
BG <4 mmol/L (72 mg/dL)	no insulin subcutaneous
BG 4–8 mmol/L (72–144 mg/dL)	2 units of subcutaneous insulin
BG 8–12 mmol/L (144–216 mg/dL)	4 units of subcutaneous insulin
BG 12–16 mmol/L (144–288 mg/dL)	6 units of subcutaneous insulin
BG >16 mmol/L (288 mg/dL)	8 units of subcutaneous insulin

Plasma TG is often increased in newly diagnosed diabetes patients, but not to that degree, and therefore an inherited (familial) hypertriglyceridemia was suspected. The most common cause of familiar hypertriglyceridemia is a defect in the lipoprotein lipase (LPL) enzyme catalyzing the cleavage of TG into free fatty acids for uptake in cells, especially muscle and fat cells.[1] Therefore, the LPL gene was analyzed and a mutation in the N291S allele was demonstrated.

The diagnosis of familial hypertriglyceridemia was confirmed, and the gene defect was found in both children, but the patient's mother did not have it. This disease often leads to diabetes, pancreatitis, myocardial infarction, and, less commonly, xanthoma of the skin.[1]

Hypertriglyceridemia seems to cause diabetes by inducing severe insulin resistance in both liver and skeletal muscle.[2] The mechanism seems to be ectopic accumulation of intracellular lipids, especially as diacylglycerol, which inhibits insulin signaling. Therefore, it is important to reduce plasma TG values with low-fat, low-carbohydrate diets and treatment with statins, but most important, with gemfibrozil or fenofibrate, which specifically inhibits TG synthesis. Along with this, insulin treatment is also needed, not only because BG must be controlled but also because insulin stimulates LPL activity and thereby reduces TG values. In the acute phase, insulin treatment is especially beneficial because it takes time before gemfibrozil and fenofibrate starts working. Therefore, insulin treatment is obligatory and lifesaving.

Our patient presented with a high fasting plasma C-peptide value of 1,100 pmol/L (normal value is ~400 pmol/L), indicating severe insulin resistance; in addition, she was GAD antibody negative.

After recovery from the episode of acute pancreatitis, the patient was discharged on a statin, gemfibrozil, and insulin treatment. A basal-bolus insulin regimen with Insuman rapid (human regular insulin) and Insulatard (intermediate action insulin) at night was chosen instead of insulin analogues because the patient was still producing insulin and the risk of hypoglycemia was low (due to her underlying insulin resistance). The patient's mealtime doses were 18-12-14 units; bedtime insulin dose was 48 units of Insulatard. The doses were adjusted based on carbohydrate counting and a correction factor before each meal and at night.

Three months after discharge, the patient was seen in the outpatient clinic and presented with an HbA$_{1c}$ value of 7% (53 mmol/L). Her fasting

plasma TG had decreased to 4 mmol/L (354 mg/dL). Testing for exocrine pancreatic insufficiency was negative. Because of the risk of arteriosclerosis, the patient was started on low-dose aspirin 75 mg/day.

The patient remained well on the recommended treatment for the next 4 years. She was readmitted to the emergency department with chest pain and a myocardial infarction was diagnosed. On admission, her BG was increased to 18 mmol/L (324 mg/dL), but no sign of ketoacidosis was noted. The patient was anticipated to spend 2–3 days in the coronary care unit, and therefore intravenous treatment with insulin and glucose were started to keep her BG stable (6–9 mmol/L; 108–162 mg/dL).

Treatment of BG values in patients with diabetes during critical illness, for example, myocardial infarction, has been greatly debated. For many years, BG control was not thought to be beneficial in these situations, but a recent study showed that BG control in myocardial infarction patients improved their prognosis. Subsequent studies, however, indicated that strict control may increase the risk of hypoglycemia, and therefore a therapeutic window around 6–9 mmol/L (108–162 mg/dL) in BG levels has been suggested to be optimal.[3]

After 2 days the patient went back to her previous treatment with rapid (Insuman rapid) and long (Insulatard) acting insulin, and she was discharged after 3 days with her usual dose of simvastatin and gemfibrozil.

Elevated TG values for several years along with diabetes are a strong risk factor for developing a myocardial infarction, and therefore proper control of both variables is important in patients with familial hypertriglyceridemia.

REFERENCES

1. Overgaard M, Brasen CL, Svaneby D, Feddersen S, Nybo M. Familial lipoprotein lipase deficiency: a case of compound heterozygosity of a novel duplication (R44Kfs*4) and a common mutation (N291S) in the lipoprotein lipase gene. *Ann Clin Biochem* 2013;50(Pt.4):374–379. doi:10.1177/0004563213477393

2. Boden G. Free acid-induced inflammation and insulin resistance in skeletal muscle and liver. *Curr Diab Rep* 2006;6(3):177–181

3. Rydén L, et al. ESC Guidelines on diabetes, pre-diabetes, and cardiovascular diseases developed in collaboration with the EASD: the Task Force on diabetes, pre-diabetes, and cardiovascular diseases of the European Society of Cardiology (ESC) and developed in collaboration with the European Association for the Study of Diabetes (EASD). *Eur Heart J* 2013 34(39): 3035–3087. doi:10.1093/eurheartj/eht108

No Effect of Gluten-Free Diet in Prevention of Autoimmune Type 1 Diabetes and Other Autoimmune Disorders in a Child with Celiac Disease

Sandro Muntoni, MD, PhD,[1] and Mauro Congia, MD[2]

An 11-month-old Sardinian female infant was brought to our clinic in March 2000 for 3 weeks of diarrhea (4–5 bowel movements daily), associated with weight loss from 9.0 kg to 7.5 kg. She was naturally born at the 39th week of gestation and breast-fed until 1 month of age when baby formula milk was introduced. At the end of the sixth month, she started the weaning until the progressive onset of the diarrhea. Clinical examination showed abdominal distension and emaciation with evidence of recent weight loss, including loose skin folds (see Fig. 76.1). A complete blood count, serum iron, transferrin, and ferritin showed an iron deficiency anemia. Celiac disease (CD) was suspected. Immunoglobulin G (IgG) and immunoglobulin A (IgA) gliadin antibodies and IgA endomysium antibodies were positive. CD was confirmed by duodenal biopsy showing Marsh 3c intestinal damage.[1] HLA typing showed a DR3/DR4 genotype conferring not only a genetic risk for CD but also for type 1 diabetes (T1D).[2] The gluten-free diet (GFD) was therefore administered. After a couple of months, she regained weight and in about 12 months antigliadin and endomysium antibodies became negative. At 4 years of age serum thyroid peroxidase (TPO) and thyroglobulin antibodies started to increase with the maintenance of a normal thyroid function until 10 years of age when overt hypothyroidism appeared. Therapy with levothyroxine was started and maintained for 1 year.

When she was 11 years old, she presented with weight loss from 32 kg to 27 kg in about 1 month. Hematological analysis and clinical signs suggested not only T1D (400 mg/dL of glucose in the serum and glycosuria) but also thyrotoxicosis (tachycardia). Therefore, levothyroxine therapy was stopped and insulin therapy started. Complete thyroid function, including thyroid stimulating hormone (TSH), free thyroxine (FT4), free thriiodothyronine (FT3), together with TPO, thyroglobulin, and TSH receptor antibodies (TRAb) were determined. High values of TRAb (5.6 units/L) and of FT3 (6.58 pg/mL) and strong suppression of TSH (0.001 μUI/mL), requiring methimazole therapy, were found. Therefore, our patient developed almost simultaneously T1D and Graves' disease at 11 years of age.

Insulin therapy at 1 units/kg (about 30 units/day) was administered as follows: insulin aspart before breakfast, lunch, and dinner according to the

[1]Department of Biomedical Sciences, University School of Cagliari and Centre for Metabolic Diseases and Atherosclerosis, The ME.DI.CO. Association, Cagliari, Italy. [2]Pediatric Gastroenterologic Unity, Microcitemic Hospital, Cagliari, Italy.

DOI: 10.2337/9781580405713.76

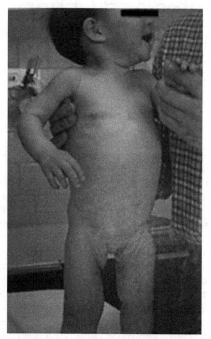

Figure 76.1—Abdominal distension and emaciation.

glycemia and isophane insulin 3–4 units at night. Methimazole was initially administered at 0.5 mg/kg/day and progressively reduced at 0.4, 0.3, 0.2, 0.1 mg/kg/day; finally, after about 18 months, methimazole was suspended and substituted with levothyroxine sodium for the onset of hypothyroidism. Both serum glucose and thyroid hormones were unstable and needed frequent adjustments. At the present time, the patient is on GFD, insulin, and levothyroxine therapy.

A typical form of CD presenting with gastrointestinal symptoms was suspected. These typical forms characteristically appear at age 9–24 months with symptoms that may begin at various times after the introduction of foods that contain gluten (in our case after only 5 months).[3] Infants and young children typically present with chronic diarrhea, anorexia, abdominal distension, abdominal pain, poor weight gain or weight loss, and vomiting. Severe malnutrition can occur if the diagnosis is delayed.[3] This case, in which the gluten exposure lasted for a very short period of time, is in contrast with a previous observation showing that the prevalence of autoimmune disorders in CD is related to the duration of exposure to gluten.[4]

The HLA typing we usually perform in CD patients and their relatives to establish a genetic risk for the disease showed a DRB1*0301, DQA1*0501, DQB1*0201/DRB1*0405, DQA1*0301, DQB1*0302 genotype conferring not only a strong genetic risk for CD but also for T1D in Sardinians.[2] Our CD patients are screened annually for autoimmune thyroiditis with serum TPO, thyroglobulin, and TSH receptor antibodies. Autoimmune thyroiditis has a frequency of 10% in Sardinian CD patients, an age of onset before puberty at 10.5 years, and a female-to-male bias similar to that reported in adults.[5] Our patient had a very early onset of autoimmune thyroiditis (4 years of age).

This case illustrates that although GFD is the most effective therapy for CD, it is not able to prevent the appearance of additional autoimmune disorders in children presenting with high-risk HLA genotypes for CD and T1D.

REFERENCES

1. Oberhuber G. Histopathology of celiac disease. *Biomed Pharmacother* 2000;54(7): 368–372

2. Cucca F, et al. The distribution of DR4 haplotypes in Sardinia suggests a primary association of type I diabetes with DRB1 and DQB1 loci. *Hum Immunol* 1995;43(4): 301–308

3. Fasano A. Clinical presentation of celiac disease in the pediatric population. *Gastroenterology* 2005;128(4 Suppl. 1):S68–S73

4. Ventura A, Magazzu G, Greco L. Duration of exposure to gluten and risk for autoimmune disorders in patients with celiac disease. SIGEP Study Group for Autoimmune Disorders in Celiac Disease. *Gastroenterology* 1999;117(2): 297–303

5. Meloni A, et al. Prevalence of autoimmune thyroiditis in children with celiac disease and effect of gluten withdrawal. *J Pediatr* 2009;155(1):51–55

Case 77

What Does It Take to Keep Glucose Normal?

Lawrence S. Phillips, MD[1,2]

T he U.S. Diabetes Prevention Program (DPP) and other studies have shown that in patients with prediabetes, the development of diabetes could be reduced by lifestyle change programs or glucose-lowering medications. After the studies ended, the cumulative incidence of diabetes in patients who previously had received the active interventions remained lower than in the control patients,[1] consistent with a change in their natural histories. Moreover, during follow-up after the end of the DPP, patients who had attained normal glucose levels at least once had a 56% decrease in subsequent development of diabetes, and the benefit was comparable in patients who had previously been in the lifestyle change, metformin, or control arms;[2] it didn't matter how normal glucose levels were attained. In combination, such findings indicate that keeping glucose levels normal may help to prevent or delay the development and progression of diabetes, and to change the natural history of the disease.

To translate such observations into practice, clinicians may wish to attempt to normalize glucose levels in some of their patients. However, there is little understanding of the management regimens that might be required. We describe three patients in whom glucose levels were kept in the normal range for a prolonged period.

PATIENT A

Patient A was first seen in 2005 (Fig. 77.1). At age 65 years, he had valvular heart disease, congestive heart failure, and atrial rhythm abnormalities, and his BMI was 27.3 kg/m². A previous HbA$_{1c}$ was 6.1%, with fasting glucose 152 mg/dL (8.4 mmol/L). With lifestyle change, repeat HbA$_{1c}$ was 5.9% with average home glucose 108 mg/dL (6 mmol/L) before meals, but up to 200 mg/dL (11.1 mmol/L) after meals; nateglinide was begun. In 2006, HbA$_{1c}$ was 5.6%, with home glucose 98 mg/dL (5.4 mmol/L) before and 121 mg/dL (6.7 mmol/L) after meals. Exenatide was begun, allowing nateglinide to be used mainly before large meals. Over several years, his BMI fell to 25 kg/m², HbA$_{1c}$ was about 5.6%, and home glucose was about 95 mg/dL

[1]Atlanta VA Medical Center, Decatur, GA. [2]Division of Endocrinology and Metabolism, Department of Medicine, Emory University, School of Medicine, Atlanta, GA.

The author is supported in part by the Department of Veterans Affairs (VA). This work is not intended to reflect the official opinion of the VA or the U.S. government.

DOI: 10.2337/9781580405713.77

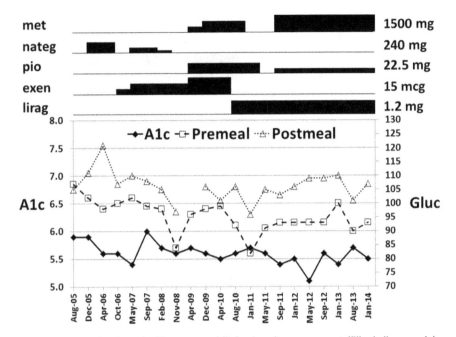

Figure 77.1 — Patient A. Shown are HbA$_{1c}$ levels as percent (filled diamonds), average premeal glucose levels as mg/dL (open boxes) based on home glucose monitoring, and average postmeal glucose levels (open triangles) recorded at office visits from August 2005 through January 2014. Above the glucose-related information, use of medications is shown by dark columns at different dates for metformin, nateglinide, pioglitazone, and liraglutide, with maximum dosages shown to the right of the columns.

(5.3 mmol/L) before and 105 mg/dL (5.8 mmol/L) after meals. In 2009, he was begun on pioglitazone (0.5–1 45 mg tablet every other day), and extended-release metformin. In 2010, he was switched from exenatide to liraglutide 1.2 mg daily. He was stable on these dosages for the next 4 years.

PATIENT B

Patient B was first seen in 2004 (Fig. 77.2). At age 64 years, she was a homemaker with BMI 36.9 kg/m² and HbA$_{1c}$ 5.9%. Attempted lifestyle change was ineffective, and in 2005, HbA$_{1c}$ was 6.2% with home glucose 117 mg/dL (6.5 mmol/L) before and after meals. Metformin and nateglinide were begun, but in 2006, HbA$_{1c}$ was 6.5%. Exenatide was begun, and nateglinide was stopped. In 2006, HbA$_{1c}$ was 5.9% with home prebreakfast

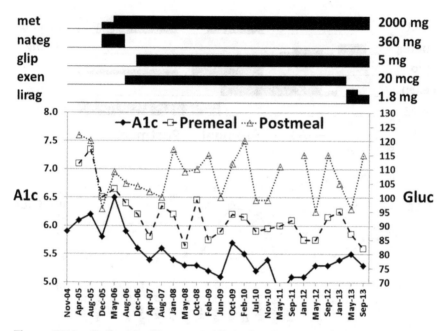

Figure 77.2—Patient B. Shown are HbA$_{1c}$ levels and glucose levels as in Figure 77.1, recorded at office visits from November 2004 through September 2013. Use of medications is shown by dark columns at different dates for metformin, nateglinide, glipizide, and liraglutide, with maximum dosages shown to the right of the columns.

glucose 110 mg/dL (6.1 mmol/L), so glipizide was added at bedtime, 2.5–5 mg to keep prebreakfast glucose <100 mg/dL (5.6 mmol/L). This regimen was maintained for the next 7 years, with a gradual fall in BMI to 30.2 kg/m², HbA$_{1c}$ levels 5.0–5.5%, and glucose levels stable. Nocturnal hypoglycemia was rare. In 2013, she was switched from exenatide to liraglutide.

PATIENT C

Patients C was first seen in 1999 (Fig. 77.3). At age 62 years, he was a physician with BMI 27.2 kg/m² and HbA$_{1c}$ 6.8%. Metformin was begun. In 2001, HbA$_{1c}$ was 5.6% with home glucose 117 mg/dL (6.5 mmol/L) before breakfast and 126 mg/dL (7 mmol/L) after meals; pioglitazone was added. In 2002, HbA$_{1c}$ was 5.9% with home glucose 118 mg/dL (6.6 mmol/L) before breakfast and 121 mg/dL (6.7 mmol/L) after meals; nateglinide was added. In 2003, HbA$_{1c}$ was 5.9% with home glucose 118 mg/dL (6.6 mmol/L) before breakfast and 107 mg/dL (5.9 mmol/L) after meals;

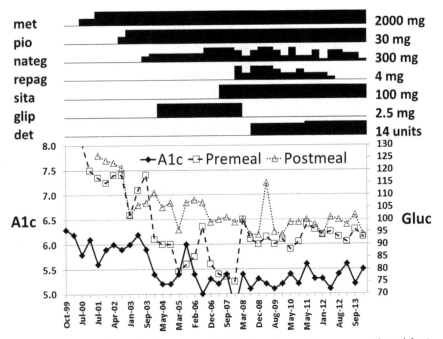

Figure 77.3—Patient C. Shown are HbA$_{1c}$ levels and average prebreakfast and postmeal glucose levels as in Figure 77.1, recorded at office visits from October 1999 through February 2014. Use of medications is shown by dark columns at different dates for metformin, pioglitazone, nateglinide, repaglinide, sitagliptin, glipizide, and detemir, with maximum dosages shown to the right of the columns.

glipizide 2.5 mg was added at bedtime. Subsequently, HbA$_{1c}$ was generally 5.0–5.5%, with home glucose <100 mg/dL (5.6 mmol/L) before breakfast and about 110 mg/dL (6.1 mmol/L) after meals. He had hypoglycemia during the night about every other month, when his evening meal was small. His weight declined gradually, and in 2006, his BMI was 23.9 kg/m². Sitagliptin 100 mg was added, with the goal of taking less nateglinide. In 2007, repaglinide was added at lunch, the nateglinide was reduced, and bedtime glipizide was stopped. In 2008, HbA$_{1c}$ was 5.4% with home glucose 100 mg/dL (5.6 mmol/L) before breakfast and 100 mg/dL (5.6 mmol/L) after meals, and detemir insulin was begun at bedtime. Over the next 6 years, HbA$_{1c}$ and glucose levels were controlled, but he had intermittent hypoglycemia after lunch, with hypoglycemia unawareness. Avoiding hypoglycemia was emphasized, and the repaglinide was reduced and then stopped. In 2014, he was taking nateglinide only before lunch, and HbA$_{1c}$ was 5.5% with home glucose 96 mg/dL (5.3 mmol/L) before breakfast and 94 mg/dL (5.2 mmol/L) after meals.

These patients' treatment was aimed at achieving normoglycemia—prebreakfast glucose <100 mg/dL (5.6 mmol/L) and 2-h postprandial glucose <130 (7.2 mmol/L) and ideally <120 mg/dL (6.7 mmol/L)—and their management was based on glucose patterns with home monitoring. To control fasting glucose, we used metformin with or without small doses of plain glipizide or detemir insulin at bedtime. To control postprandial glucose, we used a dipeptidyl peptidase 4 (DPP-4) inhibitor or glucagon-like peptide 1 (ˉGLP-1) agonist, with or without pioglitazone and/or glinides; sodium-glucose cotransporter 2 (SGLT-2) inhibitors were not available during most of the period when these patients were managed, but agents also would be useful for this purpose. In our experience, such tight control cannot be achieved with long-acting sulfonylureas, or mealtime or premixed insulin. Although "secondary failure" can be a problem with sulfonylureas or other drugs used as monotherapies,[3,4] we have not seen it with glipizide or glinides as used here. Our approach generally provides HbA_{1c} levels of about 5.5%, which in the Norfolk study were not associated with increased mortality.[5]

The management requirements of our patients illustrate what might be needed to maintain normoglycemia at different stages of the early natural history of diabetes. Our patients appeared to be ordered A earlier than B, and B earlier than C, based on their highest HbA_{1c} levels; the highest HbA_{1c} was 6.1% in patient A and 6.5% in patient B, while patient C had had an HbA_{1c} of 6.8%. Patient A was able to maintain prebreakfast glucose levels <100 mg/dL (5.6 mmol/L) with metformin, while patient B required additional bedtime glipizide, and patient C required insulin. Such needs might reflect differences in residual β-cell function.

These patients have little evidence of progression of their diabetes, and they also have no diabetic retinopathy or nephropathy. These examples show that combination therapies can be used safely to maintain near-normoglycemia for years. It might be possible to use combination therapies such as these to test the hypothesis that such a strategy can change the natural history of diabetes.

REFERENCES

1. Knowler WC, Fowler SE, Hamman RF, Christophi CA, Hoffman HJ, Brenneman AT, Brown-Friday JO, Goldberg R, Venditti E, Nathan DM. 10-year follow-up of diabetes incidence and weight loss in the Diabetes Prevention Program Outcomes Study. *Lancet* 2009;374:1677–1686

2. Perreault L, Pan Q, Mather KJ, Watson KE, Hamman RF, Kahn SE. Effect of regression from prediabetes to normal glucose regulation on long-term reduction in diabetes risk: results from the Diabetes Prevention Program Outcomes Study. *Lancet* 2012;379:2243–2251

3. UK Prospective Diabetes Study Group. Intensive blood-glucose control with sulphonylureas or insulin compared with conventional treatment and risk of complications in patients with type 2 diabetes (UKPDS 33). *Lancet* 1998;352:837–853

4. Kahn SE, Haffner SM, Heise MA, Herman WH, Holman RR, Jones NP, Kravitz BG, Lachin JM, O'Neill MC, Zinman B, Viberti G. Glycemic durability of rosiglitazone, metformin, or glyburide monotherapy. *N Engl J Med* 2006;355:2427–2443

5. Pfister R, Sharp SJ, Luben R, Khaw KT, Wareham NJ. No evidence of an increased mortality risk associated with low levels of glycated haemoglobin in a non-diabetic UK population. *Diabetol* 2011;54:2025–2032

Case 78

Psychosocial Stressors and Management in an Adolescent with Type 2 Diabetes

RADHA NANDAGOPAL, MD,[1] AND KRISTINA I. ROTHER, MD, MHSc[2]

A 13-year-old African American girl presented to the pediatric emergency department at an urban hospital with complaints of vaginal pruritus and dysuria. She also noted that she has been drinking more water throughout the day and was awakening at night to urinate for the past month. Her BMI was 39 kg/m². On examination, she was found to have severe cervical acanthosis nigricans and copious white vaginal discharge. Workup revealed a vaginal candida infection, 4+ urine glucose, 1+ urine ketones, and blood glucose (BG) of 563 mg/dL (31.3 mmol/L), but otherwise normal serum chemistries, including normal renal and liver function.

The prevalence of insulin resistance and symptomatic hyperglycemia is rising in parallel with increasing obesity rates in adolescents. Patients with type 2 diabetes represented only up to 16% of new cases of childhood diabetes in urban diabetes centers in 1994.[1] By 1999, depending on geographic location, type 2 diabetes accounted for 8–45% of new cases of childhood diabetes, with a disproportionately high prevalence among minority populations.[2]

The girl was accompanied by her maternal grandmother who reported that she herself had diabetes and was currently on dialysis; the child's 16-year-old sister was recently diagnosed with type 2 diabetes by one of our colleagues. In addition, their father was reportedly obese and had "sugar problems," while their mother's medical history was reportedly significant for gestational diabetes and obesity. Unfortunately, the mother also used illicit drugs and was only occasionally present in the children's lives. The child's older brother had recently died in the pediatric intensive care unit of the same hospital due to methicillin-resistant staphylococcus aureus (MRSA) sepsis. He had acanthosis nigricans, severe hyperglycemia, and insulin resistance associated with obesity.

A family history of type 2 diabetes is a strong risk factor for development of type 2 diabetes in children, more so than for type 1 diabetes.[2] Although

[1]Pediatric Endocrinology, Providence Medical Group, Spokane, WA. [2]Section on Pediatric Diabetes and Metabolism, Diabetes, Endocrinology, and Obesity Branch, NIDDK, National Institutes of Health, Bethesda, MD.

DOI: 10.2337/9781580405713.78

monogenic forms of diabetes need to be included in the differential diagnosis; in this case, type 2 diabetes is clearly the most likely etiology because both the paternal and maternal sides of the family are affected. In addition, gestational diabetes is a predictor of childhood overweight and obesity, which are strong risk factors for type 2 diabetes, especially in minority populations.[3]

Twice daily split-mixed insulin therapy was started for simplicity and supervision purposes, and the patient was asked to return to the outpatient clinic 2 weeks later. Her HbA$_{1c}$ at presentation had been 13.5%, and her GAD65, islet cell, and anti-insulin antibodies were negative. Her grandmother supervised her injections when possible, which was about once a day when the grandmother was not at the dialysis center. Otherwise, the 13-year-old girl was expected to check her BG and administer her insulin independently. Her school nurse had been checking her BG daily at lunchtime and had sent the report. When downloading the patient's blood glucose meter, it was noted that she had checked her BG on average less than once a day. The current BG in the clinic was 480 mg/dL (26.7 mmol/L) ~2 h after breakfast. Her lunch BG ranged from 121–475 mg/dL (6.7–25 mmol/L), suggesting sporadic morning insulin administration. When addressing these concerns, the girl appeared sullen and withdrawn. After taking her aside to speak with her alone, she became tearful and stated that she did not feel she could handle everything on her own. She thought that since her brother had died in this hospital, she "probably will too." Also, because she saw that her grandmother was on dialysis, she "figured [she] was headed there too, so why bother?" She had lost interest in activities that used to give her pleasure, often arguing with her sister, and wanted to sleep all day. She revealed that she had considered ending her life, but she did not have an active plan to do so.

Depression and anxiety are known to be more common in children with chronic medical disorders. In this child's case, her situation was complicated by a family with complex medical issues, recent loss of a sibling, tension with her other sibling, and a feeling of fatalism and hopelessness. Baseline data in youth with type 2 diabetes[4] suggest that these youths are at increased risk for lower quality of life and mood disorders as compared with other children. Adherence to medical therapy is an especially important issue in children with chronic illnesses, in particular when supervision is limited or unavailable. In this patient's case, her primary caregiver (her grandmother) had major medical issues herself requiring time-consuming therapy.

The patient was assessed by child psychiatry and admitted to the inpatient adolescent psychiatry unit at the hospital. After 10 days of intensive inpatient counseling and initiation of antidepressant medication, she was discharged to daily outpatient therapy. Child protective services were briefly involved, but she was able to return to her home and to her grandmother's care. Her state insurance did not cover ongoing psychotherapy, but ongoing counseling was arranged through a charity service. Unfortunately, she stopped attending the sessions after 2 visits, and discontinued her antidepressant medication. Her follow-up in the endocrinology clinic

remained sporadic as well, and she continued to struggle with her diabetes management.

The ongoing care and management of youth with type 2 diabetes is challenging from a psychosocial standpoint, as issues of poverty, access to care, family dynamics, and trust in the medical profession all come to the forefront. Social services are not often capable of standing in for caregivers with regard to medical adherence to therapy, and families struggle with the ongoing need for chronic therapy. Additional or alternative therapies, such as bariatric surgery should be discussed, but are controversial in light of the psychosocial circumstances.[5]

REFERENCES

1. Pinhas-Hamiel O, Dolan LM, Daniels SR, Standiford D, Khoury PR, Zeitler P. Increased incidence of non-insulin dependent diabetes mellitus among adolescents. *J Pediatr* 1996;128:608–615

2. Dabelea D, Pettitt DJ, Jones KL, Arslanian SA. Type 2 diabetes mellitus in minority children and adolescents. An emerging problem. *Endocrinol Metab Clin North Am* 1999;28:709–729

3. Kim SY, Sharma AJ, Callaghan WM. Gestational diabetes and childhood obesity: what is the link? *Curr Opin Obstet Gynecol* 2012;24(6):376–381

4. TODAY Study Group, Wilfley D, Berkowitz R, Goebel-Fabbri A, Hirst K, Ievers-Landis C, Lipman TH, Marcus M, Ng D, Pham T, Saletsky R, Schanuel J, Van Buren D. Binge eating, mood, and quality of life in youth with type 2 diabetes: baseline data from the TODAY study. *Diabetes Care* 2011;34(4):858–860

5. Nandagopal R, Brown RJ, Rother KI. Resolution of type 2 diabetes following bariatric surgery: implications for adults and adolescents. *Diabetes Technol Ther* 2010;12(8):671–677

Case 79

Suicide, Homicide, or Diabetes-Related Incident?

JOHN N. CARTER, BSc (MED), MBBS, FRACP, MD[1]

I was recently contacted by the police department from a western New South Wales town to assist in their determination of the cause of death of a 51-year-old male. The specific question I was asked was:
"Is the cause of death suicide, homicide, or a diabetes-related incident?"
The patient had been a farmhand and tractor driver who was reported missing by his partner on September 2, after she had last seen him at 5:00 A.M. on September 1. On September 29, 4 weeks after he was last seen, the owner of a sheep station 18 km east of the town where the patient lived was checking the water level of his dam when he noticed a submerged utility vehicle. The dam was 100 meters from the highway. The police were notified and subsequently a deceased male was discovered in the driver's section of the cabin. The sheep station was in the "exact opposite direction" of the route that the patient would have taken to work. The driver would have had to negotiate numerous obstacles, including several trees and channels and a fence, to reach the dam.

The police noted that the ignition key and windscreen wipers were switched on and the vehicle was in second gear. The patient was not wearing a seat belt, and he was slumped over a cooler box containing Coca-Cola, yogurt, and fruit packs.

The incident was treated as suspicious, and the man was identified by dental records. At autopsy, features consistent with decomposition and immersion were noted, but there were no obvious external or internal injuries. His serum insulin level was 14 µU/mL and blood alcohol was 0.047 g/dL, a common finding at 28 days postmortem and not necessarily indicative of alcohol intake. Severe coronary artery disease was also noted. The postulated cause of death was drowning.

PAST HISTORY

The patient had been diagnosed with type 1 diabetes at the age of 25 years (26 years' duration) and was being treated with twice-daily short- and intermediate-acting insulin. He previously had suffered from numerous hypoglycemic comas.

[1]Clinical Professor of Endocrinology, Sydney Medical School, University of Sydney, Australia.

DOI: 10.2337/9781580405713.79

His will and life insurance policies were reviewed by the police, but no suspicious factors were noted. He had a current court action against a former employer, which was described as "quite nasty," but otherwise he was not known to have any so-called enemies.

A review of his past history indicated that he suffered from an unrecognized nocturnal hypoglycemic event at least once per month. He had spent one night in jail for presumed alcohol intoxication, but he was actually hypoglycemic. He had numerous incidents when driving: on one occasion he drove directly across a T-intersection through signposts and into a fence. On another occasion he "took a bit of a turn" after cutting wood but he reported being "okay" after eating cream cakes and jubes. He then drove his car in the wrong direction, snaked across a paddock, and through trees with a branch spearing through the front windscreen and out of the back window. Six months before his death, he was reported as having a "diabetic seizure" while driving a tractor, and he had crashed into an irrigation channel.

Thus, the real question being asked by the police was: *Could hypoglycemia induce a man to drive 18 km in the wrong direction and then drive off the road avoiding various obstacles such as tree trunks, boulders, and a fence, and end up in a dam?*

DISCUSSION

Hypoglycemia can cause a clouding of consciousness in which confused, semipurposeful acts can occur. Patients in this twilight state can carry out complex automatic acts, known as automatism, for a significant period of time before either becoming unconscious or recovering sufficiently to take oral glucose. Hypoglycemia is a well-recognized cause of automatism, the definition of which is that behavior is involuntary, there is no conscious control, the behavior is inappropriate to the circumstances, the act can be seemingly quite complex and purposeful, and the individual has no recollection or only partial memory of his or her actions. Automatism due to hypoglycemia has been implicated as a contributing factor in numerous incidents, such as shoplifting, theft, assault, murder, and motor vehicle accidents. Although rare, there are numerous reports of insulin-treated subjects driving on the wrong side of the road due to hypoglycemia; this has even been noted in patients with hypoglycemia secondary to an insulinoma.

Important factors to be considered if hypoglycemia is to be implicated in automatism include the following:

1. Taking a drug known to potentially cause hypoglycemia (e.g., insulin), with the offense occurring at a time when hypoglycemia was likely in view of the known time course of the drug.
2. Documentation of hypoglycemia around the time of the offense, although this is not always possible.
3. Presence of precipitating factor(s) for the hypoglycemia, such as missing a meal or increased exercise.

4. History of mental changes during previous hypoglycemic episodes, especially if the subject had become aggressive or developed antisocial behavior.
5. Evidence that the subject's behavior normalized shortly after eating and that he/she was surprised about, and had total amnesia for, the alleged offense.

With respect to this patient, his actions on September 1 were consistent with automatism. His diabetes was treated with twice-daily intermediate- and short-acting insulin, but what dose(s) he took on September 1 is unknown. He was known to have had numerous other episodes consistent with automatism associated with driving a vehicle or tractor; he had a history of aggression, including being jailed for "being drunk" but subsequently having been shown to have hypoglycemia; and he demonstrated evidence of total amnesia for numerous accidents when driving.

From the evidence provided, it would be impossible to unequivocally rule out suicide or homicide as the cause of death, but on the balance of probabilities and for reasons summarized in this case, I believed the cause of death to be a "diabetes-related incident" (i.e., hypoglycemia-induced automatism) that resulted in drowning.

REFERENCES

1. Guide to obtaining specimens at post mortem or analytical toxicology [article online]. Available from http://www.toxlab.co.uk/postmort.htm

2. On the diagnosis of hypoglycemia in car drivers—including a review of the literature. *Forensic Sci Int* 2001;115:89–94

3. Marks V. Murder by insulin: suspected, purported and proven—a review. *Drug Test Anal* 2009;1:162–176

4. Beaumont G. Automatism and hypoglycemia. *J Forensic Leg Med* 2007;14:103–107

5. American Diabetes Association. Diabetes and driving. *Diabetes Care* 2012;35(Suppl. 1):S81

Case 80

The Case of an Older Woman with Diabetes on Insulin Pump Therapy, Struggling with Cognitive Decline, Hypoglycemia, and Loss of Autonomy

JENNIFER M. HACKEL, DNP, GNP-BC, CDE;[1] LISELLE DOUYON, MD;[2] AND JEFFREY B. HALTER, MD[3]

A woman with longstanding type 2 diabetes (T2D), received an insulin pump upon enrollment in a research study at age 69 years. At age 74 years, she began receiving primary care at a geriatric clinic where a gerontological nurse practitioner (GNP), geriatrician, and social worker saw her as a team.

INITIAL GERIATRIC EVALUATION

When the patient presented for her initial geriatric evaluation she was 74 years old. Her medical history included hypertension and T2D for 33 years, insulin therapy for 23 years, coronary artery disease, stage 3 chronic kidney disease, and background retinopathy. She denied any peripheral vascular disease or stroke. She reported good corrected vision following laser therapy in the past. She reported a mechanical fall the year before, followed by a head computed tomography (CT) scan (no acute changes), and no problems on annual visits to her private cardiologist and nephrologist.

She lives independently, has weekly contact with her children, and reports no difficulty driving, managing her pump, or remembering appointments and bills. She expressed keen desire to continue with the insulin pump, enjoying the flexibility it allowed her with her frequent social outings. Her blood glucose levels fluctuated between 50 and 350 mg/dL (2.8–19.4 mmol/L).

Her physical exam revealed an overweight, friendly, and articulate woman. Her mini mental state exam (MMSE) was 29/30. She had moderate hypertension with asymptomatic orthostasis and peripheral sensory neuropathy.

Notable lab results included an HbA_{1c} of 8.5% and serum creatinine of 1.5 mg/dL (stable for several years). Download of her meter indicated that she was checking her glucose 3.2 times daily.

The GNP referred her to the endocrinologist, who verified a low C-peptide level of 1.3 ng/dL. In the context of moderate chronic kidney

[1]University of Massachusetts Boston, Boston, MA. [2]University of Michigan, Endocrinology and Metabolism, Ann Arbor, MI. [3]University of Michigan Geriatrics Center, Ann Arbor, MI.

DOI: 10.2337/9781580405713.80

disease the C-peptide was low enough to confirm β-cell failure necessary for pump eligibility under Medicare guidelines. The endocrinologist agreed to continue the pump at the patient's request. The endocrinologist's goal was to bring her HbA$_{1c}$ in the 7% range without hypoglycemia. Over ensuing years, patient A. showed greater interest in her social life than attending to her diabetes care and refused to consider any other insulin program than her pump therapy.

FOLLOW-UP

At age 78 years, despite an increasing tendency to omit glucose measurements or use the "wizard" to calculate meal boluses, the patient's HbA$_{1c}$ declined to 7.5%. Concurrently, the patient's daughter reported concern about two episodes of hypoglycemia, which the patient denied. The endocrinologist then adjusted her insulin pump settings, and the team consulted neurology about possible dementia.

The patient scored 27/30 on the MMSE, but her Montreal Cognitive Assessment (MoCA) was significantly lower at 20/30. Brain imaging showed multiple old strokes (of which the patient and her family were unaware), comparable to previous outside films. Neuropsychological test scores were consistent with mild cognitive impairment. It was recommended she discontinue driving, but the patient refused. As for many seniors, driving was critical to her autonomy. Her children agreed to take her for a road test, which she ultimately failed.

The social worker moderated a family meeting in which the patient denied difficulty with living alone, managing her diabetes, or driving. Her children expressed inability to operate her pump. The endocrinologist was again consulted, especially in light of new guidelines suggesting it is appropriate to relax HbA$_{1c}$ goals for older adults with multimorbidity, particularly those with cognitive and functional decline.[1,2] But the patient did not want to give up her pump.

The endocrinologist justified continuing the pump, given that interrogation of the device at each clinic visit offered the team more reliable information about the patient's daily insulin dosing than the patient could report. For diabetes management data see Fig. 80.1, in which the patient's glucose log and pump download show concerning discrepancies. For instance, careful examination reveals she logged breakfast bolus insulin daily, whereas the pump readout indicates no bolus given.

The endocrinologist noted several advantages of the insulin pump. The pump uses only one type of insulin, thus avoiding dosing mix-ups. Hypoglycemia can be treated with food and immediate discontinuation of insulin. Insulin delivery limits could be programmed into her pump to minimize stacking. Most important, it would be easier to confirm adherence to her medical regimen (insulin use, glucose checks, meal times) and to see the temporal effects of meals, insulin, and exercise on glucose. She was able to

Info recorded by patient

Info recorded by pump

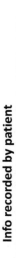
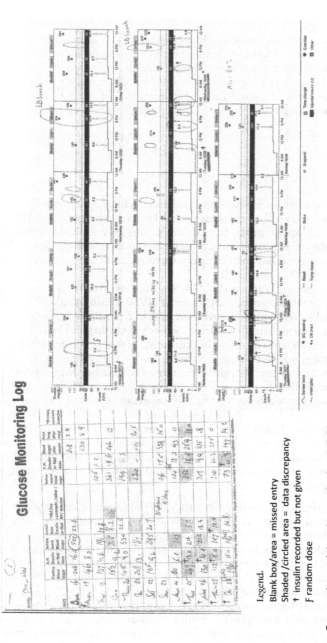

Legend:

Blank box/area = missed entry

Shaded /circled area = data discrepancy

† insulin recorded but not given

F random dose

Figure 80.1—Comparison of the glucose logbook (LB) to the insulin pump (IP) data set. The patient manually records all the data (glucose, insulin, meal) in the LB. Only the carbohydrate content of meals is manually placed in the IP. The IP glucose values (target range in gray), carbohydrate intake (black shaded area), insulin boluses (spikes), and basal rates are plotted relative to time. Exercise and other events can be added. The temporal effects of meals, insulin, and exercise on glucose levels are readily apparent. Both charts show missed glucose levels or insulin (10/16–24, 27, 29). Elevations follow missed doses. Insulin in the LB was not given per the IP (10/25–28)†. An IP insulin bolus (not in LB) appeared to be random (no paired glucose or carbohydrate) 10/17f. Data discrepancies were noted between the LB (shaded areas) and IP (circled areas). Other information not shown (regarding adherence, programmed insulin delivery, reminder alarms, infusion site changes, detailed data analysis) obtained from the IP differed from patient's reported self-management behavior. The chart findings are consistent with her history of increasing cognitive decline and loss of executive function with complex tasks. The IP provided objective confirmation of adherence (or lack of) to her medical regimen.

safely operate the device. Patient A and her family received intensive pump and diabetes education to assist her at home. Patient A has been able to maintain HbA$_{1c}$ of <8.5% with no severe hypoglycemia.

The patient is now 82 years old and still lives in her own home with her daughter, despite patient A's continued insistence that she would be fine living alone. A hired driver takes her to her social functions and the gym. A caretaker assists her 4–5 days/week when family is unavailable.

IMPLICATIONS

This case highlights several issues critical to optimal geriatric diabetes care. Older adults often have complex medical history; cognitive decline can be insidious and may not be recognized by health professionals. Strokes can be silent. Organizing safe care quickly, especially when the patient resists the involvement of caregivers, is challenging; a coordinated geriatric team is much more suitable than a single provider. Enlisting the family in the team is crucial.

Although the insulin pump is not a common treatment modality for an older adult with T2D and relaxed HbA$_{1c}$ goals, it offered a more reliable way to assess insulin use and ensure dose changes and also allowed patient A some choice in her diabetes care.

This patient's cognitive decline is not atypical for an older adult with hypertension and diabetes.[3] The MMSE, once considered the gold standard for screening for cognitive loss, is not as sensitive as the MoCA in detecting the loss of executive function commonly seen in vascular dementia.[4] Executive function is critical for determining insulin adjustments for glucose correction and exercise. Patient A's relatively good MMSE scores were even more misleading in combination with her lack of stroke-like symptoms and of lateralized findings on her neurologic exam, despite extensive old strokes on her brain imaging. Ironically, the patient's anosognosia, or lack of comprehension of her own deficits, which is not uncommon in poststroke patients, further derailed efforts to engage her in protective self-care behaviors that would have helped her preserve her autonomy.

This case exemplifies the complexity of respecting autonomy, not with an all-or-none approach, but in a stepwise fashion. Person-centered care is critical to the growing demand for geriatric diabetes management.[2]

REFERENCES

1. Kirkman SM, Briscoe VJ, Clark N, et al. Diabetes in older adults: a consensus report. *J Am Geriatr Soc* 2012;159:262–274

2. Halter JB. Diabetes mellitus in an aging population: the challenge ahead. *J Gerontol A Biol Sci Med Sci* 2012;67:1297–1299

3. Kravitz E, Schmeidler J, Schnaider Beeri M. Type 2 diabetes and cognitive compromise: potential roles of diabetes-related therapies. *Endocrinol Metab Clin North Am* 2013;42:489–501

4. Alagiakrishnan K, Zhao N, Mereu L, Senior P, Senthilselvan A. Montreal Cognitive Assessment is superior to Standardized Mini-Mental Status Exam in detecting mild cognitive impairment in the middle-aged and elderly patients with type 2 diabetes mellitus. *Biomed Res Int* 2013;1–5;186106

Case 81

Somnambulism (Sleepwalking) Caused by Nocturnal Hypoglycemia

David S.H. Bell, MB[1]

A 26-year-old white woman developed type 1 diabetes at the age of 17 years and had been reasonably controlled (HbA$_{1c}$ 7.5–7.9%) on two injections of premixed 70/30 human insulin. Some details of this case history have been previously published.[1] Because she intended to become pregnant, her regimen was changed to a basal-bolus regimen with bedtime glargine and preprandial lispro insulin: 1 unit/10 g of carbohydrate. On this regimen, she achieved an HbA$_{1c}$ of 6.1%, but achieving this level of HbA$_{1c}$ led to frequent albeit mild hypoglycemia during the day. In addition, once or twice a week, she would awake with a headache accompanied by nausea, which suggested that she had slept through a period of severe hypoglycemia.

A more serious problem was that once or twice a week, on awakening, she would recognize that during the night she had left her home because her socks, which were clean when she went to bed, were covered in dirt. She had no memory of being outside and neither her departure nor her return had been witnessed by her "heavy sleeping" husband. Since she had a strong family history of "sleepwalking," she recognized that this was the likely reason for her dirty socks. Even as a child, however, she had never been a "sleepwalker."

This patient was able to be controlled on twice daily premix insulin because even though she was GAD positive, she had residual pancreatic β-cell activity as evidenced by a fasting C-peptide level of 2.1 ng/dL. Retention of endogenous insulin production results in better glycemic control because of the ability to release endogenous insulin following meal ingestion, which reduces postprandial glucose levels. In addition, there is, with retention of the ability to produce endogenous insulin, a lower frequency and severity of hypoglycemia. As glucose levels decrease, her endogenous insulin release is suppressed, which cannot occur when exogenous insulin is the only insulin source. In spite of the protective effect of retaining the ability to produce endogenous insulin, she developed frequent and severe hypoglycemia with intensive basal–bolus insulin therapy.

Nocturnal hypoglycemia is in many cases not recognized and patients "sleep through" the event. This has been shown to be the case in even nondiabetic children made hypoglycemic with intravenous insulin. A symptom of severe and unrecognized nocturnal hypoglycemia is the presence of a morning headache accompanied by nausea, which resolves with eating. In this particular

[1]Clinical Professor of Medicine, University of Alabama, Birmingham, AL.

DOI: 10.2337/9781580405713.81

case, a rare manifestation of nocturnal hypoglycemia (i.e., somnambulism, or sleepwalking) occurred.

Somnambulism is defined as a parasomnia of non-rapid-eye-movement (NREM) sleep during which movement behaviors that normally occur only in the awake state occur during sleep. Somnambulism occurs when slow wave sleep is either prolonged or disrupted and delta-wave activity increases.[1] Somnambulism is mainly a disease of childhood but can occur in adults in which case it can be precipitated by changes in sleep schedule, such as jet lag or emotional stress, or the use of hypnotics (particularly zolpidem), sedatives, narcoleptics, and alcohol. Sleep apnea, which is very common in type 2 diabetic patients, cardiac arrhythmias, or psychiatric problems, also have been reported to cause somnambulism. As in this case, somnambulism has to be diagnosed from the clinical history as episodes seldom if ever occur during a sleep study.

New-onset somnambulism, particularly in an adult, should raise the suspicion of an underlying pathological cause. Hypoglycemia has been shown to activate arousal-related neurons in rats but not in humans. Although a sleep study of teenage subjects with type 1 diabetes did not show changes in arousal with hypoglycemia, in adults, hypoglycemia induced by intravenous insulin did show increased arousal accompanied by an increase in the amplitude of delta waves and sleep fragmentation.[2] Monitoring of interstitial glucose levels during sleep have shown that glucose levels increase during rapid eye movement sleep (REMS), which confirms that hypoglycemia is a cause rather than the result of somnambulism.[3]

Her insulin glargine was reduced to 18 units at bedtime (0.3 units/kg from the previous dose of 0.4 units/kg), which did not prevent nocturnal hypoglycemia that was being documented by 2:00 A.M. home glucose monitoring readings. When these readings were discontinued, somnambulism recurred in spite of taking precautions, such as locking the bedroom door. Only when the glargine insulin was administered twice daily (60% A.M./40% P.M.) did the nocturnal hypoglycemia and somnambulism resolve. The somnambulism did not recur, even during pregnancy, when her HbA$_{1c}$ levels were in the 4.9 to 5.5% range.

With current long-acting insulins (glargine and detemir) utilizing doses of <0.7 units/kg once daily will result in peaks that may cause hypoglycemia. Furthermore, duration of action of these insulins may be <24 h. Therefore, in many type 1 patients, these types of long-acting insulin need to be given twice daily; whereas in type 2 diabetes, for whom high per kilogram insulin doses are utilized, these types of insulin can be administered once daily, because at doses >0.7 units/kg, there are lower peaks and a longer duration of action.

REFERENCES

1. Bell DSH. Nocturnal hypoglycaemia presenting as somnambulism. *Diabetologia* 2010;53:2066–2067

2. Bendtson I, Gade J, Thomsen CE, Rosenfalck A, Wildschiødtz G. Sleep disturbances in IDDM patients with nocturnal hypoglycemia. *Sleep* 1992; 15(1):74–81

3. Bialasiewicz P, Pawlowski M, Nowak D, Loba J, Czupryniak L. Decreasing concentration of interstitial glucose in REM sleep in subjects with normal glucose tolerance. *Diabet Med* 2009;26(4):339–344

Case 82
Hypoglycemic Unawareness

Amita Maturu, MD,[1] and Neda Rasouli, MD[1,2]

A 65-year-old man was referred to our clinic for management of type 1 diabetes. He was diagnosed with type 1 diabetes at age 18 years and has developed nonproliferative diabetic retinopathy and albuminuria. His insulin regimen consisted of insulin glargine 8 units in the morning and 6 units in the evening and insulin aspart with meals (6 units with breakfast, 6 units with lunch, 8 units with dinner, and a correction factor of 1:50 >150 mg/dL; 8.3 mmol/L). He also had a past medical history of depression, hypertension, hyperlipidemia, and coronary artery disease (CAD). His family history was significant for a father with CAD. He denied any tobacco, alcohol, or illicit drug use. At the time of consultation, his weight was 100 kg. He was afebrile, blood pressure was elevated at 152/86 mmHg, and pulse was 68. His physical exam was unremarkable. His most recent hemoglobin A1c (HbA$_{1c}$) was 8.4%.

A home monitoring device download was performed and revealed frequent hypoglycemic episodes. Hypoglycemia of <70 mg/dL (3.9 mmol/L) occurred at least one or two times daily and episodes with self-monitored blood glucose levels <40 mg/dL (2.2 mmol/L) occurred two or three times weekly. Severe hypoglycemic episodes (<40 mg/dL) generally occurred at night, but occasionally occurred after exercise or following an inappropriate meal-time insulin dosing. The patient informed us that he had no adrenergic symptoms during his severe hypoglycemic episodes and was unable to self-treat his hypoglycemia. His wife confirmed that he was confused and aggressive during hypoglycemic episodes and required third-party assistance for treatment.

Hypoglycemic unawareness is defined as a severe hypoglycemia with the onset of neuroglycopenic symptoms without preceding adrenergic warning symptoms. Patients with type 1 diabetes lack the initial defense of hypoglycemia of insulin suppression and glucagon secretion, making the onset of autonomic symptoms critical to restore normoglycemia.[1] The autonomic response includes secretion of acetylcholine, norepinephrine, and epinephrine, which trigger the symptoms of anxiety, palpitations, hunger, sweating, irritability, and tremor and signal the body to ingest food. This arrests further fall in glucose

[1]Division of Endocrinology, Diabetes and Metabolism, University of Colorado, Aurora, CO. [2]Denver Veterans Affairs Medical Center, Denver, CO.

      DOI: 10.2337/9781580405713.82

that can lead to neuroglycopenic symptoms of dizziness, blurred vision, difficulty concentrating, and faintness. Patients with neuroglycopenic symptoms often fail to self-treat their hypoglycemia and require third-party assistance. If glucose continues to fall, complications can include unconsciousness, arrhythmia, and even death.

The biggest risk factor for hypoglycemic unawareness in patients with type 1 diabetes is antecedent hypoglycemia. A short episode of antecedent hypoglycemia has been shown to reduce the epinephrine levels and autonomic symptom response to a subsequent hypoglycemic episode.[2] Studies have shown that with scrupulous avoidance of hypoglycemia, subjects with hypoglycemic unawareness can regain awareness within 3 weeks. The American Diabetes Association therefore recommends raising glycemic targets for several weeks in patients with hypoglycemic unawareness to restore awareness.[3]

During his initial consultation, we spent a considerable amount of time on education about hypoglycemia and unawareness. We recommended a reduction in both his insulin glargine and aspart dose in an attempt to achieve a 3-week period without hypoglycemia to restore awareness. Patient returned for a follow-up visit in 3 months, but he had not implemented any of the changes we had made at the prior appointment. He was apologetic, but felt that the changes would cause his blood glucose levels to run too high and was unwilling to allow that to happen. We emphasized the risk of hypoglycemic unawareness and relatively safety of 3 weeks of mild hyperglycemia to restore autonomic symptoms. We again made recommendations for a reduction in his insulin doses. Unfortunately, this pattern of noncompliance with insulin dose reduction persisted for >1 year, and the patient continued to have severe hypoglycemia requiring third-party assistance and hypoglycemic unawareness.

A review of patients with hypoglycemic unawareness enrolled in a structured type 1 diabetes education program showed that at 1 year, half of the patients did not regain awareness despite a structured education program. Additionally, it has been demonstrated that patients with hypoglycemic unawareness have decreased adherence to medication changes and physician advice compared with patients with type 1 diabetes and normal awareness.[2] A role for cognitive behavioral therapy in patients with hypoglycemic unawareness has been suggested to identify and change unhelpful thoughts and incorporate motivational interviewing to minimize resistance. Preliminary results of a pilot program incorporating this strategy are encouraging, although such an intervention is not yet widely available.[4] Technology also can play a role in managing patients with hypoglycemic unawareness resistant to the standard educational strategies of hypoglycemic avoidance. Real-time continuous glucose monitoring has failed to restore awareness in adult patients with type 1 diabetes and hypoglycemic unawareness, but it has been effective in reducing the frequency of severe hypoglycemic episodes. The preliminary results of the effect of the automatic low-glucose suspension insulin infusion pumps in restoring hypoglycemic awareness are encouraging and hopefully will be confirmed by future research.[5]

At our last visit with this patient, we again spent a significant amount of time on education and recommended a reduction of his insulin dose. We then contacted him weekly over the phone to review his self-monitored blood glucose levels and to provide more education and feedback. This regular contact and encouragement has worked well in his particular case. He has adhered to the reduction in insulin doses and the frequency of his hypoglycemic episodes has reduced drastically. He is also starting to regain some awareness and has been able to self-treat his hypoglycemia.

Although it has been clearly demonstrated that scrupulous avoidance of hypoglycemia for 3 weeks can restore awareness in patients with hypoglycemic unawareness, this strategy can be challenging to implement in a clinical setting. Some patients are very resistant to medication changes and have anxiety associated with hyperglycemia. It is important to continue to educate the patient at each visit and personalize the approach to treatment in those who appear resistant to standard education and hypoglycemic avoidance.

REFERENCES

1. Cryer PE, Mechanisms of disease: mechanisms of hypoglycemia-associated autonomic failure in diabetes. *N Engl J Med* 2013;369:362–372

2. Amiel S. Hypoglycemic unawareness—from the laboratory to the clinic. *Diabetes Care* 2009;32(8):1364–1371

3. American Diabetes Association. Standards of medical care in diabetes, 2015. *Diabetes Care* 2015;38(Suppl. 1):S1–S93

4. de Zoysa N, Rogers H, Stadler M, Gianfrancesco C, Beveridge S, Britneff E, Choudhary P, Elliott J, Heller S, Amiel SA. A psychoeducational programme to restore hypoglycemia awareness: the DAFNE-HART pilot study. *Diabetes Care* 2014;37:863–866

5. Choudhary P. Insulin pump therapy with automated insulin suspension: toward freedom from nocturnal hypoglycemia. *JAMA* 2013;310(12):1235–1236

Case 83

Successful Use of Plasmapheresis in the Treatment of Hypoglycemia Due to Insulin Antibody Syndrome

Pankaj Sharda, MD;[1] Thottathil Gopan, MD;[2] Robert Zimmerman, MD;[2] and Elias S. Siraj, MD[1]

An 89-year-old man was admitted with frequent, severe hypoglycemic episodes presenting with neuroglycopenic symptoms. About 2 months before admission, he started experiencing recurrent episodes of confusion, seizures, loss of consciousness, and falls. These episodes were not preceded by adrenergic symptoms and could occur at any time, but most occurred within a few hours after meals. Blood glucose (BG) level of 30 mg/dL (1.6 mmol/L) was recorded by paramedics on two occasions, which improved after bolus injections of 50% dextrose.

Past medical history included hyperlipidemia, osteoporosis, transient ischemic attacks, and anemia. No history of diabetes, exposure to insulin, or sulfonylureas. No history of liver or kidney disease or any autoimmune disorders. No family history of autoimmune disorders. Medications included aspirin, simvastatin, and alendronate.

Physical examination was unremarkable with no vitiligo, acanthosis nigricans, or thyromegaly.

The differential diagnosis of hypoglycemia in elderly includes sepsis, chronic kidney disease, malnutrition, adrenal insufficiency, and alcoholism, but our patient did not have any evidence of these symptoms.

When recurrent severe hypoglycemic episodes with neuroglycopenic symptoms occur, additional differential diagnoses include the following:

- Surreptitious intake of insulin or sulfonylureas
- Insulinoma
- Noninsulinoma pancreatogenous hyperinsulinemic syndrome (NIPHS)
- Insulin antibody syndrome (IAS)

Although insulinomas tend to present mostly as fasting hypoglycemia, both NIPHS and IAS tend to present as postprandial hypoglycemia. This clinical distinction may be helpful to a certain degree, but the definitive diagnosis requires proper laboratory testing during a hypoglycemic episode assessing plasma glucose, insulin, C-peptide, proinsulin, and sulfonylurea assays.

[1]Section of Endocrinology, Diabetes and Metabolism, Temple University School of Medicine, Philadelphia, PA. [2]Department of Endocrinology, Diabetes and Metabolism, Cleveland Clinic, Cleveland, OH.

DOI: 10.2337/9781580405713.83

Table 83.1—Results of Initial Laboratory Tests for Hypoglycemia

Test	Reference Range	Result
Glucose (mg/dL)	65–100	21
Plasma C-peptide (ng/mL)	0.8–3.2	10.6
Plasma insulin (µU/mL)	1–24	49,261.9*
Plasma proinsulin (pmol/L)	2.1–26.8	40,450*
Serum sulfonylurea screen**	Negative	Negative

*Spurious result because of presence of insulin antibodies; measurement of free and total insulin is indicated.
**The presence of meglitinides cannot be detected in this screen, but it was thought to be unlikely.

A 72-h supervised fasting protocol was performed. BG level at the start of the fasting was 64 mg/dL (3.6 mmol/L). One hour later, the patient developed a severe hypoglycemic episode with confusion and disorientation. Bedside fingerstick BG level was 21 mg/dL (1.2 mmol/L), which was confirmed by plasma BG testing in the laboratory. Venous blood was drawn for insulin, C-peptide, proinsulin, and sulfonylureas levels (Table 83.1). BG levels improved to 55 mg/dL after administration of D-50% and glucagon.

During this episode of severe hypoglycemia, plasma insulin and proinsulin levels were extremely elevated, while the C-peptide level was elevated to a less degree. These findings speak for the presence of hyperinsulinemic hypoglycemia.[1] The presence of both proinsulin and C-peptide speak against the possibility of exogenous insulin, while the negative sulfonylurea assay rules out that etiologic possibility. Although both insulinoma and NIPHS are associated with elevated insulin, proinsulin, and C-peptide levels, the degree of elevation seen in this patient is unusual for those conditions. Insulin levels >100 µU/mL are very uncommon in insulinoma or NIPHS.[2]

Given the extreme elevation of insulin and proinsulin levels, which are uncommon in insulinomas and NIPHS, interference in the assay was suspected, and insulin antibody levels as well as free and total insulin levels were measured using polyethylene glycol (PEG) precipitation (Table 83.2). Abdominal computed tomography (CT) scan was unremarkable.

As shown in Table 83.2, the 90% insulin antibody binding (normal <5%) as well as the extremely elevated total and free insulin levels support the diagnosis of IAS. The very high insulin and proinsulin levels are likely spurious because of the interference of the endogenous IA with the assay antibody.[3] Total insulin levels depend on the binding capacity of circulating insulin antibodies and insulin availability. Insulin autoimmune syndrome (IAS) or Hirata's disease is a condition characterized by hypoglycemia associated with the presence of autoantibodies to insulin in patients with no previous exposure to insulin and no pathologic abnormalities of the islets. Since the original description of the

Table 83.2—Results of Further Workup for Hypoglycemia

Test	Reference range	Result
Insulin antibody (% binding)	<5%	90
Total insulin (μU/mL)	1–24	7,360
Free insulin (μU/mL)	1–24	1,008

condition, more than 240 IAS patients have been reported from Japan, where it represents the third leading cause of spontaneous hypoglycemia.[4] The condition, however, remains extremely rare outside Asia.

Established mechanisms for hypoglycemia in IAS include a "buffering" effect of IA, which causes desynchronized binding and the release of free insulin with respect to prevailing glucose concentration. This desynchronized behavior explains postprandial hypoglycemia, commonly seen in IAS patients, when antibody-bound insulin is released, resulting in inappropriately high circulating free insulin relative to prevailing glucose level. Other proposed mechanisms include cross-linking of insulin–insulin receptor complexes by IA, resulting in the potentiation or prolongation of insulin action, development of anti-idiotypic antibodies to IA that are capable of directly activating insulin receptors, and the direct stimulation of insulin secretion by IA.

To determine other associated autoimmune conditions, laboratory tests including serum protein electrophoresis were done. The results showed the presence of a faint monoclonal protein band; however, immunofixation electrophoresis showed normal immunoglobulin levels, but faint abnormal homogeneous bands in the immunoglobulin G (IgG) and kappa regions, suggestive of trace IgG kappa-type monoclonal gammopathy. The urine immunofixation electrophoresis was normal and skeletal survey did not show any lytic lesions.

IAS is associated with a history of autoimmune disorders like systemic lupus erythematosus (SLE) or Graves' disease, or exposure to sulfhydryl group-containing medications (e.g., methimazole). Rarely, it could be associated with plasma cell dyscrasias, including benign monoclonal gammopathies, as is seen in our patient. The majority of IA are polyclonal, belonging to IgG class, with variable kappa and lambda light chains.

The patient continued to have recurrent severe hypoglycemic events, necessitating continuous 10% dextrose infusion and intermittent 50% dextrose boluses. These interventions resulted in temporary elevation of BG to 200–400 mg/dL (11.1–22.2 mmol/L) postprandially with a precipitous drop to 30–40 mg/dL (1.7–2.2 mmol/L) 3–4 h after meals. He was started on prednisone 40 mg b.i.d. and diazoxide 50–100 mg t.i.d. Despite these interventions, he continued to have labile BG fluctuating between 30 and 400 mg/dL

(1.7–22.2 mmol/L). Hence, plasmapheresis was initiated and he underwent six sessions over the next 2 weeks. This led to significant improvement of BG levels ranging from 80 to 140 mg/dL during the second week of treatment. Dextrose infusion was weaned off after the completion of plasmapheresis with no further hypoglycemic events. The insulin antibodies decreased to 52% after plasmapheresis. Prednisone taper was stopped after 3 months. He was doing well on 1-year follow-up visit with no episodes of severe hypoglycemia.

The clinical course in IAS can be variable, with spontaneous remission seen in some within 3–6 months, whereas in others it follows a persistent course.

The role of plasmapheresis to reduce the IA titers in IAS as well as patients with diabetes who have insulin-induced antibodies has been described in the literature.[5] It is used to remove pathogenic macromolecules, such as antibodies, or immune complexes selectively from the blood. In our patient, the use of plasmapheresis was effective in treating the IAS, leading to the reduction of the IA titer and disappearance of the hypoglycemic episodes.

REFERENCES

1. Service FJ, McMahon M, et al. Functioning insulinoma-incidence, recurrence and long-term survival of patients: a 60-year study. *Mayo Clin Proc* 1991;66:711–719

2. Hirata Y, Ishizu H, Ouchi N. Insulin autoimmunity in a case of spontaneous hypoglycemia. *J Jpn Diabetes Soc* 1970;13:312–320

3. Casesnoves A, Mauri M, et al. Influence of anti-insulin antibodies on insulin immunoassays in the autoimmune insulin syndrome. *Ann Clin Biochem* 1998;35(6):768–774

4. Takayama-Hasumi S, Eguchi Y, Sato A, Morita C, Hirata Y. Insulin autoimmune syndrome is the third leading cause of spontaneous hypoglycemic attacks in Japan. *Diabetes Res Clin Pract* 1990;10:211–214

5. Yaturu S, DePrisco C, et al. Severe autoimmune hypoglycemia with insulin antibodies necessitating plasmapheresis. *Endocr Pract* 2004;10:49–54

Case 84

Postprandial Hypoglycemia, an Uncommon Presentation of Type 2 Diabetes

Muhammad W. Salam, MD,[1] and James R. Sowers, MD[1-4]

A 52-year-old white man presented to his primary care physician with neurogenic symptoms (sweating, palpitations, headache) accompanied by capillary blood glucose levels in the 40–60 mg/dL range. The symptoms would always occur 1–2 h after a meal and would resolve with ingestion of a sugar source (e.g., orange juice, regular soda). There was no history of neuroglycopenic symptoms (confusion, loss of consciousness, seizure) during any of these episodes. Patient's prior history was notable for hypertension, hyperlipidemia, and gastroesophageal reflux disease (GERD). Physical examination was remarkable for central obesity with a BMI of 32 kg/m².

Most patients with type 2 diabetes (T2D) are either asymptomatic if the diagnosis is established on routine screening or present with symptoms of hyperglycemia (polyuria, polydipsia, nocturia). A small minority, however, may present with episodes of postprandial or reactive hypoglycemia (within 4 h of meal intake). These patients typically have mild T2D or insulin resistance without evidence of overt diabetes. The symptoms are almost always neurogenic rather than neuroglycopenic in nature. The pathophysiology of this condition is closely linked with the regulation of insulin release. In normal subjects, the rapid rise in blood glucose concentration after a meal is immediately followed with a rapid burst of insulin release that lasts about 10–15 min (first-phase insulin release).[1] If the blood glucose level remains elevated, the high insulin concentration is sustained, leading to a second relatively smaller peak of insulin release lasting about 1–2 h following ingestion of a meal (second-phase insulin release).[2] A decrease in the early phase insulin secretion is an early feature of β-cell dysfunction seen in patients with impaired glucose tolerance or early T2D with fasting blood glucose in the range of 100–115 mg/dL.[3] It is hypothesized that the impaired first-phase insulin release results in supranormal blood glucose levels following a meal. This, in turn, leads to an exaggerated second-phase insulin release ultimately culminating in episodes of postprandial hyperglycemia.[4]

[1]Division of Endocrinology, Diabetes and Metabolism, Department of Medicine, University of Missouri, Columbia, MO. [2]Department of Medical Pharmacology and Physiology, University of Missouri, Columbia, MO. [3]Diabetes and Cardiovascular Center, University of Missouri, Columbia, MO. [4]University of Missouri, Harry S. Truman Memorial Veterans' Hospital, Columbia, MO.

DOI: 10.2337/9781580405713.84

The patient was prescribed a dietary regimen of frequent low-carbohydrate meals with modest improvement. During a follow-up visit, he was noted to be symptomatic with a concomitant capillary blood glucose level of 63 mg/dL. Blood work done after ingestion of 4 glucose tablets (16 g carbohydrate) revealed an elevated level of insulin and C-peptide consistent with patient's postprandial state. This, however, was mistaken as an inappropriate elevation concerning for insulinoma, and the patient was referred to endocrinology. Meanwhile, an endoscopic ultrasound (EUS) done for evaluation of chronic pancreatitis disclosed a 2 mm hypoechoic focus in the body of the pancreas. Fine-needle aspiration biopsy of the lesion was undertaken and showed inflammatory cells and fibrous tissues without evidence of any neuroendocrine tumor.

Evaluation of hypoglycemia should always start by establishing the Whipple's triad composed of hypoglycemic symptoms, a low plasma glucose measurement of <50 mg/dL, and resolution of symptoms with a rise in plasma glucose. The differential diagnosis can be narrowed based on the timing of hypoglycemia episodes. Insulinomas typically present with fasting hypoglycemia or less commonly with a combination of fasting and postprandial episodes. Exclusively postprandial hypoglycemia, however, is typically seen with β-cell hyperplasia postgastric bypass surgery (nesidioblastosis), early T2D, or less commonly in hereditary fructose intolerance or factitious hypoglycemia. The evaluation should start with biochemical testing establishing existence of endogenous hyperinsulinemic hypoglycemia (low plasma glucose, elevated insulin and C-peptide levels, negative sulfonylurea screen) before proceeding to imaging studies.

A detailed biochemical evaluation done in the endocrine clinic showed a mildly elevated fasting glucose level of 112 mg/dL. Fasting insulin, C-peptide, as well as chromogranin A and 24 h urine 5-hydroxyindole acetic acid levels were within normal limits. HbA$_{1c}$ level was elevated at 7.0%, establishing a diagnosis of T2D. The patient was started on metformin monotherapy with complete resolution of his hypoglycemic symptoms.

As expected, postprandial hypoglycemia associated with insulin resistance and early T2D tends to respond to any measure that attenuates the supranormal rise in plasma glucose following a meal. This includes lifestyle modifications, such as ingestion of small, frequent meals rich in proteins and fiber as well as avoidance of simple carbohydrates. Weight loss and exercise help by lowering insulin resistance and improving glucose utilization. If needed, pharmacotherapy with biguanide can be added and usually results in marked improvement of symptoms.[4] Experience with acarbose is limited and tolerability remains a limiting factor.

REFERENCES

1. Ferrannini E, Pilo A. Pattern of insulin delivery after intravenous glucose injection in man and its relation to plasma glucose disappearance. *J Clin Invest* 1979;64:243–254

2. McCulloch DK, Bingley PJ, Colman PG, et al. Comparison of bolus and infusion protocols for determining acute insulin response to intravenous glucose in normal humans. The ICARUS Group. Islet Cell Antibody Register User's Study. *Diabetes Care* 1993;16:911–914

3. Brunzell JD, Robertson RP, Lerner RL, et al. Relationships between fasting plasma glucose levels and insulin secretion during intravenous glucose tolerance tests. *J Clin Endocrinol Metab* 1976;42:222–226

4. Faludi G, Bendersky G, Gerber P. Functional hypoglycemia in early latent diabetes. *Ann N Y Acad Sci* 1968;148:868–871

Case 85

Factitious Hypoglycemia in a Type 2 Diabetic Patient

Stacey A. Seggelke, MS, RN, CNS, CDE, BC-ADM[1]

A 52-year-old man with a past medical history of pancreatic cancer status postpartial pancreatectomy presented to the emergency department with nausea, vomiting, and hyperglycemic hyperosmotic syndrome (HHS) on November 2, 2013. Laboratory values included a blood glucose level of 928 mg/dL (51.5 mmol/L), calculated serum osmolality of 300 mOs/kg, negative serum and urine ketones, and a hemoglobin A1c of 12%. Glucose was easily corrected with intravenous (i.v.) fluids and i.v. insulin drip. The patient was transitioned to subcutaneous insulin injections of glargine 50 units twice daily and a lispro base dose of 6 units at meals with a correction factor (CF) of 1 units for every 25 mg/dL (1.4 mmol/L) of glucose >100 mg/dL (5.6 mmol/L).

The patient reported developing diabetes after partial pancreatectomy 5 months before presentation. His home regimen was detemir 45 units b.i.d. and lispro 20 units at meals with a sliding scale to use postprandially. Patient reported blood glucose levels elevated in the 300 to >600 mg/dL (16.6 to >33.3 mmol/L) on home blood glucose monitoring. Of note, his detemir had an expiration date of March 2013 which was 9 months before admission and therefore initially was thought to be the cause of the patient's HHS.

HHS is a serious acute complication of type 2 diabetes.[1] The underlying pathogenesis of HHS is a combination of insulin resistance or deficiency and an elevation of counter-regulatory hormones, primarily glucagon. In the case of our patient, he had been using insulin that was well past its expiration date. Without the suppressive effect of effective insulin, pancreatic glucagon production increases, leading to increased gluconeogenesis and hepatic and renal glucose production, resulting in hyperglycemia. Dehydration further exacerbates hyperglycemia.

The recommended management of HHS includes the use of an i.v. insulin infusion. An i.v. insulin infusion is composed of 1 unit of regular human insulin per 1 mL of 0.9% NaCl (normal saline). When given intravenously, regular insulin has a rapid onset and short half-life, allowing for quick adjustment of insulin dose to achieve tight glycemic control. In this case, normoglycemia was quickly achieved and the patient was able to transition to a subcutaneous insulin regimen based upon the current i.v. insulin infusion rates.

[1]Adult Diabetes Program, University of Colorado Denver, School of Medicine, Denver, CO.

          DOI: 10.2337/9781580405713.85

The patient had a rapid decline in insulin requirement thought to be a result of poor oral intake. By November 2013, he had been titrated down to glargine 25 units daily with lispro remaining at 6 units at meals with a CF of 25 for glucose levels >100 mg/dL (5.6 mmol/L). On November 5, 2013, at 8:00 A.M. the patient's blood glucose level was 173 mg/dL (9.6 mmol/L) and glargine 25 units were administered with no lispro as patient was not eating breakfast. At 1:30 P.M. on the same day, patient had a blood glucose level of 38 mg/dL (2.1 mmol/L). After ingestion of 500 ml of juice (~60 grams of carbohydrates), the patient's blood glucose level normalized to 101 mg/dL (5.6 mmol/L) and remained between 101 and 158 mg/dL (5.6–8.8 mmol/L) for the rest of the day. In the morning of November 6, 2013, patient's blood glucose level was 111 mg/dL (6.2 mmol/L) at 8:00 A.M. and a reduced dose of glargine 10 units was administered. By 1:00 P.M., blood glucose level had dropped to 44 mg/dL (2.4 mmol/L). After ingestion of 750 ml of juice (~75 grams of carbohydrates) the patient's blood glucose level normalized to 144 mg/dL (8 mmol/L).

After discussion and subsequently ruling out causes of hypoglycemia (normal C-peptide level and negative vasoactive intestinal polypeptide), the patient was asked if he had any home medication with him. He denied having any medication. The patient's son who was in the room stated that was not true and located a bag of medication. Review of the medications revealed three vials of lispro insulin, two detemir insulin pens, pain medication, and sleep medication. The medications were confiscated.

Psychiatric service was consulted. On the basis of their initial interview with the patient, there was no evidence that he was purposefully mismanaging his diabetes to induce self-harm. They did note that the patient had mild cognitive delay with some difficulty understanding complex concepts, including how to accurately manage his diabetes.

There was high concern that patient was unable to use his own insulin correctly, and he may have been surreptitiously using it in the hospital, although he denied this adamantly. After confiscation of all insulin from the patient's room, he did not experience any other episodes of hypoglycemia.

Adjustment of insulin dosage to obtain factitious hypoglycemia occurs more commonly in the third and fourth decade of life and more often in women.[2] This is also increased in people who are employed in the health field and have knowledge of insulin action. Most information on induced hypoglycemia focuses more on suicide attempts than behavior-seeking events.

In our patient's case, he denied hypoglycemia events at home, took much higher doses of subcutaneous insulin at home than administered in the hospital, and stated during the initial interview that he did not want to be discharged until his abdominal pain was "figured out." Although factitious hypoglycemia can be assumed based on the patient's history, laboratory data also should be obtained to verify the diagnosis. Pancreatic β-cells produce insulin through the conversion of proinsulin to equal amounts of insulin and C-peptide. Measuring a C-peptide level can help a clinician distinguish between exogenous or endogenous insulin sources. Because insulin and C-peptide are secreted at equal rates, an elevated C-peptide level and insulin level would indicate an endogenous source of insulin. Conversely, if C-peptide is normal or low and insulin levels are elevated, the cause of hypoglycemia would more likely be from exogenous insulin.[3]

Unfortunately in our patient, an insulin level was not drawn at the same time as the C-peptide level to confirm the suspicion of excessive exogenous insulin injection.

REFERENCES

1. Kitabchi AE, Umpierrez GE, Murphy MB, Kriesberg RA. Hyperglycemic crises in adult patients with diabetes: a consensus statement from the American Diabetes Association (Consensus Statement). *Diabetes Care* 2006;29:2739–2748

2. Grunberger G, Weiner JL, Silverman R, et al. Factitious hypoglycemia due to surreptitious administration of insulin. *Ann Intern Med* 1988;108:252–257

3. Service JF. Etiology and diagnosis of factitious hypoglycemia [Internet], 2008. Available from www.UptoDate.com. Accessed 6 January 2014

Case 86

Recurrent Hypoglycemia in a Patient with Type 2 Diabetes

Pavani Srimatkandada, MD;[1] Marie E. McDonnell, MD;[1]
and Sonia Ananthakrishnan, MD[1]

A 72-year-old Somali woman was brought into the hospital for recurrent hypoglycemia, nausea, vomiting, and poor oral intake. The patient had a history of type 2 diabetes, had been on insulin therapy in the past, and more recently had been on metformin alone. A recent HbA$_{1c}$ was 6.4%. She had multiple admissions over the past year for severe hypoglycemia. The patient's family reported that she often had asymptomatic hypoglycemia at home, both fasting and postprandial.

The American Diabetes Association defines hypoglycemia as a blood sugar ≤70 mg/dL (3.9 mmol/L) with severe hypoglycemia <40 mg/dL.[1] Cognitive impairment is usually recognized with blood glucose levels ≤50 mg/dL (2.8 mmol/L); but with recurrent hypoglycemia, patients maybe asymptomatic because of an attenuated sympathoadrenal response, known as hypoglycemic unawareness. Hypoglycemia is known to predict negative outcomes, including death, in both ambulatory[2,3] and inpatient populations.[4] Death from hypoglycemia is thought to be related to triggering of arrhythmias, decreased baroreceptor sensitivity, and QT prolongation.[5]

On arrival at the hospital, the emergency management service noted a fingerstick blood glucose of 59 mg/dL (3.3 mmol/L). Despite an initial glycemic response to dextrose, the blood glucose continued to drop. On arrival at the emergency department, the plasma glucose was 38 mg/dL (2.1 mmol/L), and there was mild alteration in alertness. Again after initial improvement in mental status and glucose level with 12.5 mL of intravenous (i.v.) dextrose 50%, she continued to have hypoglycemia on the medical floor. Continuous dextrose 10% infusion was begun. Despite avoidance of insulin and all hypoglycemic agents in the hospital, the patient continued to have recurrent hypoglycemia during her hospitalization. The initial differential diagnosis by the team included poor nutritional status with low glycogen stores, sepsis secondary to urinary tract infection, and occult malignancy. The patient's prescription medication list was noncontributory, and her pharmacy confirmed she had not picked up insulin or secretagogue medications in >6 months. Renal and liver functions were normal.

[1]Boston University School of Medicine, Section of Endocrinology, Diabetes, Nutrition and Weight Management, Boston, MA.

DOI: 10.2337/9781580405713.86

The most common cause of hypoglycemia among patients presenting to the hospital is medication related.[6] Other causes of hypoglycemia include insulinoma, nesidioblastosis, noninsulinoma pancreatogenous hypoglycemia syndrome (NIPHS), and insulin autoimmune hypoglycemia. Causes not mediated by endogenous hyperinsulinemia, which may stem from altered glycogenolysis or gluconeogenesis, include liver and renal disease, sepsis, adrenal insufficiency, and islet cell tumors producing IGF-II.[5] Historical factors related to timing of the hypoglycemia (e.g., either fasting or postprandially) can sometimes assist in elucidating the diagnosis, although this classification is now considered unreliable.

Baseline adrenocortotropic hormone (ACTH) was 49 pg/mL and cortisol was 12.9 μg/dL. Sixty minutes after cosyntropin administration, the cortisol was 27.8 μg/dL, effectively ruling out adrenal insufficiency. A comprehensive plasma screen for sulfonylurea and glinide medications was negative.

Two days after i.v. fluids containing dextrose were discontinued, the patient had an episode of hypoglycemia to 46 mg/dL (2.6 mmol/L) noted on random fingerstick. Plasma glucose at that time was 59 mg/dL (3.3 mmol/L), insulin >600 μU/mL, C-peptide 1.39 ng/mL, proinsulin 17.1 pmol/L. β-Hydroxybutyrate was <0.04 mmol/L, indicating that insulin was present. Insulin antibody was undetectable, making insulin autoimmune hypoglycemia unlikely. Insulin growth factor 2 (somatomedin A) was not elevated, ruling out paraneoplastic syndrome described in large squamous cell tumors. The insulin level was further evaluated with mass spectrometry analysis, which revealed levels >300 μIU/mL and the presence of only human-type insulin. Human-type insulin suggested either endogenous or synthetic human regular insulin, which is a polypeptide structure identical to human insulin. Synthetic insulin analogs were not detected.

Service noted hypoglycemia (plasma glucose ≤45 mg/dL) associated with insulin ≥21 pmol/L, and higher levels of C-peptide ≥0.6 ng/mL and proinsulin ≥5 pmol/L was almost always diagnostic of an endogenous hyperinsulinemic state.[6] It appears that ~35% of patients with known endogenous hyperinsulinemic states had more subtle increases in insulin levels ≤21 pmol/L during documented episodes of hypoglycemia. In addition, plasma glucose levels between 45 and 59 mg/dL often had conflicting values of C-peptide and insulin, making it difficult to interpret the data at hand. This is especially true outside of a formally conducted fast, which this patient had not undergone. Proinsulin levels were the best method to diagnose endogenous hyperinsulinemic states, with levels >22 pmol/L being 98% specific for endogenous hyperinsulinemia. In this patient, given very high elevations of human-type serum insulin with low and normal levels of C-peptide and proinsulin, surreptitious exogenous human regular insulin was suspected.

Given the sociolegal implications of suspecting exogenous insulin administration, to further rule out other endogenous insulin-mediated causes, the patient underwent a formal 72-h fast under direct supervision by hospital staff assigned to her bedside (Table 86.1). She completed a full 72-h period, at which time the plasma glucose was 53 mg/dL (2.9 mmol/L). The lowest

Table 86.1—Results of a 72-h Fast

Time	Fingerstick	Plasma (mg/dL)	Insulin (µU/mL)	C-peptide (ng/mL)	Proinsulin (pmol/L)
9:20 A.M.	149	142	8	2.3	35.3
4 P.M.	110	114	3	1.26	24.4
11 P.M.	134	130	2	0.89	16
6 A.M.	—	136	3	1.04	15.1
1 P.M.	95	106	2	0.98	16.6
7 P.M.	92	83	2	0.55	10.0
1 A.M.	78	62	<1.0	0.31	<5.0
7 A.M.	67	59	2	0.46	6.0
10 A.M.	—	66	2	0.58	7.7
1 P.M.	67	57	2	0.55	7.7
4 P.M.	—	54	2	0.52	6.8
7 P.M.	—	61	2	0.46	6.8
1 A.M.	—	56	<1.0	0.26	6.5
7 A.M.	—	49	1	0.28	<5.0
End	—	53	2	0.29	6.3

plasma glucose documented during the fast was 49 mg/dL (2.7 mmol/L) at hour 70. During episodes of plasma glucose <70 mg/dL (3.9 mmol/L), the patient remained asymptomatic and all insulin values were <2 µU/mL and C-peptide levels were <0.6 ng/mL. The patient was administered glucagon at the end of the fast: 10, 20, and 30 min after receiving glucagon, her plasma glucose was 56, 57, and 59 mg/dL (~3.3 mmol/L), respectively, suggesting a lack of glycogen retention in the liver and further refuting the possibility of an endogenous hyperinsulinemic state.

The patient had a negative 72-h fast test with normal insulin and C-peptide levels at the end of the fast. Perhaps of greatest significance, she did not respond to glucagon administration. β-Hydroxybutrate was appropriately elevated at 5.77 mmol/L at the end of the fast. She was determined to have been administered exogenous human regular insulin before admission and during the hospitalization, and the family was suspected. The appropriate authorities were contacted and the patient was discharged under state-issued supervision.

This case exemplifies how factitious hypoglycemia can be difficult to confirm, and it often leads to excess testing and imaging; in some extreme cases, pancreatic exploration and resection have been performed. With proper laboratory testing and interpretation, however, the diagnosis usually can be determined.

REFERENCES

1. American Diabetes Association. Standards of medical care in diabetes, 2015. *Diabetes Care* 2015;38(Suppl. 1):S1–S93

2. The Action to Control Cardiovascular Risk in Diabetes Study Group. Effect of intensive glucose lowering in type 2 diabetes. *N Engl J Med* 2008;358:2545–2559

3. Duckworth W, Abraira C, Moritz T, Reda D, Emanuele N, Reaven PD, Zieve FJ, Marks J, Davis SN, Hayword R, Warren SR, Goldman S, McCarren M, Vitek ME, Henderson WG, Huang GD. Glucose control and vascular complications in veterans with type 2 diabetes. *N Engl J Med* 2009;360:129–130

4. Turchin A, Matheny ME, Shubina M, Scanlon JV, Greenwood B, Pendergrass ML. Hypoglycemia and clinical outcomes in patients with diabetes hospitalized in the general ward. *Diabetes Care* 2009; 32(7):1153–1157

5. Rubin DJ, Golden SH. Hypoglycemia in non-critically ill, hospitalized patients with diabetes: evaluation prevention, and management. *Hospital Practices* 2013;41(1):109–116

6. Service FJ. Hypoglycemia disorders. *N Engl J Med* 1995;1144–1152

Case 87

Munchausen Syndrome: Hypoglycemia in an Obese Woman with Type 2 Diabetes

R. Paul Robertson, MD[1]

A 53-year-old woman presented to the emergency department (ED) accompanied by her husband and her six children. She complained of recurrent hypoglycemia and reported another episode earlier in the evening just before dinner. This event was accompanied by weakness, rapid heart rate, feeling of warmth and anxiety, and mild confusion. Her husband obtained a capillary blood glucose level of 40 mg/dL. She was tired afterward but otherwise felt fine. The ED nurse obtained a point-of-care blood glucose reading of 235 mg/dL (13.1 mmol/L). The ED resident took her history and noted her medicines included glyburide, metformin, and regular insulin. His physical examination revealed a very obese woman standing 5 feet 6 inches tall weighing 264 lb (BMI 42.6 kg/m^2) with normal vital signs. Most of the exam was normal except for excessive facial hair, mild facial acne, and abdominal striae. Her muscle strength was moderately strong. The patient and family were sent back to the waiting room while the resident conferred with his attending physician. Because it was a very busy evening in the ED, the patient had to wait >3 h before the resident could return. While waiting, she visited the restroom and read magazines; her children and husband played cards. The resident returned and informed the patient he had not found any clear reason for the hypoglycemic episode, but he would order lab tests to check her urine and blood and arrange for a visit to the endocrinology clinic in 6 weeks for follow-up. The resident noted the patient seemed dissatisfied and, in fact, became somewhat distant. She started fanning herself with a magazine, complained of feelings of warmth, started to perspire, and turned to her husband saying "Get the glucometer. Honey, it's happening again." Her glucose was 35 mg/dL. The resident drew a blood sample, started an intravenous (i.v.) infusion of 10% glucose, and admitted her to the hospital.

The differential diagnosis of hypoglycemia includes excessive insulin secretion by tumors, chiefly insulinomas; adrenal insufficiency; circulating antibodies to insulin or insulin receptors; and by far the most common, overuse of drugs that stimulate insulin secretion, such as sulfonylureas, or insulin itself. The work-up for insulinoma is extensive and complicated. It initially

---

[1]Professor of Medicine, University of Minnesota, Professor of Medicine and Pharmacology, University of Washington, President Emeritus and Principal Investigator, Pacific Northwest Diabetes Research Institute.

DOI: 10.2337/9781580405713.87

involves a 72-h fast to document hypoglycemia and measurements of insulin and C-peptide as well as circulating antibodies to endogenous insulin and insulin receptors. If the results warrant further study, radiologic studies of the pancreas are performed to search for a β-cell tumor. The approach to diagnosing iatrogenic hypoglycemia is the most complicated diagnostic pursuit because the patient is the person primarily in change of taking the medicines. Testing for levels of hypoglycemia-inducing drugs and simultaneous measurements of plasma insulin and C-peptide during a hypoglycemic episode are key strategies.

In the hospital, the patient was visited by two consulting physicians. The endocrinologist found her sitting up in bed saying she felt fine and that she had had no more hypoglycemic episodes over the night. He was struck by the fact that the husband and all six children stayed overnight with the patient. He also discovered that the father worked long hours six days weekly and could not provide much information. The six children expressed varying levels of concern. One of them, a bright girl in the tenth grade, was very interested in science. She had looked up hypoglycemia on the Internet and was certain her mother had an insulinoma and wondered when she was going to get a computed tomography scan. The endocrinologist reviewed the available lab data, noting that the insulin and C-peptide values from the evening before were still pending. He suggested that no further tests be performed and that a psychiatrist be consulted. The psychiatrist found nothing unusual in his interview but did note the patient felt generally unappreciated by her family even though she worked very hard accommodating their individual schedules and serving as overall manager of the family. The psychiatrist asked her directly whether she was overdosing her medicines. She looked him in the eye with a slight smile and said, "No."

The psychiatrist was asked to see the patient because the endocrinologist was suspicious of the family interactions, suspecting the mother was overdosing on insulin to gain attention. He found in the ED nursing report that the mother had left the family to go to the restroom 3 h before her ED glucose level of 35 mg/dL and suspected she had given herself an injection of regular insulin. His working diagnosis was Munchausen's syndrome.[1-3] The next day, the urine screen showed reasonable levels of glyburide; the plasma insulin level was reported as too high to measure; and the plasma C-peptide was nonmeasureable. No insulin or insulin receptor antibodies were found.

The endocrinologist revisited the patient to explain the test results. He told her they could mean only one thing: her hypoglycemia in the ED was caused by an insulin injection because C-peptide was totally suppressed, which ruled out an insulin-producing tumor, and would be consistent with exogenous insulin, which contains no C-peptide. He asked her whether it was possible anyone in the family might be giving her excessive insulin doses, including herself. She flatly said, "No." The endocrinologist said, "Well, then, I need you to help me out. I have a major problem because I cannot think of any other explanation. I would like you to think about how you put all this together, and then we will chat again tomorrow afternoon."

The endocrinologist took the approach of indirectly letting the patient know he thought someone was manipulating her blood glucose and causing hypoglycemia. He did not flatly accuse her, hoping she might acknowledge her behavior as a starting point to correcting the psychopathology. On rounds the next day, he discovered she was not in her room and that she had signed out of the hospital. He was gratified to learn she had arranged for an appointment in the psychiatry clinic in 2 weeks.

REFERENCES

1. Spiro HR. Chronic factitious illness. Munchausen's syndrome. *Arch Gen Psychiatry* 1968;18:569–579

2. Reich P, Gottfried LA. Factitious disorders in a teaching hospital. *Ann Intern Med* 1983;99:240–247

3. Krahn LE, Li H, O'Connor MK. Patients who strive to be ill: factitious disorder with physical symptoms. *Am J Psychiatry* 2003;160:1163–1168

Case 88

The Use of Medical Technologies for the Reduction of Hypoglycemia in Type 1 Diabetes: Technology for Hypoglycemia Reduction

Viral N. Shah, MD;[1] Aaron W. Michels, MD;[1,2] and Satish K. Garg, MD[1–3]

A 37-year-old man, with type 1 diabetes for 17 years and celiac disease for 8 years, is physically very active at work (5 days/week, working in a warehouse in the morning shift between 5:00 A.M. to 1:00 P.M.). His BMI (24.8 kg/m²) is normal. He has maintained good glycemic control (A1C ranging from 7 to 7.8%) in the past 17 years with mean A1C of 7.2%. He does not have micro- or macrovascular complication. His lipid profile, thyroid stimulating hormone (TSH), and renal function are normal.

Since he was diagnosed, he has been treated with multiple daily injections of insulin, most recently with glargine and lispro. He does not follow carbohydrate counting and tries to adhere to a gluten-free diet as much as possible. He has had multiple episodes of hypoglycemia (nocturnal and daytime, especially after lunch and before dinner) resulting in several visits to the emergency room over the past 10 years.

The prevalence of type 1 diabetes (T1D) is increasing globally.[1] The Diabetes Control and Complication Trial and the Epidemiology of Diabetes Interventions and Complications Study demonstrated that intensive insulin therapy reduces micro- and macrovascular complications but increases the risk of severe hypoglycemia.[2] Hypoglycemia remains the major obstacle for achieving glycemic targets in T1D patients. Meal content, exercise duration and intensity, and insulin timing are helpful in reducing hypoglycemic events. Furthermore, the use of newer technologies, such as insulin pumps and continuous glucose monitors (CGMs) alone or in combination have been shown to reduce hypoglycemia.[3] This patient with long-standing T1D is able to achieve good A1C values, but at the cost of recurrent severe hypoglycemia. Blood glucose meter downloads document several such episodes (data not shown). The physical nature of his job adds risk for hypoglycemia during the day and lasting through the night. Because he continued to have hypoglycemic episodes, a CGM was initiated.

Fig. 88.1 shows 10 days of CGM use with several episodes of hypoglycemia (defined as blood glucose <70 mg/dL; 3.9 mmol/L). He tries to use CGM most of the time, but the use has been limited in the past because of

[1]Barbara Davis Center for Diabetes, University of Colorado Denver, Aurora, CO.
[2]Departments of Internal Medicine and Pediatrics, School of Medicine, University of Colorado, Denver, Aurora, CO. [3]Editor-in-Chief, *Diabetes Technology and Therapeutics*, Aurora, CO.

DOI: 10.2337/9781580405713.88

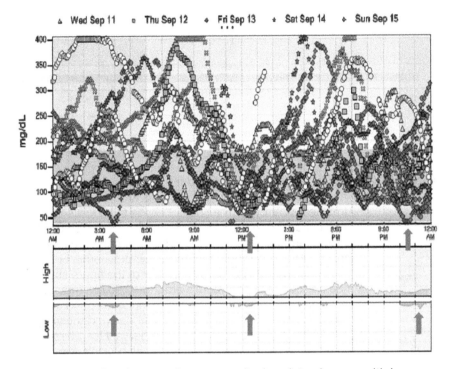

△ Wed Sep 11　　◻ Thu Sep 12　　✦ Fri Sep 13　　★ Sat Sep 14　　◆ Sun Sep 15

Figure 88.1 — Continuous glucose monitoring data shows multiple episodes of hypoglycemia (depicted by arrows) at night, after meals, and before dinner.

poor insurance coverage. He continued to have severe hypoglycemia 4% of the time despite the use of CGM in the past 1 year.

Severe nocturnal hypoglycemia can be life-threatening in patients with T1D. More than half of hypoglycemic episodes occur during the night, with 75% of hypoglycemic seizures and 4–6% of deaths attributed to nocturnal hypoglycemia in younger individuals with T1D.[4] Hypoglycemia may be associated with increased risk for cardiovascular events. In addition, hypoglycemia triggers release of catecholamine and inflammatory markers such as leukotrienes, interleukin (IL)-6, IL-8, tumor necrosis factor-α, endothelin-1, and platelet dysfunction.

Our subject experienced a significant reduction in the severe hypoglycemic episodes with modest reduction of HbA_{1c} value (7.1%) with the use of CGM. Continued visits to the emergency room prompted us to initiate the sensor-augmented insulin pump with threshold suspend (TS) in this subject.

In follow-up 20 days after initiating the TS pump, there was a significant decrease in hypoglycemic episodes. Most often, the subject corrected his

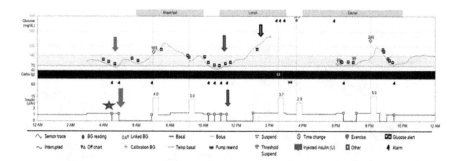

Figure 88.2A —A 24-h Care-Link download from the insulin pump
revealed episodes of hypoglycemia around 4:30 A.M.
(marked as arrows). The subject chose to have a snack
and cancel TS to suspend insulin delivery (marked as star).
After alarms continue, he allows the pump to suspend
insulin for 2 h without any further hypoglycemia or late
rebound hyperglycemia. The center of the figure shows
the episode of hypoglycemia around 10:00 A.M. (marked as
arrows), but he did not allow the pump to suspend the
insulin delivery. Hypoglycemia continues and the subject
allows the pump to suspend insulin delivery for 1 h resulting
in rebound hyperglycemia (marked as a black arrow).

hypoglycemia when alarmed by the sensor, or allowed the pump to suspend
insulin delivery using TS. The pump download on day 10 is shown in Fig.
88.2A. There was an episode of hypoglycemia starting around 4:30 A.M.
while he was asleep, but the alarm woke him up. He chose to have a snack
and canceled suspension of insulin delivery. Because his hypoglycemia continued, he then allowed the pump to suspend insulin for 2 h, and did not
have further hypoglycemia or late rebound hyperglycemia. Later that day, he
had another episode of hypoglycemia at 10:00 A.M., but he did not allow the
pump to suspend insulin delivery. Hypoglycemia continued and the subject
allowed the pump to suspend insulin delivery for 1 h, resulting in rebound
hyperglycemia.

Fig. 88.2B is a pump download from a different subject highlighting the
benefit of a TS pump in mitigating hypoglycemia at night without significant hyperglycemia. The subject was sleeping throughout the episode of
hypoglycemia.

In the sensor-augmented insulin pump with threshold suspend system, the
pump shuts off insulin delivery for 2 h if hypoglycemia is not acknowledged by
the patient. Patients, however, can override the alarm and TS to continue insulin
delivery. The Threshold Based Insulin-Pump Interruption for Reduction of
Hypoglycemia (ASPIRE) study showed that sensor-augmented insulin-pump
therapy with the TS feature reduced area under the curve (AUC) for nocturnal

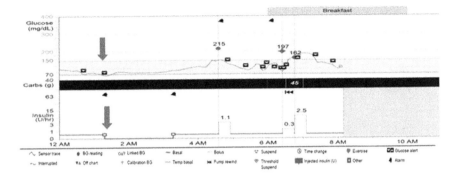

Figure 88.2B — The overnight glucose reading from another subject highlighting an episode of noctural hypoglycemia (the subject slept through the episode) mitigated by the suspension of insulin delivery by the pump without significant hyperglycemia.

hypoglycemia by 37% without any significant change in A1C levels.[5] The U.S. Food and Drug Administration (FDA) recently approved the use of the TS pump in patients with T1D, which has been available in Europe for the past 4 years. These two subjects using sensor-augmented pumps with the TS feature documented reduction in hypoglycemia with the use of the system.

The TS system is the first step in making a complete artificial pancreas (closed-loop system). Future steps in closing the loop include *1)* the use of predictive alarms and glucose threshold to suspend insulin delivery before hypoglycemia occurs, *2)* insulin delivery if the sensor glucose level is >180 mg/dl, *3)* a fully automated system in which the insulin is delivered as per sensor glucose levels, and *4)* use of glucagon or amylin along with insulin by the same pump (dual hormone closed-loop system). The use of technology like CGM and the insulin pump with the TS system reduces the severity and duration of hypoglycemia.

REFERENCES

1. Atkinson MA, Eisenbarth GS, Michels AW. Type 1 diabetes. *Lancet* 2013; 383:69–82

2. Nathan DM. DCCT/EDIC Research Group. The diabetes control and complications trial/epidemiology of diabetes interventions and complications study at 30 years: overview. *Diabetes Care* 2014;37:9–16

3. Bergenstal RM, Tamborlane WV, Ahmann A, Buse JB, Dailey G, Davis SN, et al. Effectiveness of sensor-augmented insulin-pump therapy in type 1 diabetes. *N Engl J Med* 2010;363(4):311–320

4. Seaquist ER, Anderson J, Childs B, Cryer P, Dagogo-Jack S, Fish L, et al. Hypoglycemia and diabetes: a report of a workgroup of the American Diabetes Association and the Endocrine Society. *J Clin Endocrinol Metab* 2013;98(5):1845–1859

5. Bergenstal RM, Klonoff DC, Garg SK, Bode BW, Meredith M, Slover RH, et al. Threshold-based insulin-pump interruption for reduction of hypoglycemia. *N Engl J Med* 2013;369(3):224–232

Case 89

Reversal of Insulin-Requiring Type 2 Diabetes and Development of Hypoglycemia in a Morbidly Obese Patient

DAVID S.H. BELL, MB[1]

A 50-year-old morbidly obese African American man was in good health until age 38 years when he was diagnosed as having heart failure resulting from severe hypertension. Some details of this case have been published previously.[1] He had no family history of diabetes and at age 40 years, when he weighed 166 lb (BMI 23 kg/m²), he had a normal glucose tolerance test. After age 40 years, for unknown reasons, his weight increased to 275 lb (BMI 37.5 kg/m²), and at age 43 years, type 1 diabetes was diagnosed based on a random serum glucose of 684 mg/dL accompanied by ketonemia and a metabolic acidosis (pH 7.3, PCO_2 26 mmHg, and bicarbonate 15 mEq/L). Because of the laboratory findings, he was admitted to the hospital where the ketoacidosis was treated. Because of this episode of ketoacidosis, he was assumed to have type 1 diabetes and was discharged on twice-daily NPH and regular insulin.

Because of ketoacidosis, the patient was assumed to have type 1 diabetes. If his C-peptide level had been measured at that time, it probably would have been in the normal range or even elevated. In addition, a glutamic acid decarboxylase antibody would have been negative, indicating that in spite of the ketoacidosis, the patient had type 2 and not type 1 diabetes. Especially in the African American population the stress of an illness such as a myocardial infarction (due to high stress hormone levels) or an infection (due to high cytokine levels) can, by increasing insulin resistance, result in ketoacidosis. Following the resolution of the illness, resistance to insulin decreases, and many of these ketoacidotic patients can be treated with oral agents.

Over the next 4 years, there were numerous hospital admissions for chest pain, heart failure, and urinary tract infections. During these admissions, in spite of large doses of insulin, serum glucose levels were often >300 mg/dL (16.7 mmol/L), and these high levels of glycemia did not drop until the precipitating cause of the severe insulin resistance had improved or resolved. Over this time, he continued to gain weight.

At age 49 years, he was hospitalized with a urethral stricture; on that occasion, however, while on his usual dose of insulin and a low-calorie diet, his serum glucose levels dropped to <50 mg/dL (2.8 mmol/L). His insulin therapy was discontinued and his serum glucose levels on diet alone were

[1]University of Alabama, Birmingham, AL.

DOI: 10.2337/9781580405713.89

between 90 and 120 mg/dL (5–6.7 mmol/L). He was not started on oral hypoglycemic agents and was discharged on only a low-calorie diet.

The logical conclusion for his diabetes being managed with diet alone was that due to a low-calorie diet in the absence of infection or stress, the resistance to insulin was lower and his endogenous insulin production was sufficient to maintain glycemic control. This hypothesis was only partially correct.

Following discharge from the hospital, his glucose readings remained normal without insulin or oral hypoglycemic agents. For the first 2 months, he felt well although he did not adhere to his low-calorie diet and continued to gain weight. After 2 months, however, he regularly became confused between 3:00 and 5:00 A.M. His wife recognized that his symptoms were due to hypoglycemia and administered orange juice, after which his confusion resolved. The frequency and severity of the nocturnal confusion increased and finally the confusion was so severe that his wife was unable to administer orange juice and called an ambulance. When he entered the hospital emergency room, he was found to have a blood glucose level of 22 mg/dL (1.2 mmol/L). On admission to the hospital, the intravenous glucose started in the emergency room was discontinued, the patient was fasted, and within 5 h his serum glucose dropped again to 28 mg/dL (1.6 mmol/L). At this glucose level, serum insulin should have been very low or undetectable, but it was high at 264 pmol/L, indicating the patient had hyperinsulinemic hypoglycemia.

Hyperinsulinemic hypoglycemia could have been the result of surreptitious administration of insulin in which case endogenous insulin would have suppressed. It was not, however, because the concomitant C-peptide level was 3.7 nmol/L. In addition, utilization of sulfonylureas was ruled out with a negative urine screen for sulfonlyureas. Other possible causes of hypoglycemia were ruled out with normal hepatic, thyroid, and renal function and normal cortisol, growth hormone, and glucagon levels. On the basis of this data, a pancreatic etiology for his hyperinsulinemic hypoglycemia was sought.

Ultrastenography and a computed tomography scan did not identify a pancreatic lesion. A celiac angiogram, however, showed a "blush" in the tail of the pancreas, suggesting an insulinoma in that area. During an exploratory laparotomy, a pancreatic mass was not identified and a subtotal pancreatectomy, including the tail of the pancreas where most insulin-producing β-cells are located, was performed.

Pathological evaluation of the excised pancreas showed no evidence of pancreatitis and an increase in the total number of islets, which were enlarged, varied in size and shape, and showed nuclear pleomorphism. Adjacent to the pancreatic ducts islet, cell neoformation was noted and atypically shaped islets were seen in the peripancreatic fat and pancreatic fibrous septa. All of these features are characteristic of nesidioblastosis.[1]

Although the diagnosis of nesidioblastosis is well accepted in children, it is controversial in adults. Nesidiolastosis is defined as a form of acquired hyperinsulinism associated with β-cell hyperplasia and with a characteristic microscopic appearance of β-cells budding from the ductal epithelium, and with islet cell dysplasia.[2] Multiple cases of nesidiolastosis have been described in adults, but few of these have been described in patients with diabetes. Furthermore, an insulinoma rarely if ever occurs in either type 1 or type 2 diabetes. Recently following Roux-en-Y gastric bypass surgery in morbidly obese patients, post-prandial hypoglycemia resulting from endogenous hyperinsulinemia in subjects without diabetes has been attributed to nesidioblastosis.[3]

Following surgery, the patient's diabetes was well controlled without the utilization of exogenous insulin or oral hypoglycemic medications. There was also a small but nevertheless significant weight loss. The patient believed that the surgery had cured his diabetes and wondered why more people did not have this curative surgery. He was lost to follow-up having last been seen 2 months after his subtotal pancreatectomy.

REFERENCES

1. Bell DSH, Grizzle WE, Dunlap NE. Nesidioblastosis causing reversal of insulin-dependent diabetes and development of hyperinsulinemic hypoglycemia. *Diabetes Care* 1995;18:1379–1380

2. Harness JK, Geelhoed GW, Thompson NW, Nishiyama RH, Fajans SS, Kraft RO, Howard DR, Clark KA. Nesidioblastosis in adults. A surgical dilemma. *Arch Surg* 1981;116(5):575–580

3. Service GJ, Thompson GB, Service FJ, Andrews JC, Collazo-Clavell ML, Lloyd RV. Hyperinsulinemic hypoglycemia with nesidioblastosis after gastric-bypass surgery. *N Engl J Med* 2005;353(3):249–254

Case 90

Munchausen-by-Proxy: Hypoglycemia in an Islet Autotransplantation Recipient

R. Paul Robertson, MD[1]

An 8-year-old girl was admitted to the emergency department (ED) because of profound hypoglycemia. She had a history of unrelenting, painful chronic idiopathic pancreatitis since age 2 years that led to an inability to attain normal weight, daily narcotic use, depression, and poor school attendance. At the age of 7 years, she underwent total pancreatectomy to relieve pain followed by intrahepatic islet autotransplantation to prevent diabetes. In the post-transplant period she felt much better, improved attendance at school, and discontinued narcotics within 12 months. The entire family was pleased with this result except the girl's mother, who initially had objected to the surgery. In her view, it made no sense to make her little girl develop diabetes and then treat the diabetes by removing islets from the pancreas and putting them in the liver. The husband understood that pancreatectomy was needed for pain relief, sided with the surgeons, and dismissed the mother's anxieties. Post-transplant, the mother decided she would help the girl by using her blood glucose meter to monitor her glucose levels, which pleased the father.

Total pancreatectomy and intrahepatic islet autotransplantation is not familiar to hospital personnel in most medical centers, although this procedure has been proven successful since 1980 by surgeons at the University of Minnesota. Pancreatectomy results in pain relief for 85% of patients and 70% of patients are insulin independent at 3 years post-transplant. Blood glucose control is good if >5,000 islets/kg body weight are recovered and transplanted.[1] Transplant surgeons believe in early preemptive pancreatectomy when it is clear the patient's pain is relentless. Their philosophy is that it is better to remove the pancreas early to improve quality of life and to prevent progressive islet damage that is a consequence of the chronic pancreatic inflammation that accompanies the disease. This patient had had prolongation of her clinical course for 5 years during which time she received pancreatic duct stents to no avail and partial pancreatectomy to remove a chronically inflamed area of the pancreas.

The endocrinologist who had been managing the patient and her family was puzzled by the patient's hypoglycemia, which recently had been occurring

[1]Professor of Medicine, University of Minnesota; Professor of Medicine and Pharmacology, University of Washington; President Emeritus and Principal Investigator, Pacific Northwest Diabetes Research Institute.

 DOI: 10.2337/9781580405713.90

at more frequent levels. After the most recent ED incident, the patient was admitted to the hospital for close monitoring of her glucose, insulin, and C-peptide levels. The father and mother visited the patient frequently, and the mother continued to monitor capillary glucose levels. None of the patient's hormone and glucose levels were abnormal and no symptoms of hypoglycemia were observed.

The social pathology in this family had improved somewhat because the surgery had been successful in relieving pain and because the father praised the mother in her role as monitor of glucose levels. Her records of glucose levels were fastidiously kept.

In reviewing the records, the endocrinologist noted that the patient's low glucose levels usually were preceded by mildly elevated postprandial high glucose levels. She also discovered that when the patient had the hypoglycemic episode that led to the ED admission, the insulin and C-peptide levels that were ordered had not been entered into the chart. She checked with the lab records and discovered the insulin level was very high and C-peptide was essentially zero. The endocrinologist walked to the patient's room and asked the mother if she had been giving the patient insulin. The mother became quite angry with this question and blurted out that her little girl's hypoglycemia would not have been a problem if they had listened to her in the first place and not done the pancreatectomy. The patient and her mother left the hospital. Because the relationships with the medical staff and the family were not good, the endocrinologist spoke with a social service worker in the hospital. Based on their suspicion of Munchausen-by-proxy, they decided an unannounced visit to the family home with a police officer was indicated.

Munchausen-by-proxy is a variant of the Munchausen syndrome in which a second party purposefully manipulates the patient's health status to achieve personal secondary gain.[2] In this case, the gain to the mother was suspected to be her need to recover control as a parent after she was essentially ignored when the decision to perform pancreatectomy was made by the father and the surgeons.

The endocrinologist, the social worker, and a police officer arrived at the family home and rang the doorbell, and the mother appeared at the front door. She had no choice but to admit the visitors to her living room. The endocrinologist and social worker sat down to discuss their suspicions with the mother while the police officer went into the kitchen where he found on the counter insulin syringes and in the refrigerator a vial of rapid-acting insulin. He returned to the living room and showed the evidence to the group in the living room. The mother began crying. The endocrinologist tried to console her. The social worker asked the mother whether she would come to the hospital for more discussion in a more neutral setting. The mother agreed and said she would follow them in her car in a few minutes. Back at the hospital, while waiting for the mother for what seemed to be an extensive period of time, the endocrinologist was called to the ED because of a code. There she found the father of the family who explained he had come home from work early and found the mother lying unconscious on the kitchen floor. She had injected herself with insulin and was now comatose in the ED.

The endocrinologist made the initial error of aggressively confronting the mother in the hospital of giving her daughter insulin injections,[3,4] causing the family to leave the hospital. The mother in her zeal to help the daughter and to recover control in the family dynamic had decided to treat each elevation of glucose with an insulin injection and overtreated her daughter. With the unassailable evidence found by the police officer, the mother attempted suicide, suggesting she had significant psychiatric impairment.

REFERENCES

1. Sutherland DE, Radosevich DM, Bellin MD, Hering BJ, Beilman GJ, Dunn TB, et al. Total pancreatectomy and islet autotransplantation for chronic pancreatitis. *J Am Coll Surg* 2012;214(4):409–424

2. Ayoub CC, Alexander R, Beck D, et al. Position paper: definitional issues in Munchausen by proxy. *Child Maltreat* 2002;7:105–111

3. Rosenberg DA. Web of deceit: a literature review of Munchausen syndrome by proxy. *Child Abuse Negl* 1987;11:547–563

4. Souid AK, Keith DV, Cunningham AS. Munchausen syndrome by proxy. *Clin Pediatr* 1998;37:497–503

Case 91
Treatment of a Patient with Diabetes and Severe Hypoglycemia

Henning Beck-Nielsen, DMSc[1]

A 52-year-old man was admitted to the emergency department after a car accident in which he went off the road and was found upside down in a cornfield. He was found in the driver's seat with his seatbelt on, but he was unconscious. He had been diagnosed with type 1 diabetes at age 5 years and, for several years, he had problems with hypoglycemia. He was still unconscious after arriving at the hospital, and his blood glucose (BG) was measured at 4.5 mmol/L (81 mg/dL). His blood pressure was 150/90 mmHg, his pulse 90 bpm, and his electrocardiogram (ECG) did not indicate acute myocardial infarction (MI) or arrhythmia. An examination of the patient did not reveal any peripheral paresis. He immediately underwent a computed tomography scan of the head, but it showed no intracranial hemorrhage. The conclusion was that the patient had suffered from a hypoglycemic attack despite the normal BG value. It was believed that his BG had increased due to counter-regulation (Fig. 91.1). An intravenous glucose infusion was started with isotonic glucose 250 mL/h to increase his BG values to approximately 10 mmol/L (180 mg/dL).

The patient regained consciousness after an hour and said that he had been driving his car, but he could not explain what had happened. Later on, he explained that he had had hypoglycemic attacks several years ago. They started when he was about 45 years old with nightly attacks of hypoglycemia, often after exercise in the evening. Therefore, he changed from human insulin to insulin analogues, aspart, and glargine, because it has been shown that insulin analogs, specifically long-acting analogs, induce fewer hypoglycemic events during the night.[1] In addition, his spouse was taught how to administer glucagon 1 mg intramuscularly for especially severe attacks. This was effective for a year or so, but thereafter the hypoglycemia episodes returned, especially after intake of alcohol. His diabetic neuropathy also worsened, and he developed unawareness for low blood glucose values.

Hypoglycemia unawareness can be explained by a reduction in both glucagon and norepinephrine production with repeated hypoglycemia as shown in Fig. 91.1. This figure illustrates the hormonal response to hypoglycemia in newly diagnosed patients and in patients with a duration of 14–31 years of diabetes.

[1]Department of Endocrinology, Department of Endocrinology, Odense University Hospital, Odense, Denmark.

DOI: 10.2337/9781580405713.91

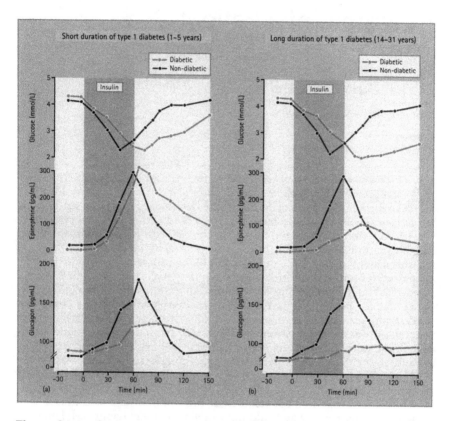

Figure 91.1 — Counter-regulatory response to hypoglycemia in T1D patients with short- and long-term duration.

With the demonstrated unawareness for hypoglycemia, the patient had been changed from basal-bolus insulin regimen via pen system to an insulin pump. He was taught to count carbohydrates and to adjust his insulin accordingly. His insulin-to-carbohydrate ratio was 1 unit for every 12 g, and his insulin sensitivity was 2 mmol/L (36 mg/dL) per 1 unit of insulin injected. His basal rate of insulin aspart was adjusted to minimize the risk of hypoglycemia, especially during the night. Furthermore he was taught specific precautions when driving, and advised to consume 6 small meals per day and to reduce his alcohol intake.

Table 91.1 provides a guideline for patients with hypoglycemia unawareness. These precautions helped, and he did not have any severe hypoglycemic events before the car accident that brought him back to our hospital for the current presentation.

Table 91.1—Advice on Hypoglycemia for Patients with Diabetes

- Take responsibility for your own diabetes.
- Stay one step ahead of your diabetes—try to figure out what can cause the blood glucose to fall.
- Always remember to have sugar on you.
- It is important to test the blood glucose before each meal and before going to bed.
- Accept all types of education regarding the regulation of diabetes; join a Facebook group.
- Always let people around you know that you have diabetes, that low blood glucose can occur, and how they should deal with it.
- Always carry your diabetes identification card.
- If low blood glucose is a problem, then it is okay to keep your average blood glucose level a bit higher for a while as it is more dangerous to have low blood glucose than high.
- You should avoid nightly hypoglycemia. Test your blood glucose before turning in. If it is <7 mmol/L (126 mg/dL), then eat a piece of bread.
- The ultimate security and helper is your partner.
- If you often use quick-acting insulin to bring down high blood glucose, then you increase the risk of hypoglycemia.
- Counting carbohydrates at each meal will help you reduce the risk of hypoglycemia as you can adjust the insulin more easily.
- Be sure to learn the correct injection technique.
- Low blood glucose while driving a car is dangerous. You have to be completely sure of your blood glucose level before and during driving.
- The insulin pump can reduce the risk of hypoglycemia.
- A glucose sensor with alarm may help.
- All people with diabetes who have severe hypoglycemia must always have a glucagon injection in the fridge.
- Increased physical activity during work or exercise is one of the most common causes for low blood glucose level.
- Alcohol can lower your blood glucose level, especially strong alcohol.
- Many fear hypoglycemia even if they do not have it. If you have this fear, then get help either through psychotherapy or a psychologist.

When he was discharged, it was decided that he should try using a glucose sensor to avoid hypoglycemia. A wireless glucose sensor was implanted in the subcutaneous tissue of his abdomen. Glucose values were transmitted to an insulin pump display, and an alarm for hypoglycemia was set at a BG level of 4 mmol/L (72 mg/dL).[2] The police decided that he should not be allowed to drive again unless he could avoid any hypoglycemic events for at least 1 year.

Our patient's 24-h glucose profile 3 months after introducing the glucose sensor is shown in Fig. 91.2. Although his BG values have not stabilized, only a few values are <4 mmol/L (72 mg/dL), and he has had few severe hypoglycemic events up to this point. In Denmark, about 20% of subjects with type 1 diabetes have two or more severe hypoglycemic attacks per year, whereas about 50% never develop severe hypoglycemia. Most of the 20% with severe hypoglycemia also develop partial or complete unawareness.[3]

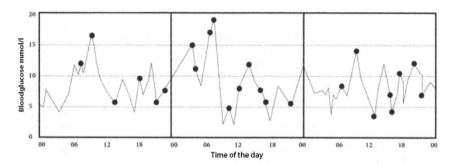

Figure 91.2—Diurnal profile of BG after intervention with insulin pump and online glucose sensor.

REFERENCES

1. Kristensen PL, Hansen LS, Jespersen MJ, Pedersen-Bjergaard U, Beck-Nielsen H, Christiansen JS, Nørgaard K, Perrild H, Parving HH, Thorsteinsson B, Tarnow L. Insulin analogues and severe hypoglycaemia in type 1 diabetes. *Diabetes Res Clin Pract* 2012;96(1):17–23. doi:10.1016/j.diabres.2011.10.046

2. Choudhary P, Ramasamy S, Green L, Gallen G, Pender S, Brackenridge A, Amiel SA, Pickup JC. Real-time continuous glucose monitoring significantly reduces severe hypoglycemia in hypoglycemia-unaware patients with type 1 diabetes. *Diabetes Care* 2013;36(12):4160–4162. doi:10.2337/dc13-0939

3. Cryer PE. Hypoglycemia-associated autonomic failure in diabetes. *Hand Clin Neurol* 2013;117:295–307. doi:10.1016/B978-0-444-53491-0.00023-7

Case 92

Hypoglycemia with Use of Glargine Insulin in the Management of Type 2 Diabetes, Occurring with Titration Aimed at Achieving Prebreakfast Glucose Levels <100 mg/dL (5.6 mmol/L)

Saira Adeel, MD,[1] and Lawrence S. Phillips, MD[2]

It is well established that intensive glycemic control in patients with type 2 diabetes (T2D) is associated with significant reductions in microvascular complications.[1] Evidence also suggests that in patients with newly diagnosed T2D, intensive glycemic control may reduce long-term cardiovascular disease rates.[2] To help achieve improved control safely, a fasting glucose level of <100 mg/dL (5.6 mmol/L) is employed as an increasingly common insulin titration target in clinical trials.[3] As add on therapy to oral antidiabetic agents, both insulin glargine and detemir have been shown to be comparable in terms of HbA$_{1c}$ (A1C) reduction with low risk of hypoglycemia.[4] We describe two cases in which hypoglycemia occurred with addition and uptitration of glargine insulin.

CASE 1

A 62-year-old man with a 7-year history of T2D had an A1C of 7.6% while taking metformin 2,550 mg daily and glipizide 5 mg twice daily. The glipizide dose was increased to a total of 27.5 mg daily. Fasting glucose levels remained suboptimal, however, so glargine insulin was added before the evening meal ("dinner"), and glipizide doses were decreased (goal prebreakfast glucose levels <100 mg/dL or 5.6 mmol/L). With uptitration of glargine, metformin was continued at the previous dose and glipizide was decreased. Eventually, the patient was instructed to take only 2.5 mg of glipizide predinner. The patient experienced postdinner hypoglycemia (glucose levels of 58 and 66 mg/dL or 3.2 and 3.8 mmol/L), which prompted discontinuation of glipizide. While using predinner glargine and metformin alone, the patient had prebreakfast glucose levels of 110–124 mg/dL (6.1–6.9 mmol/L) but experienced predinner hypoglycemia (both with and without activity during the afternoon), with glucose levels of 65–72 mg/dL (3.6–4 mmol/L) associated with typical symptoms of hypoglycemia. Therefore, predinner glargine was discontinued and

[1]Atlanta VA Medical Center, Division of Endocrinology, Emory University School of Medicine, Atlanta, GA. [2]Division of Endocrinology and Metabolism, Emory University, Atlanta, GA.

DOI: 10.2337/9781580405713.92

Table 92.1—Case 1. Profile of a Patient Who Developed Predinner Hypoglycemia

Date	Treatment regimen	Average prebreakfast BG (mg/dL) or (mmol/L)	A1C (%)	Hypoglycemia: timing/BG (mg/dL)	New regimen	Comments
Nov. 2011	Metformin 850 mg t.i.d., glipizide 5 mg b.i.d.	156 (8.7)	7.6	None	Metformin 850 mg t.i.d., glipizide 27.5 mg daily (10 mg predinner, 17.5 mg at bedtime)	Glipizide doses were adjusted over a 1-month period to 10 mg predinner and 17.5 mg at bedtime
Jan. 2012	Metformin 850 mg t.i.d., glipizide 27.5 mg daily (10 mg predinner, 17.5 mg at bedtime)	131 (7.3)	7.0	None	Metformin 850 mg t.i.d., glipizide 5 mg predinner, glargine 14 units predinner	Predinner glargine was added to attain prebreakfast BG goal <100 mg/dL; predinner glipizide dose was decreased and bedtime glipizide discontinued due to addition of glargine
Mar. 2012	Metformin 850 mg t.i.d., glipizide 2.5 mg predinner, glargine 36 units predinner	115 (6.4)	7.2	Postdinner, 58 and 66 mg/dL	Metformin 850 g t.i.d., glargine 36 units predinner	Predinner glipizide discontinued due to postdinner hypoglycemia
Apr.–Oct. 2012	Metformin 850 mg t.i.d., glargine 40 units predinner	107 (5.9)	7.0	Predinner, both with and without activity/ 65–72 mg/dL	Metformin 850 mg t.i.d., glargine 40 units predinner (decrease to 35 units if physical activity planned)	Patient advised to decrease glargine dose to 35 units in case of physical activity
Jan. 2013	Metformin 850 mg t.i.d., glargine 42 units predinner	107 (5.9)	7.0	Predinner, 79 mg/dL after yardwork with typical hypoglycemia symptoms	Metformin 850 mg t.i.d., detemir 42 units at bedtime	Predinner hypoglycemia and borderline predinner BG with and without activity likely related to prolonged duration of action of glargine, in combination with decreased insulin resistance predinner due to waning of the "dawn phenomenon"
May 2013	Metformin 850 mg t.i.d., detemir 45 units at bedtime	100 (5.6)	7.0	None	No change in regimen	

Profile of a patient who developed predinner hypoglycemia with titration of glargine insulin administered before the evening meal, aimed at achieving prebreakfast glucose levels <100 mg/dL (5.6 mmol/L). t.i.d., three times a day; b.i.d., twice a day; BG, blood glucose.

replaced by equivalent doses of detemir insulin at bedtime daily. Uptitration of detemir produced prebreakfast glucose levels of 88–114 mg/dL (4.9–6.3 mmol/L) and an A1C of 7%, without recurrence of predinner hypoglycemia.

CASE 2

A 68-year-old man with a 10-year history of T2D had an A1C of 7.7% while taking Novolin 70/30 insulin 26 units twice daily and metformin 2,500 mg daily. Because of suboptimal control, the patient was switched to a basal-bolus regimen with glargine insulin 24 units predinner and aspart insulin 4 units before each meal. Over the next 3 months, the glargine dose was increased to 50 units predinner, and the aspart was changed to 1 unit prebreakfast, 5 units prelunch, and 3 units predinner. Glipzide 2.5 mg was added with meals, permitting discontinuation of premeal aspart insulin. The predinner glipizide had to be discontinued, however, because of bedtime glucose levels in the range of 90–100 mg/dL (5–5.6 mmol/L). Subsequently, the prelunch glipizide was discontinued secondary to predinner glucose levels of 70–73 mg/dL (3.9–4.1 mmol/L). With uptitration of predinner glargine, the prebreakfast glipizide was also discontinued to avoid hypoglycemia. While the patient was taking glargine 64 units predinner and metformin 2,000 mg daily, he experienced hypoglycemia at bedtime, with a glucose level of 64 mg/dL (3.6 mmol/L). At this point, the patient was switched from predinner glargine to detemir insulin at bedtime. Uptitration of detemir produced prebreakfast glucose levels of 86–127 mg/dL (4.8–7.1 mmol/L) and an A1C of 7.1%, without recurrence of bedtime hypoglycemia.

The American Diabetes Association recommends individualization of glycemic targets and pursuit of more stringent glycemic goals in select patients as deemed appropriate, based on the duration of diabetes, age and life expectancy, comorbidities, absence of macrovascular and microvascular complications, and presence of hypoglycemia awareness.[5] A major problem in current management of T2D is inadequate use of basal insulin—starting early enough, and titrating effectively. In many practices, insulin is initiated only when glycemic control has become unsatisfactory despite the use of combinations of several alternative glucose-lowering agents, and often when A1C levels are in the range of 8–9% or higher. At such a point in the natural history, insulin may be initiated with injections of premixed insulin twice a day, or basal insulin once or twice a day along with short-acting insulin given before meals.

We believe that it is preferable to initiate basal insulin earlier in the natural history—as soon as prebreakfast glucose can no longer be maintained in a satisfactory range with alternative agents. T2D in many patients is a disorder of insulin secretion, which is insufficient to compensate for increased insulin resistance (because of overweight, inactivity, or increasing age), and the earliest manifestation of insufficient insulin may be postprandial hyperglycemia presenting as hyperglycemia during the day and at bedtime. It is a safer management strategy to use alternative agents to treat hyperglycemia during the day and to use basal insulin given in the evening to treat prebreakfast hyperglycemia. The basal insulin generally is titrated according to prebreakfast

Table 92.2—Case 2. Profile of a Patient Who Developed Nocturnal Hypoglycemia

Date	Treatment regimen	Average prebreakfast BG (mg/dL) or (mmol/L)	A1C (%)	Hypoglycemia timing/BG (mg/dL)	New regimen	Comments
Sep. 2011	Novolin 70/30 26 units every morning and every evening, metformin 2,500 mg daily	132 (7.3)	7.7	None	Novolin 70/30 24 units every morning and 28 units every evening, metformin 2,500 mg daily	
Oct. 2011	Novolin 70/30 24 units every morning and 28 units every evening, metformin 2,500 mg daily	122 (6.8)	7.7	None	Glargine 24 units predinner, aspart 4 units before each meal, metformin 2,500 mg daily	Transitioned to basal-bolus regimen with glargine and aspart due to suboptimal prebreakfast BG
Jan. 2012	Glargine 50 units predinner, aspart 1 unit prebreakfast, 5 units prelunch, 3 units predinner, metformin 2,500 mg daily	134 (7.4)	6.7	None	Glargine 54 units predinner, glipizide 2.5 mg premeals, metformin 2,500 mg daily	Glargine doses titrated up between Oct. 2011 and Jan. 2012 to target prebreakfast BG <100 mg/dL; premeal glipizide added to allow discontinuation of prandial aspart
Feb. 6, 2012	Glargine 54 units predinner, glipizide 2.5 mg before meals, metformin 2,500 mg daily	133 (7.4)	6.9	None (bedtime BG 90–100 mg/dL)	Glargine 58 units predinner, glipizide 2.5 mg before breakfast and lunch, metformin 2,500 mg daily	Predinner glipizide discontinued on account of bedtime BGs in the 90–100 mg/dL range

Date	Regimen	BG mg/dL (mmol/L)	A1C	Hypoglycemia	New regimen	Comments
Feb. 15–22, 2012	Glargine 58 units predinner, glipizide 2.5 mg prebreakfast and lunch, metformin 2,500 mg daily	121 (6.7)	6.9	Predinner, 70–73 mg/dL with typical hypoglycemia symptoms	Glargine 62 units predinner, metformin 2,500 mg daily	Prelunch glipizide discontinued due to predinner hypoglycemia; prebreakfast glipizide discontinued with uptitration of predinner glargine
Feb. 28, 2012	Glargine 64 units predinner, metformin 2,000 mg daily	100 (5.6)	6.9	Bedtime, 64 mg/dL	Detemir 58 units at bedtime, metformin 2,000 mg daily	Predinner glargine was discontinued and replaced by bedtime detemir
Mar–Apr. 2012	Detemir 68 units at bedtime, metformin 2,000 mg daily	114 (6.3)	6.9	None	Detemir 74 units at bedtime, glipizide 2.5 mg prebreakfast, metformin 2,000 mg daily	
Sept. 2012	Detemir 100 units at bedtime, glipizide 2.5 mg prebreakfast, metformin 2,000 mg daily	104 (5.8)	7.1	None	No change in regimen	

Profile of a patient who developed nocturnal hypoglycemia with titration of glargine insulin administered before the evening meal, aimed to achieve glucose levels <100 mg/dL (5.6 mmol/L). BG, blood glucose.

glucose levels, aiming to achieve glucose levels of <100 mg/dL (5.6 mmol/L) or 75–105 mg/dL (4.2–5.8 mmol/L). Hypoglycemia, if it arises at all, usually occurs prebreakfast. Practitioners, however, need to be aware that basal insulin can also cause hypoglycemia at other times.

Patient safety and avoidance of hypoglycemia are critical in the individualized approach to diabetes therapy. These cases illustrate two potential patterns of "unusual" hypoglycemia with use of insulin glargine, which occurred during titration aimed to reduce prebreakfast glucose levels to <100 mg/dL (5.6 mmol/L), an increasingly common target. In our practice, glargine is usually given before the evening meal ("dinner") to minimize the risk of nocturnal hypoglycemia. As shown in our patients, hypoglycemia can occur not only prebreakfast but also either early or late after insulin administration.

Case 1 demonstrates the potential problem of predinner hypoglycemia, which was noted both with and without prior physical activity. In this patient, we attribute this problem to the prolonged duration of action of glargine, possibly in combination with decreased insulin resistance predinner because of waning of the "dawn phenomenon" during the day.

Case 2 demonstrates the potential problem of hypoglycemia occurring shortly after administration of glargine, which we attribute to a potential early peak of action, which is consistent with the pharmacodynamic pattern described by Porcellati et al.[6]

Similar rates of hypoglycemia have been reported with use of insulin glargine and detemir.[4] In both of our patients, however, the patterns of hypoglycemia resolved after switching from glargine to detemir insulin.

REFERENCES

1. UK Prospective Diabetes Study (UKPDS) Group. Effect of intensive blood-glucose control with metformin on complications in overweight patients with type 2 diabetes (UKPDS 34). *Lancet* 1998;352(9131):854–865

2. Holman RR, Paul SK, Bethel MA, Matthews DR, Neil HA. 10-year follow-up of intensive glucose control in type 2 diabetes. *New Engl J Med* 2008; 359(15):1577–1589

3. Origin Trial Investigators, Gerstein HC, Bosch J, Dagenais GR, Diaz R, Jung H, et al. Basal insulin and cardiovascular and other outcomes in dysglycemia. *New Engl J Med* 2012;367(4):319–328

4. Rosenstock J, Davies M, Home PD, Larsen J, Koenen C, Schernthaner G. A randomised, 52-week, treat-to-target trial comparing insulin detemir with insulin glargine when administered as add-on to glucose-lowering drugs in insulin-naive people with type 2 diabetes. *Diabetologia* 2008;51(3):408–416

5. American Diabetes Association. Standards of medical care in diabetes, 2015. *Diabetes Care* 2015;38(Suppl. 1):S1–S93

6. Porcellati F, Rossetti P, Busciantella NR, Marzotti S, Lucidi P, Luzio S, et al. Comparison of pharmacokinetics and dynamics of the long-acting insulin analogs glargine and detemir at steady state in type 1 diabetes: a double-blind, randomized, crossover study. *Diabetes Care* 2007;30(10):2447–2452

Case 93

Progressive Hypoglycemia Due to Insulinoma in a Patient with Type 2 Diabetes: Treatment with Image-Guided Minimally Invasive Pancreas-Sparing Surgery

Mary-Elizabeth Patti, MD;[1,5] Mark P. Callery, MD, FACS;[2,5] Robert M. Najarian, MD;[3,5] Mandeep S. Sawhney, MD, MS;[4,5] Lyle Mitzner, MD;[1,5] Allison B. Goldfine, MD;[1,5] and A. James Moser, MD, FACS[2,5]

A 54-year-old man with type 2 diabetes (T2D) presented for evaluation of hypoglycemia. T2D was diagnosed at age 35 years, when the patient presented with recurrent urinary tract infections. Treatment with diet, metformin, and pioglitazone/rosiglitazone led to normalization of glucose, with hemoglobin A1c of 6%. He remained stable until age 54 years, when he developed an inferior wall myocardial infarction (MI). Postinfarction pericarditis required initiation of higher dose aspirin (650 mg t.i.d.). Patient markedly improved diet and increased exercise in the post-MI setting, achieving a rapid 24-lb weight loss. Metformin and rosiglitazone were discontinued.

Episodic hypoglycemia was noted within 1 month post-MI. Hypoglycemia typically occurred within 1 h after meals, if meals were delayed, and in response to exercise, with no fasting or nocturnal episodes. Patient began consuming additional carbohydrate snacks before exercise to prevent hypoglycemia. The patient experienced both adrenergic and neuroglycopenic symptoms, which promptly resolved after glucose ingestion.

In retrospect, over the past year, he noted that during a long shift at work without meals, he would feel "grumpy" and eat candy for relief. A random glucose 6 months previously was 66 mg/dL (while taking metformin and rosiglitazone). Family history was negative for hypoglycemia or multiple endocrine neoplasia but was positive for T2D, obesity, and hypothyroidism.

Physical examination revealed BMI 28 kg/m², BP 134/76 mmHg supine, and 118/78 mmHg standing. Mild abdominal obesity was present. Exam was negative for hyperpigmentation, vitiligo, acanthosis, hepatomegaly, or abdominal masses. Retinal and neurological examinations were normal.

Home glucose monitoring demonstrated fasting glucose 70–90 mg/dL (3.9–5 mmol/L), postbreakfast 44–60 mg/dL 2.4–3.3 mmol/L), and postlunch 50–60 mg/dL (2.8–3.3 mmol/L). Continuous glucose monitoring was performed to help to define patterns of glycemic excursions and revealed some nocturnal (12:00–2:00 A.M.) and daytime hypoglycemia (2:00–4:00 P.M.), with minimum sensor value of 46 mg/dL (2.6 mmol/L) and 27% of all values <70 mg/dL (3.9 mmol/L). Venous blood sampling obtained during a spontaneous episode of

[1]Joslin Diabetes Center, Boston, MA. [2]Institute for HepatoBiliary and Pancreatic Surgery, Beth Israel Deaconess Medical Center, Boston, MA. [3]Department of Pathology, Beth Israel Deaconess Medical Center, Boston, MA. [4]Department of Medicine, Beth Israel Deaconess Medical Center and Dana Farber Harvard Cancer Center, Boston, MA. [5]Harvard Medical School, Boston, MA.

DOI: 10.2337/9781580405713.93

Table 93.1 — Results of Metabolic Testing during Extended Overnight Fast

Time	Plasma Glucose (mg/dL)	Insulin (µU/mL)	C-Peptide (ng/mL) (1.1–4.2 ng/mL)	Proinsulin (pmol/L) (<18.8 pmol/L)	BOHB (mmol/L) (<0.4 mmol/L)	Cortisol (µg/dL) (3–22 µg/dL)
9:00 A.M. (fasting)	70	33	3.9	270	0.1	11
11:00 A.M.	68	15	2.4	91	0.1	10
12:55 P.M.	56	13	2.6	104	0.1	8
1:23 P.M.	50	36	4.4	310	0.2	12
Glucagon 1 mg administered; capillary glucose increased to 80 at 10 min, 111 at both 20 and 30 min.						

hypoglycemia (at 1:00 P.M.) showed plasma glucose 61 mg/dL (3.4 mmol/L), insulin 13 µU/mL, C-peptide 2.4 ng/mL, proinsulin 287 (normal <19), and cortisol 18, and a negative screen for sulfonylureas, repaglinide, and nateglinide. Anti-insulin antibodies were negative. TSH, prolactin, cortisol, calcium, parathyroid hormone PTH, and chromogranin A were normal. Discontinuation of high-dose salicylates did not alter the frequency or severity of hypoglycemia.

Overall impression was that of postprandial hypoglycemia in a patient with T2D, who had recently adopted healthy eating and exercise patterns, achieving rapid weight loss. Insulin levels were inappropriately nonsuppressed during hypoglycemia, however, and proinsulin levels were high. This raised concern for autonomous insulin secretion by an insulinoma or noninsulinoma pancreatogenous hyperinsulinemia syndrome.

An extended overnight fast was conducted. As seen in Table 93.1, hypoglycemia (venous glucose 50 mg/dL or 2.8 mmol/L) developed after a 15-h fast, with impaired cognition and sweating. Laboratory evaluation confirmed inappropriate insulin secretion (elevated insulin, C-peptide, proinsulin) and inappropriately low β-hydroxybutyrate. Glycemic response to glucagon was robust (>25 mg/dL or 1.4 mmol/L increase), suggesting adequate hepatic glycogen stores.

Computed tomography during the arterial phase of contrast administration (Fig. 93.1*A*) demonstrated a 9 × 8 mm hypervascular solid lesion in the pancreatic neck anterior to the superior mesenteric artery and abutting an adjacent cystic lesion consistent with intraductal papillary mucinous neoplasm. The hypervascular lesion became isodense with the surrounding parenchyma during the portal venous phase. The lesion was redemonstrated during magnetic resonance imaging (Fig. 93.1*B*), which demonstrated its proximity to the adjacent main pancreatic duct.

During preoperative preparation, diazoxide was administered at 50 mg every 8 h. Glucose values markedly improved, but the patient continued to have mild hypoglycemia with exercise.

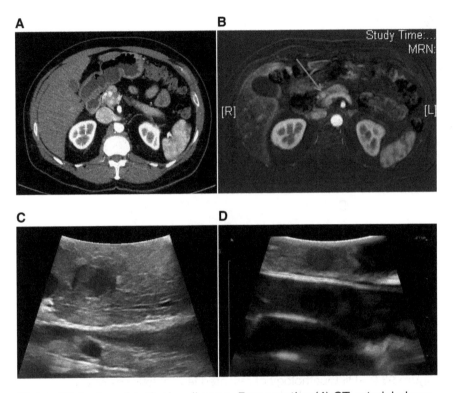

Figure 93.1 — Imaging the insulinoma. Preoperative (A) CT, arterial phase, demonstrating hypervascular lesion behind gastroduodenal artery, and (B) MRI, arterial phase. Lesion is indicated by arrow. Intraoperative ultrasound of (C) pancreas in vivo and (D) resected specimen.

Robot-assisted minimally invasive central pancreatectomy[1] was performed to resect the pancreatic neck containing the insulinoma and to reconstruct the remnant pancreas to preserve the pancreatic body and tail, while minimizing the risk of pancreatic leak. Intraoperative ultrasound (Fig. 93.1C) clearly demonstrated a solid lesion adjacent to the gastroduodenal artery. The gastroduodenal artery was ligated and the neck of the pancreas was resected under direct vision using robotic cautery scissors. The presence of the entire solid mass was confirmed by specimen ultrasound (Fig. 93.1D). Frozen sections demonstrated the lesion and negative surgical margins. Hypoglycemia resolved immediately without medication. The patient was discharged home with a surgical drain in place on day 6 eating regular food.

Pathologic exam of the resected lesion (Fig. 93.2) was consistent with a well-differentiated insulinoma, 0.9 cm, grade 1 of 3 (World Health Organization

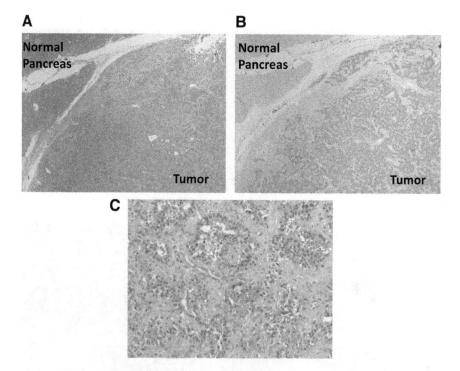

Figure 93.2—Histopathology of resected lesion: low-power view of tumor and adjacent normal pancreas, stained with H & E (*A*) and anti-insulin antibody (*B*), and high-power view showing tumor nests and vascularity (*C*).

classification), with focal low-grade pancreatic intraepithelial neoplasia (PanIN1). Insulin staining was positive diffusely throughout the tumor.

Postoperatively, as the patient began to increase his oral intake, fasting and postprandial glucose values increased, and metformin and prandial insulin were initiated. No further hypoglycemia was experienced.

Hypoglycemia developing in patients with T2D is usually attributable to insulin or oral medications (especially insulin secretagogues), typically in the setting of reduced food intake, altered meal schedules, weight loss, increased exercise, interactions with prescription or alternative medications, alcohol, or intercurrent systemic illness. Patient education and adjustment of medications to better match food intake and activity is usually sufficient to reduce or eliminate hypoglycemia. When hypoglycemia persists despite complete withdrawal of medications, suspicion should be raised for excessive endogenous insulin secretion.

In our patient, hypoglycemia persisted despite withdrawal of medications. Continued hypoglycemia was initially attributed to abrupt adoption of an improved lifestyle following MI. Reduced calorie intake, weight loss, and increased exercise, all of which enhance insulin sensitivity, could have contributed to a mismatch between insulin sensitivity and secretion, leading to postprandial or "reactive" hypoglycemia. However, hypoglycemia did not respond to low–glycemic index diet, was observed in response to exercise, and was persistent and progressive, prompting evaluation for autonomous insulin secretion.

Biochemical evaluation during spontaneous hypoglycemia demonstrated inappropriately high plasma C-peptide, high proinsulin levels, and a negative screen for hypoglycemic agents, indicating autonomous insulin secretion. These patterns were confirmed during an extended overnight fast, during which the patient became hypoglycemic, again with inappropriately high insulin, C-peptide, and proinsulin. Low β-hydroxybutyrate levels with fasting and robust response to glucagon also confirmed insulin-mediated suppression of lipolysis and stimulation of glycogen synthesis. Imaging demonstrated a neuroendocrine tumor in the pancreatic neck, and pathological examination confirmed that this was an insulinoma. Image-guided, minimally invasive pancreatic resection maximized the volume of remnant β-cell mass and minimized the impact of surgical intervention on the patient's quality of life. Postoperative resolution of hypoglycemia and recurrence of hyperglycemia, requiring reinstitution of medications for diabetes, indicates successful resection of tumor and absence of autonomous insulin secretion.

Prior reports have described the development of insulinoma in a total of 36 patients with T2D. These cases share similar gender and age distribution to overall demographic patterns of insulinoma.[2] Although hypoglycemia resulting from insulinoma is most likely to occur with fasting, it can be exclusively postprandial (6% of insulinoma patients without diabetes) or in both fasting and postprandial conditions (21%).[2] A similar distribution of hypoglycemia timing is also present in individuals with diabetes and insulinoma. Notably, many patients had T2D for more than a decade and required medical therapies, often in combination, before the development of progressive hypoglycemia. In most cases, hypoglycemia persisted despite medication withdrawal, and successful tumor resection resulted in recurrence of hyperglycemia.

The coexistence of diabetes and insulinoma may simply reflect that a rare condition can occur in individuals with a highly prevalent disease, such as T2D. Given that the estimated incidence of insulinoma is ~4 cases per 1 million persons per year,[3] and the prevalence of diagnosed T2D is 18 million in the U.S., these data suggest there could be up to 72 patients with T2D developing insulinoma per year. Not surprisingly, case reports are likely to substantially underestimate prevalence. Symptoms of hypoglycemia in patients with diabetes are likely to be attributed by both patients and physicians to medications, reducing the suspicion for autonomous insulin secretion. It is intriguing to speculate that in rare patients, sustained insulin resistance could contribute to islet proliferation, as has been observed in mouse models of insulin resistance, who have increased islet mass in parallel with increases in novel β-cell trophic factors.[4,5]

We report a patient with long-standing T2D in whom postprandial hypoglycemia developed after substantial lifestyle changes and weight loss, and persisted despite withdrawal of all antihyperglycemic medications. Diagnostic evaluation demonstrated autonomous endogenous insulin secretion resulting from an insulinoma. With successful resection of the tumor, diabetes recurred. This case underscores the importance of considering the rare possibility of insulinoma even in patients with preexisting diabetes.

REFERENCES

1. Abood GJ, Can MF, Daouadi M, et al. Robotic-assisted minimally invasive central pancreatectomy: technique and outcomes. *J Gastrointest Surg* 2013; 17(5):1002–1008

2. Placzkowski KA, Vella A, Thompson GB, et al. Secular trends in the presentation and management of functioning insulinoma at the Mayo Clinic, 1987–2007. *J Clin Endocrinol Metab* 2009;94(4):1069–1073

3. Service FJ, McMahon MM, O'Brien PC, Ballard DJ. Functioning insulinoma— incidence, recurrence, and long-term survival of patients: a 60-year study. *Mayo Clin Proc* 1991;66(7):711–719

4. Yi P, Park JS, Melton DA. Betatrophin: a hormone that controls pancreatic beta cell proliferation. *Cell* 2013;153(4):747–758

5. El OA, Kawamori D, Dirice E, et al. Liver-derived systemic factors drive beta cell hyperplasia in insulin-resistant states. *Cell Rep* 2013;3(2):401–410

Case 94

Managing Pain and Paralysis in Chronic Inflammatory Demyelinating Polyneuropathy in Diabetes

Aaron I. Vinik, MD, PhD, FCP, MACP, FACE[1]

A 61-year-old Caucasian man with poorly controlled type 2 diabetes presented to our clinic with a 5-month history of right foot drop and severe excruciating pain in the right leg that progressed to the right buttock, left buttock, and left leg resulting in left foot drop. Before the visit, a neurologist had diagnosed him with diabetic amyotrophy and ganglioside GM1 antibody–mediated autoimmune neuropathy. Magnetic resonance imaging (MRI) of the brain was unremarkable. Nerve conduction studies showed absent sural, ulnar, and radial potentials with a right peroneal motor nerve conduction velocity of 19.6 m/sec, and a right posterior tibial conduction velocity of 32.9 m/sec. The patient could walk a few steps using a cane but mainly used a wheelchair. He complained of numbness and burning sensations in his feet and legs. Pain control was inadequate using duloxetine 60 mg/d, pregabalin 75 mg in the morning and 150 mg in the afternoon and evening, gabapentin 300 mg as needed, tramadol 50 mg three times daily, and hydrocodone acetaminophen 7.5/750 mg as needed.

Physical examination revealed quadriceps and foot muscle wasting, thigh adduction and leg extension weaknesses, and a total loss of ankle dorsiflexion and great toe extension bilaterally. Knee and Achilles' reflexes were absent. Sensory exam showed a bilateral decrease in soft touch perception to 30 cm as measured from the great toes, prickling pain reduction to 34 cm, absent vibration sense in the great toes using a 128 Hz tuning fork, and absent 1- and 10-g monofilament sensation and joint proprioception in the great toes.

Biochemical workup was normal. An in-house lab called a NINA assay was used to test the patient's serum toxicity to our N1E-115 neuroblastoma cell line in vitro (compared with the serum toxicity of pooled human serum) over 4 d growth. The test revealed the patient's serum to be highly toxic to the nerve cells, resulting in complete apoptosis and cell death of the nerve cells by day 2.

We diagnosed this patient with chronic inflammatory demyelinating polyneuropathy (CIDP), which is a progressive and symmetrical immune-mediated peripheral neuropathy resulting in weakness of the proximal and distal muscles.1 First-line treatment in CIDP is intravenous immunoglobulin (IVIg),

[1]Eastern Virginia Medical School, Strelitz Diabetes Center, Norfolk, VA.

DOI: 10.2337/9781580405713.94

so we began with a course of Gamunex 1 g/kg/day 2 days/week for 3 consecutive weeks (a total of 6 treatments).

After the first round of IVIg therapy, he discontinued using the wheelchair and could even occasionally walk short distances without his cane. Small gains in muscle strength were noted in the thighs. The treatments made the patient very weak and he needed 24-h assistance with activities of daily living for three weeks after finishing IVIg. The follow-up NINA assay demonstrated no change in toxicity with all neuroblastoma cells apoptosed by day 2. The treatment provided a short-term mild improvement in pain during which time the patient rarely needed either hydrocodone/APAP or tramadol. His leg pain returned 1.5 months after finishing the treatments, and he resumed his regular pain medicine regimen.

We ordered a second course of IVIg treatment. Once again, the patient experienced profound weakness and required 24-h assistance at home. He then developed metabolic acidosis with the serum lactic acid level reaching 7.1 mmol/L (normal 0.5–2.2 mmol/L). This returned to normal after rehydration at the emergency department. He was able to discontinue hydrocodone/tramadol, but the gabapentin was increased to 600 mg four times daily. He could ambulate for longer distances without a cane, but he had little energy to do so. Movement of the right great toe was observed (previously absent), and he returned to functional activities 1 month after treatment. A repeat NINA assay showed only moderate toxicity with neuroblastoma cells surviving all the way to day 4, although in a markedly reduced number compared with the pooled human serum.

Four months after the second IVIg treatment, the patient developed leg pain again and began using a cane and taking hydrocodone and tramadol once more. Repeat NINA assay was highly toxic with 100% neuroblastoma apoptosis by day 4. He tolerated four out of six IVIg treatments in the third course of therapy having stopped because of weakness requiring hospitalization and uncontrolled blood glucose levels >550 mg/dL (30.5 mmol/L). His blood glucose levels improved after discharge but were still poorly controlled with nightly insulin glargine.

At that time, he developed abdominal pain in both upper quadrants. He was found to have cholelithiasis, and a laparoscopic cholecystectomy was performed. The surgery resolved the right-sided colicky pain but a residual band of pain developed in the left lateral abdominal region in the T9/T10 distribution along with a roll of fat protrusion. This was consistent with a mononeuropathy because entrapment at the thoracic spine was ruled out by MRI. His NINA assay returned to being highly toxic with all neuroblastoma cells undergoing apoptosis by day 3.

We considered another course of IVIg but had doubts about the patient's ability to tolerate another round or treatment. Corticosteroids are also first-line therapy for CIDP with expected responses comparable to IVIg. The patient's hemoglobin A1C at 8.9% (normal 4.8–5.9%), however, indicated poor glycemic control and chronic steroid use would surely exacerbate that. The European Federation of Neurological Societies Task Force supports these considerations and also adds plasmapheresis if IVIg and corticosteroids are ineffective.

A fourth option in those guidelines was adding an immunosuppressant. Data are limited and inconclusive about the immune-modulator azathioprine's potential use in CIDP, but it was an attractive option given its activity against immune responses, availability in oral form, side-effect profile, and low cost. After his complete blood count (CBC) proved to be normal, a trial of azathioprine 50 mg/d was started.

This patient's CIDP had a notable response to IVIg, yet he still developed the mononeuropathy while under treatment. There had been a precedent in our initial treatment with IVIg and subsequent use of an immune-modulating agent for autoimmune-mediated neuropathy. In that patient, we formerly used IVIg and then etanercept to successfully mitigate the effects of an acetylcholine receptor antibody-induced autonomic neuropathy.[2]

Seven months into treatment, the current patient no longer has leg pain and there is no biochemical evidence of abnormalities on CBC or transaminase elevation. He has regained 50% of strength in the ankle dorsiflexors and great toe extensors. The knee and ankle reflexes are still absent. His only pain medication now is gabapentin 300 mg twice daily. Functionally, he is able to walk more than several blocks at a time, needs a cane only for stability (not support), and is able to sail on his boat nearly every weekend. His current NINA assay demonstrates moderate toxicity with the neuroblastoma cells present in reduced numbers to day 4 when compared with pooled human serum, similar to his best response after the second round of IVIg. Additionally, the pain from the mononeuropathy at T9/T10 is almost completely resolved. Because the mononeuropathy may be autoimmune related, it is reasonable to question whether azathioprine may have had a beneficial effect on shortening its course and severity.

REFERENCES

1. Vinik AI, Anandacoomaraswamy D, Ullal J. Antibodies to neuronal structures: innocent bystanders or neurotoxins? *Diabetes Care* 2005;28(8):2067–2072

2. Bourcier ME, Vinik AI. A 41-year-old man with polyarthritis and severe autonomic neuropathy. *Ther Clin Risk Manag* 2008;4(4):837–842

Case 95

Neuropathy in Metformin-Treated Type 2 Diabetes

Aaron I. Vinik, MD, PhD, FCP, MACP, FACE[1]

A 68-year-old woman with a 3-year history of type 2 diabetes had been treated with metformin 500 mg b.i.d. since her diagnosis. Hemoglobin A1c (HbA$_{1c}$) was 6.5%, and she had no evidence of diabetic retinopathy or nephropathy. She complained of progressive numbness in her extremities for the past 3 months. The symptoms started in her feet and progressed to affect her lower legs up to her knees as well as her hands bilaterally. She denied pain or tingling but complains of mild weakness in her legs.

On examination, she has decreased sensation to pin prick to her knees and mid-forearms bilaterally, decreased vibration detection using a 128-Hz tuning fork and loss of 1 g monofilament but not 10 g in toes. Proprioception was reduced slightly in toes to ankles. She had 5/5 muscle strength proximally and 4/5 distally, with slight weakness of dorsiflexion of the big toes bilaterally. There was no evidence of entrapment. Her ankle reflexes were absent, but the rest were intact.

Development of diabetic polyneuropathy is related to duration of diabetes and degree of hyperglycemia. It is unusual to see significant diabetic polyneuropathy in the absence of retinopathy or nephropathy. Diabetic polyneuropathy progresses over years, not months. Motor symptoms generally are mild and tend to be a late finding.[1,2]

Encountering a patient with polyneuropathy and diabetes, one must answer the following questions: 1) What is the differential diagnosis of diabetic polyneuropathy? 2) Are there some nondiabetic neuropathies that are more common in people with diabetes? 3) What is the most appropriate workup?

The importance of glycemic control for prevention and development of diabetic neuropathy was clearly established by the Diabetes Control and Complication Trial.[3] This randomized trial with 1,440 patients with type 1 diabetes revealed that patients without preexisting neuropathy had 64% lower incidence of neuropathy when their glycemia was treated intensively. Patients in the intensive therapy group who entered the trial with neuropathy had an increase in nerve conduction velocity as compared with the conventionally treated group.[4] Incidence of neuropathy in type 1 diabetes is associated with the duration of diabetes, degree of glycemic control as assessed by the HbA$_{1c}$, level of triglycerides, hypertension, and smoking. Differential diagnosis of

[1]Eastern Virginia Medical School, Strelitz Diabetes Center, Norfolk, VA.

DOI: 10.2337/9781580405713.95

diabetic neuropathy can be challenging. No characteristics of diabetic neuropathy are unique. In fact because some nondiabetic neuropathies are equally, if not more, common in patients with diabetes, the diagnosis of diabetic neuropathy always requires exclusions of all other causes.

If sensory symptoms predominate consider the following etiology:

- Metabolic that includes neuropathy of uremia, hypothyroidism, folate/B_{12} deficiency, acute intermittent porphyria
- Toxic that develops under the influence of alcohol, heavy metals, industrial hydrocarbons
- Inflammatory or infectious origin that can be seen in patients with connective tissue diseases, vasculitis, celiac disease, sarcoidosis, Lyme disease, HIV, hepatitis B/C
- Others that include hereditary, monoclonal gammopathies (MGUS), paraneoplastic syndromes, amyloidosis

If motor symptoms and signs predominate consider the following:

- Chronic inflammatory demyelinating polyneuropathy (CIDP), MGUS, Guillain-Barre syndrome, myopathies

Several nondiabetic neuropathies are more common in diabetes. Among them are the following:

- CIDP, which is 11-fold more frequent in diabetes
- Uremia
- Vitamin B_{12}/folate/B_6 deficiencies
- Hypothyroidism

The workup for patients with typical presentation should include the following

- Blood urea nitrogen/creatinine (BUN/Cr)
- Thyroid-stimulating hormone (TSH)
- Vitamin B_{12}

For those with atypical presentation, the workup should include the following:

- Electromyography (EMG) /nerve conduction study (NCS)
- Further evaluation depends on predisposing factors
- Physical exam, EMG/NCS findings
- Comprehensive metabolic profile (CMP), CBC, TSH, B_{12}, folate, methylmalonic acid (MMA), serum protein electrophoresis (SPEP)/urine protein electrophoresis (UPEP), HIV
- Hepatitis B/C, Lyme disease, erythrocyte sedimentation rate (ESR), antinuclear antibody (ANA), rheumatoic factor (RF), ACE level, porphyrins, heavy metals, malignancy workup, antiparaneoplastic Ab screen, anti-GM1

In our patient, laboratory findings were as follows:

- **Normal CMP, CBC, TSH**
- **Vitamin B_{12} was 260 pg/mL**
- **Folate 10 pg/mL**

- MMA 70 pg/mL
- SPEP/UPEP no monoclonal gammopathy
- Negative ANA/RF, Lyme disease, HIV, and hepatitis B/C
- EMG/NCS—reduction in amplitudes in tibial, sural, and peroneal sensory and motor nerves, median and ulnar normal
- QAFT normal, sudoscan abnormal

Low level of vitamin B_{12} is an apparent abnormality in this patient. There is now clear evidence that people treated with metformin develop a B_{12} malabsorption. In the older person with diabetes, it has been shown that the threshold for development of neurological symptoms and signs is not 250 pg/mL but ~460 pg/mL.[5] Replacement therapy with B_{12} given as oral supplements and even administration of cyanocobolamin fail to adequately replace B_{12}, and this is best achieved with methylcobolamin in a dose of 3,000 µg/day, which will achieve blood levels of close to 1,000 pg/mL. Our patient received this replacement, and over the course of the next 6 months, the numbness improved. She had mild weakness of dorsiflexion of the big toe, and this is a major concern for tripping and falling with traumatic fractures and brain injury. With strength and balance training, she regained strength, and in the interim, she was given the CDC STEADI (Centers for Disease Control and Prevention: Stopping Elderly Accidents, Deaths and Injuries) guidelines on reducing risk of falling.

REFERENCES

1. Vinik AI, Strotmeyer ES. Chapter 65, Diabetic neuropathy. In *Principles and Practice of Geriatric Medicine*, 5th ed. Sinclair AJ, Morley JE, Vellas B, Eds. New York, Wiley-Blackwell 2012, p. 751–767

2. Fonseca VA, Lavery LA, Thethi TK, Daoud Y, DeSouza C, Ovalle F, Denham DS, Bottiglieri T, Sheehan P, Rosenstock J. Metanx in type 2 diabetes with peripheral neuropathy: a randomized trial. *Am J Med* 2013;126(2):141–149

3. The DCCT Research Group. The effect of intensive treatment of diabetes on the development and progression of long-term complications in insulin-dependent diabetes mellitus. *New Engl J Med* 1993;329:977–986

4. The DCCT Research Group. The effect of intensive diabetes therapy on the development and progression of neuropathy. *Ann Inten Med* 1995;122:561–568

5. Leishear K, et al. Relationship between vitamin B12 and sensory and motor peripheral nerve function in older adults. *J Am Geriatr Soc* 2012;60:1057–1063

Case 96

A Case of Acute Sensory Neuropathy in Type 1 Diabetes

ANDREW J.M. BOULTON, MD, DSc, FACP, FRCP[1]

A 22-year-old woman attended the diabetes clinic complaining of increasingly severe pain in both legs and feet over the past 2 weeks. She found it difficult to describe the pain but said that it was of a burning, stinging character with occasional electrical shock sensations shooting down the lower legs to the feet. She stated that it felt as if her feet were on fire and that the pain was much worse at night: in fact, she was finding it increasingly difficult to sleep and found that the bedclothes and even her socks were irritating the skin of her feet.

Until recently, her glycemic control had been poor; in her past history, she had frequent hospital admissions as a teenager with ketoacidosis and admitted that she had omitted insulin on occasions in the past to assist with her weight control. Four months previously, hemoglobin A1c (HbA$_{1c}$) had been 10.1% (87 mmol/mol).

The described symptoms are typical of neuropathic pain in the lower extremities. Unlike nociceptive pain (e.g., a fracture or toothache), patients typically find it difficult to describe the painful symptoms of neuropathy.[1,2] Distal symmetrical polyneuropathy (DSP) is a very common complication of diabetes, but the symptoms of chronic DSP tend to be gradual in onset.[1] This patient has a typical history of acute DSP.

It transpired that after discussion with a nurse educator 3 months previously, she had decided to change her therapy to continuous subcutaneous insulin infusion (CSII). She was starting a new job and was keen to avoid hospital admissions with hyper- or hypoglycemia. She was self-monitoring up to seven times daily and, in the last 8 weeks, her control had rapidly improved. Recent fasting glucose levels had been in the range of 3.5–6.5 mmol/L (63–117 mg/dL), and at other times, readings were <9 mmol/L (162 mg/dL). An HbA$_{1c}$ checked by the nurse 1 week before this visit was 6.8% (50 mmol/mol).

Further support for the clinical diagnosis of acute sensory neuropathy is provided by the previously noted information. Acute DSP often follows a period of metabolic instability, such as poor control, ketoacidosis, or, as in the

[1]University of Manchester, UK; University of Miami, Miami, FL; Manchester Royal Infirmary, Manchester, UK; President, European Association for the Study of Diabetes, Dusseldorf, Germany.

DOI: 10.2337/9781580405713.96

present case, rapid improvement of glycemic control over a short period of time. One example of this is so-called insulin neuritis, originally described by Ellenberg, which refers to the onset of neuropathic pain following the initiation of insulin therapy and followed by rapid improvement of control.[1] This condition also has been described in patients on oral hypoglycemic drugs, suggesting that it is not the insulin itself, but rather it is the change in blood glucose levels that results in the acute DSP. Blood glucose flux may be important in the genesis of neuropathic pain,[1,2] and one study using continuous glucose monitoring confirmed that patients with neuropathic pain had less stable control than those with painless neuropathy.[3] There were more excursions to hyper- and hypoglycemic levels in the former group, confirming increased blood glucose flux in such patients. It is believed that sudden improvement in blood glucose control results in reduced nerve blood flow, rendering the endoneurium ischemic.[4]

It also has been reported that acute DSP may be seen in young people with eating disorders and erratic glycemic control.[5] In the present case, the patient did report omitting insulin to promote weight loss.

Although the diagnosis of acute DSN is usually suggested by the history alone, a careful clinical examination is essential in the diagnosis of any neuropathy in a diabetic patient.

On examination, the patient had a BMI of 24 kg/m² and was normotensive. The only abnormalities were found in the neurologic exam of the lower limbs: peripheral pulses were all intact. Motor assessment in the legs was normal, and all reflexes were present and equal. On clinical sensory assessment, there was a decrease in pinprick sensation in both feet and reduced appreciation of the difference between hot and cold rods was detected in both feet. Vibration perception using a 128-Hz tuning fork was intact bilaterally. She demonstrated allodynia (when a non-noxious stimulus such as touch gives rise to a painful sensation) in both feet.

These findings are compatible with a diagnosis of acute DSP. In contrast to the chronic DSP, in which abnormalities of small- and large-fiber dysfunction together with absent ankle reflexes are typically found, the neurologic exam in acute DSN may reveal decreased small-fiber sensory function (pain and temperature perception) or, in some cases, may be virtually normal (Table 96.1).[1,2]

Investigations were all normal, including renal function, urinalysis and microalbuminuria screening, and a complete blood count. A diagnosis of acute DSP was made. In the first instance, her basal rates of CSII were reduced, and for the next 2 weeks, target blood glucose levels were as follows: fasting 7–10 mmol/L (126–180 mg/dL) and other times <13 mmol/L (<234 mg/dL). Treatment with pregabalin 150 mg b.i.d. was started.

Unfortunately, there is little evidence base upon which to plan the management of acute painful DSP. On the assumption that sudden improvement of glycemic control had precipitated the pain, it was decided to reduce her insulin doses to enable blood glucose control to be less rigid and thereafter to gradually improve control over the next 2 months. Additionally, those with painful DSP need pharmacological treatment for their neuropathic pain. Both pregabalin

Table 96.1 — Contrast between Acute Sensory and Chronic Sensorimotor Painful Neuropathies

	Acutesensory	Chronic Sensorimotor
Mode of onset	Relatively rapid	Gradual, insidious
Symptoms	Severe burning pain Aching; weight loss usual	Burning pain, paresthesiae, numbness; weight loss unusual
Symptom severity	+++	0 to ++
Signs	Mild sensory in some; motor unusual	Stocking and glove sensory loss; absent ankle reflexes
Other diabetes complications	Unusual	Increased prevalence
Electrophysiological investigations	May be normal or minor abnormalities	Abnormalities unusual in motor and sensory nerves
Natural history	Complete recovery within 12 months	Symptoms may persist intermittently for years; at risk of foot ulceration

Source: Reprinted with permission from Boulton.[1]

and duloxetine are recommended as first-line agents. On this occasion, pregabalin was chosen as the patient was very anxious, and this drug also has antianxiolytic properties.

Three months later, glycemic control was excellent having improved gradually over the 2 months. The neuropathic pain was controlled on pregabalin 150 mg b.i.d., and the troublesome sleep disturbance had resolved. After another 6 months, the pregabalin dosage was reduced gradually and eventually stopped.

The natural history of acute painful DSP is that of resolution of symptoms within 1 year.[1] What is unknown, however, is whether these patients have a greater history of later developing chronic DSP.

REFERENCES

1. Boulton AJM, Malik RA, Arezzo JC, Sosenko J. Diabetic somatic neuropathies. *Diabetes Care* 2004;27:1458–1486

2. Tesfaye S, Boulton AJM, Dickenson AH. Mechanisms and management of diabetic painful distal symmetrical polyneuropathy. *Diabetes Care* 2013;36; 2456–2465

3. Oyibo S, Prasad YD, Jackson NJ, Jude EB, Boulton AJM. The relationship between blood glucose excursions and painful diabetic peripheral neuropathy. *Diabetic Med* 2002;19:870–873

4. Tesfaye S, Malik RA, Harris N, Jakubowski JJ, Mody C, Rennie IG, Ward JD. Arterio-venous shunting and proliferating new vessels in acute painful neuropathy of rapid glycemic control (insulin neuritis). *Diabetologia* 1996; 39:329–335

5. Steel JM, Young RJ, Lloyd GG, Clarke BF. Clinically apparent eating disorders in young diabetic women: associations with painful neuropathy and other complications. *Brit Med J* 1987;294:859–862

Case 97

Nondiabetic Neuropathy in a Patient with Type 2 Diabetes

DAVID S.H. BELL, MB[1]

A 72-year-old white man with an 8-year history of type 2 diabetes under excellent glycemic control (HbA$_{1c}$ in the 5.5–6.5% range) on metformin monotherapy suddenly developed tingling in his feet, which he thought was due to diabetes. Some of the details of this case have been published previously.[1] As a result, he delayed reporting his new symptom to his endocrinologist. At a scheduled office visit, he reported these symptoms and, on examination, was found to have decreased pinprick sensation bilaterally without the loss of vibration or joint position sense. Ankle jerks were brisk bilaterally.

The presentation of intact ankle jerks in the presence of marked pinprick loss is not typical of diabetic neuropathy and suggests that the neuropathy could be due to vitamin B$_{12}$ deficiency.[1]

The vitamin B$_{12}$ level was low at 121 pg/mL (normal range 211–911 pg/mL). The serum gastrin level was normal at 78 pg/mL (normal range 0–115 pg/mL), and the antiparietal antibody level was 3.3 (normal range 0–20 units). Vitamin B$_{12}$ replacement was initiated with 1,000 mcg daily for 1 week, weekly for 4 weeks, and monthly thereafter.

Metformin is currently widely recommended as initial therapy for type 2 diabetes and is the most widely utilized antidiabetic oral agent. The most feared complication of metformin therapy is lactic acidosis, which will never occur unless metformin is utilized in an inappropriate situation such as a creatinine clearance of <30 ml/min. A common, well-documented, yet largely unrecognized complication of metformin therapy is vitamin B$_{12}$ deficiency resulting from metformin-induced malabsorption of vitamin B$_{12}$. In this case, pernicious anemia resulting from autoimmune gastric atrophy was ruled out by normal gastrin and antiparietal antibody levels.

Vitamin B$_{12}$ deficiency is associated with a macrocytic and megaloblastic anemia. The anemia, however, is often preceded by neurological damage: an initial demyelination is followed by axonal degeneration and neuronal death. This occurs not only in peripheral nerves but also in the posterior and lateral columns of the spinal cord and cerebrum. Clinically the earliest symptoms are numbness and paresthesias in the feet. If the vitamin B$_{12}$ deficiency is not

[1]University of Alabama, Birmingham, AL.

DOI: 10.2337/9781580405713.97

corrected, this can be followed by muscle weakness, ataxia, sphincter disturbance, and dementia.

**With correction of the metformin-induced vitamin B$_{12}$ deficiency, the
patient's neuropathic symptoms neither improved nor worsened over the
next year. More advanced neurological damage that could have occurred
from prolonged vitamin B$_{12}$ deficiency was avoided. The patient had
researched data on metformin-induced vitamin B$_{12}$ deficiency on the Internet and inquired whether his vitamin B$_{12}$ deficiency and subsequent neuropathy could have been avoided.**

For many years, it has been recognized that malabsorption of vitamin B$_{12}$
occurs in 30% of the patients who utilize metformin. This long-term effect, however, was not generally recognized in the U.S. when metformin became available
in 1994 or even after the publication of the U.K. Prospective Diabetes Study when
the utilization of metformin increased exponentially. In 2006, metformin-induced
B$_{12}$ deficiency was reintroduced after a case-control study revealed a correlation
between the dose and duration of metformin therapy and B$_{12}$ deficiency.[2]

Metformin interferes with the absorption of the B$_{12}$-intrinsic factor complex through its action on the calcium-dependent membrane in the terminal
ileum. Indeed, dietary calcium supplements can reverse metformin-induced
vitamin B$_{12}$ malabsorption.[2,3]

**The patient was informed that the only way that his metformin-induced
vitamin B$_{12}$ deficient neuropathy could have been avoided would have been
through the use of dietary calcium supplements or an annual assessment of
his serum vitamin B$_{12}$ level, or the annual administration of a prophylactic
vitamin B$_{12}$ injection.**

**The patient also inquired, again based on his Internet research, whether
his metformin-induced vitamin B$_{12}$ deficiency had occurred at an earlier
time than would have been predicted.**

The risk of metformin-induced vitamin B$_{12}$ deficiency increases with the
time of exposure to metformin. After removal of intrinsic factor through partial gastrectomy, 12–15 years usually elapses before vitamin B$_{12}$ malabsorption
results in clinically significant vitamin B$_{12}$ deficiency. However, it may occur at
an earlier time with metformin.

**The patient's last question, again based on his Internet research, was
whether peripheral nerve damage from diabetes could be amplified by
metformin-induced vitamin B$_{12}$ deficiency.**

Wile et al. have clearly shown an accelerated progression of diabetic neuropathy in the presence of metformin-induced vitamin B$_{12}$ deficiency.[4]

REFERENCES

1. Bell DS. Nondiabetic neuropathy in a patient with diabetes. *Endocr Pract*
1995;1(6):393–394

2. Bell DS. Metformin-induced vitamin B12 deficiency presenting as a peripheral neuropathy. *South Med J* 2010;103(3):265–257

3. Bailey CJ, Wilcock C, Scarpello JH. Metformin and the intestine. *Diabetologia* 2008;51(8):1552–1553

4. Wile DJ, Toth C. Association of metformin, elevated homocysteine, and methylmalonic acid levels and clinically worsened diabetic peripheral neuropathy. *Diabetes Care* 2010;33(1):156–161

Case 98

Severe Distal Symmetrical and Autonomic Neuropathy in a Patient with a Short Duration of Type 1 Diabetes

DAVID S.H. BELL, MB[1]

A 17-year-old woman had had type 1 diabetes for 2 years when she developed restless legs, which was followed by paresthesias in her lower limbs, and soon after by the development of nocturnal diarrhea, fecal incontinence, early satiety, weight loss, and dizziness on standing. Some of the details of this case have been published previously.[1]

On examination there was a decrease in pinprick sensation to thigh level in the lower limbs and in the upper limbs to above the elbows. In addition, there was a loss of vibration sense and complete areflexia in both the upper and lower limbs. Furthermore, she had a fixed tachycardia, which did not respond to a Valsalva maneuver indicating that cardiac vagal denervation had occurred. Blood pressure was 110/70 mmHg lying, dropped to 70/undetectable on standing and after 2 min remained at this level.

It is unusual for neuropathy to occur with a short duration of type 1 diabetes, especially in younger patients. When neuropathy does occur in this group, it is almost always due to acute autoimmune demyelinating process. This diagnosis can be confirmed with neuroelectrophysiological studies, which will show evidence of severe demyelination. If demyelination is shown on neuroelectrophysiological studies, therapy with immunosuppressive medications and intravenous immunoglobulin should be utilized to at least prevent disease progression and hopefully result in at least some reversal of the disease process.

In this case, the neuroelectrophysiological studies showed evidence of axonal sensory and motor neuropathy but did not show evidence of demyelination. Therefore, each of the components of her neuropathy was treated symptomatically. She responded reasonably well to gabapentin and clonazepam for her paresthesias, metaclopramide for her gastroparesis, metronidazole and cholestyramine for her diarrhea, and fludrocortisone for her postural hypotension.

On a follow-up visit, it was noted that her total cholesterol (90 ng/dL), calculated low-density lipoprotein (LDL) cholesterol (42 ng/dL), and non–high-density lipoprotein (HDL) cholesterol (50 ng/dL) were low. It was also noted that she was taking a statin. On inquiring why she was taking a statin,

[1]University of Alabama, Birmingham, AL.

DOI: 10.2337/9781580405713.98

her mother said that it was because her primary care doctor thought that it would be "good for her diabetes." Her mother also remembered that her neuropathic symptoms had not been present when the statin was started. The statin was discontinued and within a week her symptoms began to improve. Within 6 months her postural hypotension, gastroparesis, diarrhea, and fecal incontinence had resolved. In addition, the signs of distal symmetrical polyneuropathy ameliorated so that after 6 months the only remaining signs were areflexia and loss of pinprick sensation to the wrist and ankle. All of her medications, with the exception of insulin, were discontinued. Unfortunately, resolution of her neuropathic symptoms was accompanied by the return of a vigorous appetite, weight gain, and worsening of glycemic control.

Statin-induced neuropathy, while much less common than statin-induced myopathy, does occur. European epidemiological and case-control studies suggest a two- to fourfold increase in the incidence of idiopathic neuropathy while on a statin, and the development of neuropathy seems to be a class effect with both polyneuropathy and mononeuropathy being described.[2,3] As in this case, improvement or even complete resolution is frequently described with cessation of statin therapy. There are no clinical, biochemical, or electrophysiological characteristics from which a diagnosis of statin-induced neuropathy can be made so that awareness of statin-induced neuropathy and a trial of statin withdrawal with careful observation for the development of a clinical improvement is the only way that statin-induced neuropathy can be diagnosed.

Proposed mechanisms for statin-induced neuropathy include an alteration in cholesterol synthesis, changes in the cholesterol-rich neuronal membrane, or a statin-induced decrease in ubiquinone coenzyme Q10 (CoQ10) activity. CoQ10 is an enzyme in the mitochondrial chain, which is inhibited by statins and, as a result, may cause neuronal damage.[1]

Statins may infrequently cause an acute idiosyncratic somatic or autonomic neuropathy that in the patient with diabetes almost invariably will be attributed to diabetes. Awareness of the possibility of a statin-induced neuropathy and removal of the statin for a short period of time as a diagnostic test may result in restoration of neurological function and an improved quality of life for the patient with diabetes.[4]

REFERENCES

1. Vaughan TB, Bell DS. Statin neuropathy masquerading as diabetic autoimmune polyneuropathy. *Diabetes Care* 2005;28(8):2082

2. Otruba P, Kanovsky P, Hlustik P. Treatment with statins and peripheral neuropathy: results of a 36-month prospective clinical and neurophysiological follow-up. *Neuro Endocrinol Lett* 2011;32(5):688–690

3. Corrao G, Zambon A, Bertù L, Botteri E, Leoni O, Contiero P. Lipid lowering drugs prescription and the risk of peripheral neuropathy: an exploratory case-control study using automated databases. *J Epidemiol Community Health* 2004;58(12):1047–1051

4. Backes JM, Howard PA. Association of HMG-CoA reductase inhibitors with neuropathy. *Ann Pharmacother* 2003;37(2):274–278

Case 99

Diabetic Amyotrophy and Neuropathic Cachexia

DAVID S.H. BELL, MB[1]

A 65-year-old white man with type 2 diabetes of 6 years' duration initially was treated with metformin for 2 years and a combination of metformin and sitagliptin. His C-peptide was 6.1 ng/mL and his HbA$_{1c}$ was 7.3%. He later presented with lower-limb parathesias, muscle weakness (difficulty arising from a chair), and severe pain in his thighs. In addition, his weight had dropped from 268 lb to 178 lb over the previous 6 months. He denied alcohol use.

Diabetic amyotrophy (DA) is a rare but well-established clinical entity initially described by Ludwig Burns in 1890. DA usually occurs in men in their fifth or sixth decade with well-controlled type 2 diabetes.[1] Classically, the initial symptom is severe somatic pain in the thigh muscles, followed by weakness in these muscles, which can initially be unilateral but invariably becomes bilateral. Another key feature of DA is the presence of involuntary weight loss (with the average weight loss being 18 kg). The cachexia is thought to be due to excess production of cytokines, especially tumor necrosis factor-α.

He reported that he got "dizzy" on rising from a chair or getting out of bed.[2] On examination, he had severe weakness and atrophy of the quadriceps, gluteus minimus and maximus, iliopsoas, hamstrings, adductor, and abductor muscles that was more severe on the right than the left. Ankle and knee jerks were absent, and vibration and pinprick sensation were decreased to the midthigh bilaterally. His heart rate did not respond to a Valsalva maneuver and his blood pressure dropped from 150/90 mmHg after lying for 10 min to 60/undetectable upon standing, and increased slightly to 85/20 mmHg after standing for 2 min. His hypotension was accompanied by patient report of lightheadedness.

DA is most often accompanied by the manifestation of distal symmetrical polyneuropathy and autonomic neuropathy. The postural hypotension was successfully treated with fludrocortisone 0.3 mg daily and the parasthesias associated with distal symmetrical polyneuropathy were treated with amitryptyline and clonazepam.

Plasma protein electrophoresis was normal as were both the vitamin B$_{12}$ and methylmalonic acid levels. Nerve conduction and electromyogram

[1]University of Alabama, Birmingham, AL.

DOI: 10.2337/9781580405713.99

studies showed severe widespread denervation with lumbosacral polyradic-ulopathy (findings are typical of diabetic amyotrophy). Based on the characteristic, clinical, and electrodiagnostic findings, neither muscle nor nerve biopsy was recommended.

The diagnosis of DA is one of exclusion and based on clinical and electro-diagnostic findings. The differential diagnosis includes lumbosacral plexopathy polyradiculopathy, focal quadriceps myopathy, inclusion body myositis, and diabetic mononeuropathy multiplex. As with all diabetic neuropathies, a plasma cell dyscrasia or vitamin B_{12} deficiency should be ruled out because they are correctable causes of neuropathy.

The cause of DA is not known but has been postulated to be due to multiple infarcts in the proximal nerve trunks and lumbosacral plexus, probably due to occlusions of the vasa nervorum. Interestingly, the cerebrospinal fluid has been reported to contain an excess of both protein and myoinositol in DA.[3]

The patient was started on an intensive physical therapy program after his symptoms from distal symmetrical polyneuropathy and autonomic neuropathy were under control.

DA will resolve spontaneously in 1–3 years, but recovery is not always complete. Generally, severe symptoms persist for >6 months, weight loss resolves within a year, and muscle strength is maximized in 2–3 years. Patients need to be reassured that they will recover from DA but that the recovery will take time.

REFERENCES

1. Bell DSH, Ward J. Peripheral and cranial neuropathy in diabetes. In *Clinical Diabetes Mellitus*, 3rd ed. Davidson JK, Ed. New York, NY, Thieme, 2000, p. 621–635

2. Vinik AI, Park TS, Stansberry KB, Pittenger GL. Diabetic neuropathies. *Diabetologia* 2000;43(8):957–973

3. Albright ES, Bell DSH. Diabetic amyotrophy associated with hepatic virus C infection. *Endocrinologist* 2003;13:445–448

Case 100

High GAD Antibody Levels and Cerebellar Atrophy in a Patient with Type 1 Diabetes

DAVID S.H. BELL, MB[1]

A 27-year old white woman had well-controlled type 1 diabetes (HbA$_{1c}$ ranging from 5.5 to 6.6%). Some details of this case have been published previously.[1] She had used an insulin pump for the past 10 years of her 16-year history of diabetes, and she had no neuropathy, nephropathy, retinopathy, or macrovascular disease. Her type 1 diabetes was accompanied by other autoimmune diseases, including Hashimoto's thyroiditis leading to hypothyroidism and pernicious anemia. On a routine visit, she reported problems with balance and vertigo. On examination, she had unilateral difficulty with the heel-to-shin test on the right. In addition, she had difficulty with tandem walking and had a broad-based gait. Ankle and knee deep tendon reflexes were present and brisk. Vibration sense and pinprick sensation were intact.

When a patient with type 1 diabetes presents with a balance problem, it is usually due to severe distal symmetric polyneuropathy. The finding of unilateral ataxia with intact peripheral sensation suggests a brainstem lacunar infarct.[2] In a well-controlled, young patient with type 1 diabetes, a cerebrovascular event is highly unlikely, and the clinical diagnosis of unilateral cerebellar dysfunction of unknown etiology was made.

Magnetic resonance imaging was performed and showed cerebellar parenchymal loss on the left side with cerebellar atrophy. An antibody screen for paraneoplastic antigens was negative. The thyroid peroxidase antibodies were strongly positive as was the antiparietal antibody, but both vitamin B$_{12}$ and thyroid-stimulating hormone levels were normal. The anti-GAD antibody titer was 3,558 nmol/L (reference range <0.02 nmol/L).

GAD catalyzes the conversion of glutamate to γ-aminobutyric acid (GABA) and is the dominant antigen in type 1 diabetes and in stiff man syndrome. A link between cerebellar dysfunction and high GAD antibodies has also been described with type 1 diabetes and polyendocrine autoimmunity (Hashimoto's thyroiditis and pernicious anemia).[3,4]

Why would a high anti-GAD antibody level be associated with cerebellar atrophy? To cause cerebellar atrophy, the GAD antibody must enter the neuron. The likely explanation for entry of GAD antibody into the neuron is that

[1]University of Alabama, Birmingham, AL.

DOI: 10.2337/9781580405713.100

when anti-GAD antibody levels are extremely high, the Purkinje cells take up the GAD antibody and transfer the antibody to the neuron, where an interaction with the GAD antigen occurs. This in turn leads to neural destruction and dysfunction. Another possible explanation is that the high anti-GAD antibody levels are simply a marker for damage to the GAD antibody-containing neurons by a T-cell–mediated immune attack on GAD antigens in the central nervous system (CNS) neurons, which is similar to the T-cell–mediated attack on the pancreatic β-cell that leads to type 1 diabetes.

A second question is that with GAD residing exclusively in the CNS and the pancreatic β-cell, why don't more patients with type 1 diabetes develop CNS pathologies? A comparison of GAD antibody-associated CNS pathologies and the GAD antibody associated with type 1 diabetes reveals the following:

1. HLA antigens differ in the CNS and the pancreatic β-cell; the DQB10201 type is most prevalent in CNS pathologies, and the DR34DQ302 type is most prevalent in type 1 diabetes.
2. GAD antibodies are directed against GAD segments 161 to 143 and 473 to 455 in type 1 diabetes, but against GAD segments 81 to 171 and 323 to 403 in the CNS.
3. GAD 65 and 67 antigens predominate in the CNS and are the major antigens in CNS lesions, whereas GAD 65 is the predominate antigen in the pancreatic β-cell.
4. In type 1 diabetes, β-cell damage is caused by a Th1 response. In a Th1 response, T-helper cells secrete interferon and interleukin-2, which inhibit the type 2 T-helper cells that are involved in cell-mediated immunity. The latter do this by activating macrophages and cytotoxic (CD8) T cells, which recognize complexes of major histocompatibility-complex molecules on the target cell membrane. With CNS pathologies, there is a Th2 response in which helper T cells secrete interferons 4, 5, 6, and 10 that inhibit type 1 T-helper cells involved in humoral immunity by stimulating B-lymphocytes to produce antibodies.
5. Most important, when the level of GAD antibody is high, GAD antibodies have the ability to enter the neuron and interfere with the synthesis of GABA.[5]

No further CNS damage occurred in this patient, although her ability to work as a registered nurse was impaired, and she had to accept that she was too disabled to continue working in her profession.

REFERENCES

1. Bell DSH. Stroke in the diabetic patient. *Diabetes Care* 1994;17:217–219

2. Bell DSH, Ovalle F, Shadmany S. Cerebellar ataxia associated with high levels of anti-glutamic acid decarbosylase antibodies. *Endocrinologist* 2001;11(3):233–235

3. Saiz A, Arpa J, Sagasta A, Casamitjana R, Zarranz JJ, Tolosa E, Graus F. Auto-antibodies to glutamic acid decarboxylase in three patients with cerebellar ataxia, late-onset insulin-dependent diabetes mellitus, and polyendocrine auto-immunity. *Neurology* 1997;49(4):1026–1030

4. Tobias L, Hawa M, Leslie DG, Lane R, Picard J, Londer M. Immune reactivity to glutamic acid decarboxylase 65 in stiff-man syndrome and type 1 diabetes mellitus. *Lancet* 2000;356:33–35

5. Levy LM, Dalakas MC, Floeter MK. The stiff-person syndrome: an autoimmune disorder affecting neurotransmission of gamma-aminobutiric acid. *Ann Intern Med* 1999;131:522–530

Case 101

Resolution of Infertility with Diabetes Therapy

David S.H. Bell, MB[1]

A 46-year-old Eurasian woman presented with new-onset type 2 diabetes. She had a long history of polycystic ovary disease (PCO) and for the previous year had been treated with metformin alone. Some details of this case have been presented previously.[1] Because she had two fasting blood glucose levels >126 mg/dL while she was taking metformin, she was diagnosed as having diabetes and referred for further assessment and treatment.

PCO is associated with insulin resistance and the features of the metabolic syndrome such as a high fasting triglyceride to high-density lipoprotein (HDL) ratio, hypertension, and visceral obesity. Because of the insulin resistance associated with the metabolic syndrome and the inability to produce enough insulin to overcome the insulin resistance, at least 40% of women with PCO develop diabetes after age 50 years. In addition, because of the presence of the cardiac risk factors of the metabolic syndrome, as well as the other cardiac risk factors of the metabolic syndrome (increased inflammation, increased oxidative stress, endothelial dysfunction, increased platelet aggregation, and decreased fibrinolysis), there is a 7.5-fold increased risk of a cardiac event in postmenopausal women with PCO.

Her menarche had occurred at age 12 years, but she had never had more than three menstrual periods per year except for two occasions during her twenties when she had dieted and lost around 20 lb. On both of these occasions, the weight loss resulted in her periods becoming regular, and the achievement of pregnancy and delivery of two healthy infants.

In PCO, high insulin levels stimulate the adrenal cortex and the ovaries to produce more testosterone. Hyperinsulinemia also results in an increased release of leutenizing hormone (LH) from the anterior pituitary, which further stimulates ovarian testosterone production. In addition, hyperinsulinemia decreases the hepatic production of sex hormone binding globulin so that free testosterone levels rise. Dependent on the levels of free testosterone, signs of virilization, such as acne, hirsuitism, temporal recession of the hairline, crown baldness, increased muscle bulk, and cliteromegaly may occur.

[1]University of Alabama, Birmingham, AL.

DOI: 10.2337/9781580405713.101

Hyperandrogenemia, however, also results in suppression of ovulation, disturbances in the menstrual cycle, and infertility. In this patient, reductions in weight had resulted in greater insulin sensitivity, decreased insulin and free testosterone levels, the return of ovulation, a regular menstrual cycle, and pregnancy.[2]

At the initial consultation, therapy with metformin was continued and a thiazolidinedione (rosiglitazone 4 mg daily) was added to her regimen. Not only did this result in well-controlled diabetes (HbA$_{1c}$ 5.8%) but also in the return of regular menstruation for 4 months. Subsequently, she again became amenorrheic but because of her age and history of amenorrhea, this did not cause concern. She did not have hot flashes, vaginal dryness, decreased libido, or other symptoms of menopause. Six months after her last menstrual period, she presented in an emergency room with abdominal pain and on abdominal ultrasonography was found to be 30 weeks' pregnant.

Spontaneous pregnancy in the mid- to late-40s is very unusual. In populations such as the Hudderites where contraception is not practiced, the average age of the last conception is 40.9 years.[1] Age-related decreases in fertility are thought to be due to a decreased number of available oocytes following years of regular ovulation. In those with PCO, however, anovulation over many years may result in a "stockpiling" of follicles that are available for ovulation and fertilization at an older age.[3] This patient possibly had a large store of oocytes, and this along with the increase in insulin sensitivity and the decrease in free testosterone may have led to ovulation and fertilization.

With the discovery of a 30-week pregnancy, metformin and rosiglitazone were discontinued by the obstetricians and insulin therapy was commenced. Six weeks later, she became hypertensive and an induced parturition occurred at 37 weeks. The baby girl was healthy and experienced no neonatal complications.

Metformin is not contraindicated during pregnancy. In fact, many endocrinologists believe that in women with PCO metformin should be continued for at least the full first trimester to decrease the risk of a spontaneous abortion. Whether metformin should be continued throughout the pregnancy, which could result in the avoidance of gestational diabetes, preeclamptic toxemia, and antipartum hemorrhage, is still disputable. Data on the effects of rosiglitazone on the outcome of pregnancy are lacking.[4] In this case, the outcome was positive, and several reports have indicated that accidental thiazolidinedione exposure during pregnancy does not result in abnormal fetal outcomes.[1]

Following the birth of her baby girl, insulin therapy was discontinued, and the patient was again treated with a combination of metformin and a thiazolidinedione. In addition, to avoid further pregnancies, the patient had a tubal ligation.

Although pregnancy is rare in the fifth and sixth decade, it can occur in patients with PCO where stockpiling of oocytes may occur. Care should be taken in all patients with type 2 diabetes who are potentially fertile to avoid undesired pregnancy by utilizing contraception measures when drugs such as thiazolidinedione and metformin that increase insulin sensitivity, decrease insulin resistance and free testosterone levels, and have the ability to restore regular ovulation are utilized.

REFERENCES

1. Vaughan TB, Bell DSH. Stockpiling of ovarian follicles and the response to rosiglitazone. *Diabetes Care* 2005;28(9)2333–2334

2. Randeva HS, Tan BK, Weickert MO, Lois K, Nestler JE, Sattar N, Lehnert H. Cardiometabolic aspects of the polycystic ovary syndrome. *Endocr Rev* 2012;33(5):812–841

3. Maciel GA, Baracat EC, Benda JA, Markham SM, Hensinger K, Chang RJ, Erickson GF. Stockpiling of transitional and classic primary follicles in ovaries of women with polycystic ovary syndrome. *J Clin Endocrinol Metab* 2004;89(11):5321–5327

4. Kalyoncu NI, Yaris F, Ulku C, Kadioglu M, Kesim M, Unsal M, Dikici M, Yaris E. A case of rosiglitazone exposure in the second trimester of pregnancy. *Reprod Toxicol* 2005;19(4):563–564

Case 102

The Initial Pregnancy Visit of a Woman with Type 1 Diabetes and Diabetes Complications

Aidan McElduff, MD[1]

A 31-year-old woman with a 20-year history of type 1 diabetes presents with 6 weeks of amenorrhea in her second pregnancy. The current glycemic control is good as determined by a hemoglobin A1c (HbA$_{1c}$) of 6.1% and the absence of major hypoglycemia. There is a history of Graves' disease. A preliminary prepregnancy counseling session had taken place but advice about active contraception, until a definite start date had been selected, was not followed. The patient has active proliferative retinopathy requiring laser therapy and moderate diabetic nephropathy with a recent albumin excretion rate of 58 μg/min and an estimated glomerular filtration rate (eGFR) of 55 mL/min/1.73 m^2 (creatinine 105 μmol/L or 1.2 mg/dL). There is no evidence of peripheral neuropathy. The pedal pulses are palpable, and there are no bruits.

Women with type 1 diabetes who received prepregnancy counseling have better pregnancy outcomes. Achieving 100% success with prepregnancy counseling has proven difficult. Understanding a woman's decision making when planning a pregnancy is an area that warrants further research.

An assessment for diabetes complications at the onset of pregnancy is important as pregnancy can affect complications and complications can influence pregnancy outcomes.

In the Diabetes Control and Complications Trial (DCCT), the likelihood of worsening retinopathy was significantly greater during pregnancy and in the first year postpartum in the 180 women who became pregnant (270 pregnancies) compared with 500 women who did not become pregnant. The odds ratio of developing retinopathy was higher in the conventionally treated group in which treatment was intensified during pregnancy, than in the intensively treated group although the confidence intervals overlapped: 2.48 (1.56–3.94) versus 1.63 (1.01–2.64) for the intensively treated group.[1]

The Diabetes in Early Pregnancy study found that, among 140 women who did not have proliferative retinopathy at the time of conception, progression of retinopathy occurred in 10% of those who had no retinopathy, 21% of those with mild background retinopathy, and 55% of those with severe nonproliferative retinopathy. The risk for progression of diabetic retinopathy during pregnancy was increased in those with the highest initial HbA$_{1c}$ values and in those with the greatest reduction in HbA$_{1c}$ value.[2]

[1]Discipline of Medicine, Sydney University, Sydney, NSW, Australia.

DOI: 10.2337/9781580405713.102

In the DCCT, the long-term risk of progression (over an average of 6.5 years of follow-up) was not different among the women who did or did not become pregnant.[1]

In summary, retinopathy may worsen in pregnancy per se and the risk is greater in women with more severe retinopathy at baseline and in those in whom glycemic control improves markedly in early pregnancy.

Ideally, glycemic control should be optimized before conception; laser therapy, if required, should be administered before conception; and the intensity of monitoring during pregnancy can be related to the degree of risk.

The information for long-term effect of pregnancy on nephropathy is clear although the acute effects are less well defined.

In the DCCT, the long-term risk of progression of albumin excretion rate (over an average of 6.5 years of follow-up) was not different among the women who did or did not become pregnant.

Rossing et al.[3] demonstrated pregnancy had no adverse long-term impact on kidney function and survival. From 93 women, 26 had pregnancies (advised against) and were followed for 16 years on average. Thirty-five percent died due to cardiovascular disease and end-stage raised renal failure. Pregnancy had no effect on the outcomes.

The DCCT and the EURODIAB IDDM Complications Study found that pregnancy was not a risk factor for development of microalbuminuria or long-term progression of nephropathy in woman with *no* nephropathy or microalbuminuria at baseline.[1,4]

Women with mild renal dysfunction creatinine < 124 µmol/L, CrCl >80 mL/min, before pregnancy are likely to maintain stable renal function throughout pregnancy. Women with moderate to severe renal insufficiency typically show rising creatinine concentrations by the third trimester that may persist postpartum.

Overt nephropathy is associated with a variety of pregnancy complications, such as fetal growth restriction, nonreassuring fetal status, and preeclampsia. Preterm delivery and caesarean are often required for maternal or fetal indications.

Medications included insulin detemir insulin 13 units at 8:00 A.M. and 8 or 9 units at 9:00 P.M.; insulin aspart usually 4 units before breakfast, 5 units before lunch, and 5 units before dinner adjusted as required for variations in carbohydrate content of the meals and any correction dose; irbesarten 150 mg once a day; and thyroxine 100 µg on Wednesday and Sunday, and 50 µg on the other 5 days. Initial therapy involved ceasing irbesarten and commencing methyldopa 250 mg three times a day and increasing the thyroxine to 100 µg on 4 days, 50 µg on 3 days each week.

At the initial pregnancy visit medication should be reviewed for safety in pregnancy. The commonly used antihypertensive agents, ACE inhibitors, or angiotensin receptor blockers can cause renal damage when used in the second or third trimester. It has been suggested that they cause an increased incidence of congenital malformations, although this work has been criticized. A risk benefit assessment of continuing ACE inhibitors or angiotensin receptor blockers into early pregnancy needs to be undertaken for the individual woman. Statins or other lipid-lowering agents should be ceased before conception.[5]

Incidental diseases need to be considered. Autoimmune thyroid problems are common in women with type 1 diabetes. In women receiving thyroxine replacement therapy, careful monitoring of thyroid function through the pregnancy is required as the dose of thyroxine may need to be increased. Many clinicians increase the thyroxine dose before conception. In women with Graves' disease, a plan for measuring the anti-thyroid-stimulating hormone receptor antibody early in the third trimester should be established to determine the risk of transplacental passage of the Graves' disease.

During the initial visit, the anticipated variation in insulin requirements was discussed.

The pregnancy proceeded relatively smoothly. A healthy 3,500-g baby girl was delivered by cesarean section at 37 weeks. Nearly 4 years later, a spot urine albumin-creatinine ratio was 1 mg/mmol with an eGFR of 62 mL/min/1.73 m² (creatinine 100 µmol/L or 1.1 mg/dL).

REFERENCES

1. Diabetes Control and Complications Trial Research Group. Effect of pregnancy on microvascular complications in the diabetes control and complications trial. *Diabetes Care* 2000;23:1084–1091

2. Chew EY, Mills JL, Metzger BE, Remaley NA, Jovanovic-Peterson L, Knopp RH, Conley M, Rand L, Simpson JL, Holmes LB, et al. Metabolic control and progression of retinopathy. The Diabetes in Early Pregnancy Study. National Institute of Child Health and Human Development Diabetes in Early Pregnancy Study. *Diabetes Care* 1995;18:631–637

3. Rossing K, Jacobsen P, Hommel E, Mathiesen E, Svenningsen A, Rossing P, Parving HH. Pregnancy and progression of diabetic nephropathy. *Diabetologia* 2002:45;36–41

4. Chaturvedi N, Stephenson JM, Fuller JH, EURODIAB IDDM Complications Study Group. The relationship between pregnancy and long-term maternal complications in the EURODIAB IDDM Complications Study. *Diabet Med* 1995;12:494–499

5. Blumer I, Hadar E, Hadden DR, Jovanovic L, Mestman JH, Murad MH, et al. Diabetes and pregnancy: an endocrine society clinical practice guideline. *J Clin Endocrinol Metab* 2013;98(11):4227–4249

Case 103

Gastroparesis and Pregnancy

Carl Peters, MB, ChB,[1] and Roy Taylor, MD[1]

Type 1 diabetes was diagnosed in a 13-year-old girl in 1990. Blood glucose control remained poor during adolescence. Proliferative retinopathy was identified by retinal screening 7 years later, and bilateral panretinal photocoagulation was applied. Persistent proteinuria was first noted in 2004. Insulin therapy was continued as twice-daily Mixtard 30.

Management of type 1 diabetes during adolescence can be challenging. Various coping strategies, personality traits, and mental health have all been implicated in long-term metabolic control and complication rates. Management during this difficult period requires a coordinated effort from an experienced multidisciplinary team.

The development and progression of microvascular complications strongly correlates with glycemic control, as originally demonstrated in the Diabetes Control and Complications Trial (DCCT). Analysis of the adolescent cohort in the DCCT (ages 13–17 years at entry) showed intensive glycemic control achieved a 53% reduction in risk of developing retinopathy in those without retinopathy at baseline (primary prevention), and a 70% risk reduction in risk of progression of retinopathy in those with mild retinopathy at baseline (secondary prevention).[1] Importantly, there is also an effect of previous metabolic control on subsequent microvascular complications, as shown in the follow-up Epidemiology of Diabetes Interventions and Complications (EDIC) study.[2] Despite intensifying glycemic control in patients previously randomized to conventional treatment targets, the rates of development or progression of microvascular complications remained higher than in those intensively managed from the outset.

In 2006, she presented at 7 weeks' gestation in her first pregnancy. HbA$_{1c}$ at the time was 9.5% and blood pressure was 118/62 mmHg. The insulin regime was replaced with once daily insulin glargine and meal-time insulin aspart. HbA$_{1c}$ was 6.2% by 20 weeks' gestation and thereafter averaged 6.1% until delivery.

An onset of vomiting began during the first trimester. Cyclizine and prochlorperazine had been prescribed without effect. Although at first this was assumed to be hyperemesis gravidarum, careful history elicited that she

[1]Newcastle Magnetic Resonance Centre, Campus for Ageing and Vitality, Newcastle upon Tyne, England.

 DOI: 10.2337/9781580405713.103

could frequently recognize the previous day's food in the vomitus. A clinical diagnosis of diabetic gastroparesis was made. Metoclopramide 10 mg t.i.d. resulted in the disappearance of unaltered food in the vomitus but did not prevent vomiting completely and was continued until successful delivery.

Hyperemesis gravidarum is a condition of intractable vomiting during pregnancy. Women with diabetes have a relative risk of 2.7 of developing hyperemesis gravidarum compared with people without diabetes. Not surprisingly, gastroparesis presenting in pregnancy can be mistaken for hyperemesis gravidarum, as the clinical distinction can be difficult and the latter is more common. The distinction is important, as severe hyperemesis (weight loss >5% of prepregnancy weight) responds dramatically to high-dose steroid therapy.[3] Evaluation typically is recommended in patients with suspected gastroparesis as accelerated gastric emptying and functional dyspepsia can present with similar symptoms that may be worsened by prokinetics and to rule out mechanical obstruction.

Published clinical guidance states a high risk of maternal morbidity and poor perinatal outcome for woman known to have gastroparesis preconception.[4] The effect of gastroparesis per se on pregnancy outcome is difficult to separate from other known risk factors for adverse pregnancy outcomes, such as poor metabolic control. Many patients usually benefit from prokinetic agents, such as metoclopramide, a drug considered to be safe for use throughout pregnancy, and erythromycin in more severe cases. Evidence regarding the effect of improving glycemic control on gastric emptying is controversial, but in the setting of pregnancy it is irrelevant as the best possible glycemic control is vital for the fetus.

After delivery, the vomiting continued unabated. Metoclopramide exerted a modifying influence upon symptoms, and domperidone brought about no additional effect. Thorough gastrointestinal investigation included endoscopy, which revealed the presence of unaltered food in the stomach despite overnight fasting. During the next 6 years, the diabetic gastroparesis followed a typical course. Exacerbations with vomiting up to 8 times per day lasted several months, and relative remissions, with vomiting only once or twice per day, lasted a similar period.

As with other symptoms attributable to autonomic neuropathy, gastroparesis tends to fluctuate with periods of severe bloating, nausea, and vomiting interspersed with intervals of diminished or absent symptoms. To date, gastric electrical stimulation has been examined only in a blinded fashion in a single, short duration study with unchanged objective measurement of gastric emptying despite subjective improvement.[5] The remainder of studies have been open label with results subject to a high degree of bias.

Renal function remained normal during her first pregnancy, but serum creatinine rose steadily from that time despite tight blood pressure control. In January 2012, she sought prepregnancy advice regarding her diabetes and renal function. At that time, serum creatinine was 137 μmol/L (1.55 mg/dL). She was additionally under the care of the nephrology clinic and blood pressure fluctuated between 124 to 140 mmHg systolic and 65 to 84 mmHg diastolic. HbA$_{1c}$ was 7.3% and weight was 59.7 kg.

Women with severe renal impairment have the greatest difficulty conceiving, the highest rate of miscarriage, and the poorest pregnancy outcome. Ideally all women should be counseled on risks before conception.

Once achieved, pregnancy is accompanied by glomerular hyperfiltration and a relative decrease in serum creatinine such that previously normal values may be considered abnormal in pregnancy. Women with serum creatinine values >124 μmol/L have an increased risk of deterioration in renal function and poor pregnancy outcome. Most women have mild renal dysfunction and pregnancy continues uneventfully. Preexisting proteinuria and hypertension increase the risk of accelerated decline in renal function. Controlling hypertension reduces the risk. Because of concerns of possible teratogenic effects, ACE inhibitors are usually continued until pregnancy is confirmed and then discontinued or replaced with another agent, if required. Calcium channel antagonists and methyldopa are commonly used agents. Urinary tract infection should be treated promptly as this has an independent negative effect on pregnancy outcome.

When she was seen for her second pregnancy at 7 weeks' gestation, the gastroparesis had become less troublesome. Vomiting ceased from the end of the first trimester until after delivery. The pregnancy progressed well, although by 24 weeks, the fetus was noted to be small for gestational age. Renal function steadily deteriorated during pregnancy to serum creatinine of 194 μmol/L (2.2 mg/dL). Good blood pressure control was maintained on nifedipine 40 mg daily together with methyldopa rising to 250 mg t.i.d. Because of declining renal function, elective cesarean section was performed at 33 weeks' gestation, and the female baby was on the fifth centile for weight (1.73 kg). During the pregnancy, she had experienced 6 months of freedom from symptomatic gastroparesis. Within 2 days of delivery, vomiting returned and she was unable to eat solids. She was managed with high-energy liquids together with metoclopramide and basal glargine only. As the symptomatic gastroparesis had returned, severe postural hypotension developed. On nifedipine alone, supine blood pressure was 162/94 mm Hg, falling to 89/57 mmHg on standing.

By careful adjustment of daily routine, she was able to manage her symptoms while maintaining weight and caring for her family. The autonomic neuropathy has continued to follow the characteristically intermittent course. Postural hypotension remitted within 6 weeks of delivery. She remains able to cope with the frequent vomiting.

To date, there have been no reports in the literature of remission of gastroparesis symptoms during pregnancy. The mechanism underlying their improvement remains unclear and requires further evaluation. Fluctuations of gastroparesis symptoms are common, although the strong relationship to pregnancy reported in this case is noteworthy.

REFERENCES

1. Diabetes Control and Complications Trial Research Group. Effect of intensive diabetes treatment on the development and progression of long-term

complications in adolescents with insulin-dependent diabetes mellitus: Diabetes Control and Complications Trial. *J Pediatr* 1994;125:177–188

2. The Diabetes Control and Complications Trial/Epidemiology of Diabetes Interventions and Complications Research Group. Retinopathy and nephropathy in patients with type 1 diabetes four years after a trial of intensive therapy. *N Engl J Med* 2000;342:381–389

3. Moran P, Taylor R. Management of hyperemesis gravidarum: the importance of weight loss as a criterion for steroid therapy. *Q J Med* 2002;95:153–158

4. American Diabetes Association. Managing preexisting diabetes for pregnancy: summary of evidence and consensus recommendations for care. *Diabetes Care* 2008;31:1060–1079

5. Abell T, McCallum R, Hocking M, Koch K, Abrahamsson H, LeBlanc I, Lindberg G, Konturek J, Nowak T, Quigley EMM, Tougas G, Starkebaum W. Gastric electrical stimulation for medically refractory gastroparesis. *Gastroenterology* 2003;125:421–428

Index

A

acanthosis nigricans, 50, 99, 290
acarbose, 75, 186, 188, 312
ACE inhibitors, 193, 265, 276, 376, 380
acromegaly, 51, 190–191
ADA. *See* American Diabetes
    Association
Addison's disease (AD)
    APS-2, 149–152, 153–154
    characterization of, 142
    type 1 diabetes, 141–144, 145–147
adiponectin, 115–117, 219
adolescents. *See* children and
    adolescents
adrenal insufficiency, 69, 141–142,
    149–150, 151
adrenal tumor, causing severe insulin
    resistance, 124–128
AGS (American Geriatrics Society),
    275–276
AIH. *See* autoimmune hepatitis
albuminuria, 137–140
alopecia, 118–119, 149–151
α-glucosidase inhibitors, 34, 109, 188
American Diabetes Association (ADA)
    classifications of ketosis-prone
        diabetes, 40
    guidelines for diagnosis of
        diabetes, 2, 86
    screening T1D patients for
        thyroid and celiac disease,
        146
American Geriatrics Society (AGS),
    275–276
ANA (antinuclear antibodies), 50,
    180–182

Angervall, L., 165
angiotensin receptor blockers, 276, 376
1,5-anhydroglucitol (1,5-AG), 92–93
anion gap metabolic acidosis, 223–224
antinuclear antibodies (ANA), 50,
    180–182
antismooth muscle antibody (ASMA),
    180–182
APECED (autoimmune
    polyendocrinopathy candidiasis
    ectodermal dystrophy) syndrome,
    181, 183
APS-1 (autoimmune polyglandular
    syndrome type 1), 143, 146, 150,
    151
APS-2 (autoimmune polyglandular
    syndrome type 2), 143, 146,
    149–152
    features of, 151
    slow progression of T1D and,
        153–154
ASMA (antismooth muscle antibody),
    180–182
aspart insulin
    atypical T2D with profound
        dyslipidemia, 156–157
    glucolipotoxicity, 121–122
    hypoglycemic unawareness,
        304–305
    insulin allergy, 253–255
    ketosis-prone diabetes, 36–37
    LADA, 64
    MODY, 3
    severe hypoglycemia, 335–336,
        341–342
    severe insulin resistance, 110, 119,
        124–125

translating hospital regimen to
home regimen, 240–242
atypical diabetes, 24. *See also* ketosis-
prone diabetes
autoimmune hepatitis (AIH), 174,
180–183
diagnosis of, 181–182
types of, 181
autoimmune polyendocrinopathy
candidiasis ectodermal dystrophy
(APECED) syndrome, 181, 183
autoimmune polyglandular syndrome
type 1 (APS-1), 143, 146, 150, 151
autoimmune polyglandular syndrome
type 2 (APS-2), 143, 146, 149–152
features of, 151
slow progression of T1D and,
153–154
automatism, 293–295
azathioprine, 171, 353
autoimmune hepatitis, 182
type B insulin resistance, 116

B

baclofen, 171, 173
Balasubramanyam, A., 24, 37
Banerji, M.A., 37
benzodiazepines, 171, 173–174
β-blockers, 193–194
Botazzo, G.F., 65
botulinum toxin A, 171
bromocriptine, 109
burns, 204–207
Burns, L., 367

C

CAD (coronary artery disease),
192–194
calcium channel blockers, 193, 380
canagliflozin, 244–246, 248, 276–277
cardiac arrest, 211–213
cardiac surgery, 196–198
cardiovascular disease, 244, 272, 339,
376
carvedilol, 193–194
catecholamines, 184, 204, 257, 325

celiac disease (CD), 146, 172, 281–283,
324
cerebellar atrophy, 369–370
CGMs (continuous glucose monitors),
87, 96, 185, 258, 324–325, 327
children and adolescents
Addison's disease and T1D,
141–144, 145–147
autoimmune hepatitis and T1D,
180–183
glycogenic hepatopathy and T1D,
175–178
metabolic syndrome-related
comorbidities and
ketoacidosis, 26–31
MODY, 1–3, 5–7, 8–10
nonobese, with T1D, 70–72
psychosocial stressors and T2D,
290–292
cholestyramine, 364
chronic inflammatory demyelinating
polyneuropathy (CIDP), 351–353
defined, 351
treatment for, 351–352
clonazepam, 162–163, 364, 367
cognitive behavioral therapy, 305
cognitive decline, 296–299
colesevelam, 109
continuous glucose monitors (CGMs),
87, 96, 185, 258, 324–325, 327
continuous subcutaneous insulin
infusion (CSII), 70, 110, 130–131
continuous veno-venous
hemofiltration (CVVH), 46
coronary artery disease (CAD),
192–194
corticosteroids, 119, 127–128, 171,
180, 182–183, 255, 352
cortisol, 128, 250, 257
Addison's disease, 141–143,
146–147, 150
hypercortisolism, 125, 128
C-peptide
defined, 63
exogenous versus endogenous
insulin sources, 315–316
CSII (continuous subcutaneous insulin
infusion), 70, 110, 130–131

Cushing's syndrome (CS), 98–99, 125, 127, 133
CVVH (continuous veno-venous hemofiltration), 46
cyanocobolamin, 356
cyclizine, 378
cyclophosphamide, 116–117, 119
cyclosporine, 116, 119
cytokines, 204, 218, 220, 329, 367

D

DA (diabetic amyotrophy), 351, 367–368
Dalakas, M.C., 171
dapsone, 90–91, 95–96
dawn phenomenon, 185, 257–258, 344
demyelination, 351–353, 361, 364
detemir insulin, 376
    allergy and noninsulin components, 254–255
    dawn phenomenon, 258
    LADA, 55
    once daily doses and hypoglycemia, 302
    type 1 diabetes, 376
    type 2 diabetes, 109–110, 339, 341
diabetes. *See also* late autoimmune diabetes in adults; maturity onset diabetes of the young; type 1 diabetes; type 2 diabetes
    ADA guidelines for diabetes diagnosis, 2
    clinical categories of, 2
diabetic amyotrophy (DA), 351, 367–368
diabetic ketoacidosis (DKA), 20–21
    APS-2, 149
    defined, 23
    growth hormone excess-induced, 189–191
    hemodialysis in patient with, 222–224
    hyperglycemic hyperosmolar syndrome, 45
    ketosis-prone diabetes, 32–34, 36–37

    metabolic syndrome-related comorbidities, 26–31
    mild to moderate severity, 15
    recurrent, 15–18
    reevaluation after presentation of, 23–25
    in T1D patient on low-calorie diet, 19–21
diabetic myonecrosis, 164–167
diacylglycerol, 279
diazepam, 162
    stiff person syndrome, 170–171, 173
diazoxide, 309, 346
dipeptidylpeptidase (DPP)-4 inhibitors, 55
    hypocaloric diet and, 247–248
    LADA, 66
    MODY, 6
    prevention of diabetes development, 288
    type 2 diabetes, 109
distal symmetrical polyneuropathy (DSP), 357–359, 364–365, 369
divalproex, 162
DKA. *See* diabetic ketoacidosis
DPP-4 inhibitors. *See* dipeptidylpeptidase-4 inhibitors
DSP (distal symmetrical polyneuropathy), 357–359, 364–365, 369
duloxetine, 351, 359
dyslipidemia, 109, 124, 156–159

E

Ellenberg, M., 83, 358
endocrine disorders, 49–51, 150, 154
end-stage renal disease (ESRD), 222–224
enteral tube feedings (TF)
    glycemic control on continuous, 200–203, 205
    after ventricular assist device placement, 219–220
ESRD (end-stage renal disease), 222–224
exenatide, 113, 245, 253–254, 265, 284–286

F

familial juvenile nephronophthisis (FJN), 140
fenofibrate, 279
ferritin, 135
FJN (familial juvenile nephronophthisis), 140
Flatbush diabetes, 24. *See also* ketosis-prone diabetes
fludrocortisone, 142, 144, 146, 153, 364, 367
fructosamine, 86–88, 92–94, 96

G

GABA. *See* γ-aminobutyric acid
gabapentin, 8, 109, 351–353, 364
GAD antibodies. *See* glutamic acid decarboxylase antibodies
gadolinium, 165–166
γ-aminobutyric acid (GABA)
GAD and, 369
hemichorea-hemiballismus, 162–163
stiff person syndrome, 170
gastric bypass surgery, 312, 331
gastroparesis, 186, 251, 364–365
pregnancy and, 378–380
GCK (glycolytic enzyme glucokinase), 2–3, 10, 13, 78, 80–82
GDH-PQQ (glucose dehydrogenase pyrroloquinoline quinone), 251
gemfibrozil, 109, 279–280
GFD (gluten-free diet), 281–283
GH (growth hormone), 189–191
ghrelin, 190
GHRH (growth hormone-releasing hormone), 190
glargine insulin
Addison's disease, 150–151
allergy and noninsulin components, 255
atypical T2D with profound dyslipidemia, 156–157
autoimmune hepatitis and T1D, 183

cardiac surgery in patient with T2D, 196–198
complex enteral tube feedings, 201
factitious hypoglycemia, 314–315
gastroparesis and pregnancy, 378, 380
glucolipotoxicity, 121–122
ketoacidosis, 23–24
ketosis-prone diabetes, 36–37
LADA, 55, 58, 60
MODY, 3
once daily doses and hypoglycemia, 302
peritoneal dialysis and T1D, 250–251
severe insulin resistance, 50, 109–110, 124–125, 128
somnambulism, 301–302
subcutaneous delivery, 233–234, 236
translating hospital regimen to home regimen, 241–242
type 2 diabetes, 110, 257–258, 339–344
ventricular assist device placement, 218–220
gliclazide, 6
glipizide, 8, 92, 94, 109–110, 286–288, 339, 340–343
glucagon secretion, effect of peripheral delivery of insulin on, 20–21
glucagon-like peptide 1 (GLP-1) agonists, 55
combination therapy with SGLT-2 inhibitors, 245–246, 248–249
insulin reduction and, 248
ketosis-prone diabetes, 157, 159
prevention of diabetes development, 288
glucagon-like peptide 1 (GLP-1) analogs, 113
LADA, 66
type 2 diabetes, 109
glucocorticoids, 24, 127–128, 173, 204
Addison's disease, 142–143
allergy, 254
glucolipotoxicity, 121–123

glucose dehydrogenase pyrroloquinoline quinone (GDH-PQQ), 251
glucotoxicity
  C-peptide level, 71
  ketoacidosis, 33
  ketosis-prone diabetes, 36
  profound dyslipidemia, 157, 159
glulisine insulin
  insulin allergy, 254–255
  ketoacidosis, 23–24
glutamic acid decarboxylase (GAD) antibodies
  associated CNS pathologies, 370
  cerebellar atrophy and high levels of, 369–370
  LADA, 53, 55, 59, 67–68, 83–84
  MODY, 6–7
  nonobese young people with T1D, 70–71
  stiff person syndrome, 170, 173
  type 1 diabetes, 61–63, 67–68, 139–140, 266
gluten-free diet (GFD), 281–283
glycated albumin, 92–94
glycolytic enzyme glucokinase (GCK), 2–3, 10, 13, 78, 80–82
Graves' disease, 172, 281, 309, 375, 377
Groop, L.C., 65
growth hormone (GH), 189–191
growth hormone-releasing hormone (GHRH), 190

H

HAIR-AN syndrome (hyperandrogenism, insulin resistance, and acanthosis nigricans), 50, 99
HAMP gene, 134
HbA$_{1c}$. *See* hemoglobin A1C
HD (hemodialysis), 222–224
heart transplant, extreme insulin resistance following, 214–216
hemichorea-hemiballismus (HHH), 160–163
  characterization of, 162
  differential diagnosis of, 161

treatment for, 163
hemochromatosis (*HFE*) gene, 134
hemodialysis (HD), 222–224
hemoglobin A1C (HbA$_{1c}$), 95–97
  factors affecting value, 96
  fructosamine and glycated albumin versus, 92–94
  limitations of evaluating, 86–88
  unexplained decline in spite of persistent hyperglycemia, 90–91
hepatic glycogenosis, 175–178
hepatitis, 355–356
  autoimmune, 174, 180–183
  non-alcoholic steatohepatitis, 106
hepatocyte nuclear factor (HNF)-1α, 2–3, 7, 9–10, 13, 78
hepatocyte nuclear factor (HNF)-1β, 2, 10, 78, 138
hepatocyte nuclear factor (HNF)-4α, 2–3, 6, 10, 78, 138
hepcidin, 134
hereditary hemochromatosis (HH), 99, 133–135
  characterization of, 134
  comorbidities, 134–135
  genetic forms of, 134
HFE (hemochromatosis) gene, 134
HFE2 gene, 134
HH. *See* hereditary hemochromatosis
HHH. *See* hemichorea-hemiballismus
HHS. *See* hyperglycemic hyperosmolar syndrome
Hirata's disease (insulin antibody syndrome; insulin autoimmune syndrome [IAS]), 307–310
HKA (hyperosmolar ketoacidosis), 45
HNF (hepatocyte nuclear factor)-1α, 2–3, 7, 9–10, 13, 78
HNF (hepatocyte nuclear factor)-1β, 2, 10, 78, 138
HNF (hepatocyte nuclear factor)-4α, 2–3, 6, 10, 78, 138
"honeymoon" phase, 17, 68, 147, 266
hormone sensitive lipase (HSL), 159
hospital settings
  burns in patient with T1D, 204–207

cardiac surgery in patient with
T2D, 196–198
complex enteral tube feedings,
200–203
DKA in patient on hemodialysis,
222–224
extreme insulin resistance
following heart transplant,
214–216
intravenous and subcutaneous
insulin in patient with severe
insulin resistance, 208–210
rhabdomyolysis in patient in
hyperglycemic hyperosmolar
coma, 226–230
therapeutic hypothermia in
patients with cardiac arrest,
211–213
transferring from intravenous to
subcutaneous insulin,
232–236
transitions from inpatient to
outpatient
failure to coordinate care,
237–238
inpatient self-management
education, 242
transition guide for
medications, 242–243
translating hospital regimen
to home regimen,
240–243
ventricular assist device
placement, 218–220
HSL (hormone sensitive lipase), 159
hydrocodone, 351–352
hydrocortisone
Addison's disease, 142–144,
146–147, 150, 153
adrenal tumor, 128
hyperandrogenemia, 373
hyperandrogenism, insulin resistance,
and acanthosis nigricans
(HAIR-AN syndrome),
50, 99
hyperchloremia, 223
hypercortisolism, 125, 128
hyperemesis gravidarum, 378–379

hyperglycemia
cardiac surgery, 196–197
following heart transplant, 214
glycogenic hepatopathy, 177
hemodialysis, 223
ketoacidosis, 23
ketosis-prone diabetes, 18, 36
MODY, 2–3
newly diagnosed, asymptomatic,
77–79
persistent fasting, continuous
monitoring for, 257–260
predominant mechanism
responsible for, 24
rhabdomyolysis, 226–230
severe burns, 204
steroid-induced, 24–25
symptomatic postprandial, 73–75
therapeutic hypothermia, 212
transitions for hospitalized
patients, 237–238
unexplained decline in HbA_{1c},
90–91
hyperglycemic hyperosmolar
syndrome (HHS), 43–48
criteria for, 45
rhabdomyolysis in patient in
coma, 226–230
treatment for, 46
type 2 diabetes, 314–316
hyperinsulinemia, 318, 331, 372
hyperkalemia
Addison's disease, 141
hemodialysis, 223–224
hypernatremia
hyperglycemic hyperosmolar
syndrome, 46
ketoacidosis, 28
rhabdomyolysis, 228
hyperosmolar ketoacidosis
(HKA), 45
hypertriglyceridemia, 278–280
hypocaloric diet. See low-calorie diet
hypoglycemia
Addison's disease, 141
causes of, 318
cognitive decline and loss of
autonomy, 296–299

conditions contributing to
recurrent, 250
dizziness, lightheadedness, and
syncope, 184–185
factitious, 314–316, 319
implicated in automatism, 293–295
islet autotransplantation, 332–334
ketosis-prone diabetes, 36–37
LADA versus T1D, 58–59
MODY, 6
Munchausen's syndrome, 321–323
plasmapheresis and IAS, 307–310
postprandial, 311–312
progressive, due to insulinoma,
345–350
recurrent, 317–320
reversal of insulin-requiring T2D
and development of, 329–331
somnambulism, 301–302
T1D patient on low-calorie meal
replacement diet, 19–20
T2D patient with glargine insulin
management, 339–344
technologies for reduction of,
324–327
therapeutic hypothermia, 212–213
transitions for hospitalized
patients, 237–238
treatment of severe, 335–338
type B insulin resistance, 116, 119
hypoglycemia unawareness, 304–306,
335–337
guideline for patients with, 337
LADA, 59–60
peritoneal dialysis, 250–251
type 2 diabetes, 247–248, 317
hypogonadism, 134–135, 151
hypokalemia
adrenal tumor, 124–125
hemodialysis, 224
hyponatremia
Addison's disease, 141, 145–147
hemodialysis, 223
hypoparathyroidism, 72, 143, 150–151
hypophosphatemia
hyperglycemic hyperosmolar
syndrome, 48
rhabdomyolysis, 228

hypophysitis, 151
hypothyroidism, 64, 66, 72, 146,
149–152, 153, 281–282, 355

I

IAS (insulin antibody syndrome;
insulin autoimmune syndrome;
Hirata's disease), 307–310
icodextrin, 250–252
idiopathic thrombocytopenic purpura
(ITP), 151
idiopathic type 1 diabetes, 24. *See also*
ketosis-prone diabetes
immunoglobulin A (IgA) deficiency, 151
incretins, 34, 245
infertility, 372–374
insulin. *See also names of specific types of
insulin and methods of delivery*;
severe insulin resistance
intravenous
cardiac surgery and, 197
severe insulin resistance and,
208–210
transferring to subcutaneous,
232–236
peripheral delivery, 20–21
poor injection techniques,
261–263
use of during surgery, 197
insulin allergy, 253–255
insulin antibody syndrome (IAS;
insulin autoimmune syndrome;
Hirata's disease), 307–310
insulin neuritis, 358
insulin pens, poor injection
techniques, 261–263
insulin promoter factor-1 (IPF-1), 2–3,
10, 78
insulin pumps
cognitive decline and loss of
autonomy, 296–299
hypoglycemic unawareness, 305
insulin allergy, 255
pregnant patient with T2D,
130–131
with threshold suspend feature,
325–327

use of insulin U-500 via, 102–104,
105–108
insulin receptor antibodies, 115–117,
118–120
insulin staircase and cliff effect, 106–107
insulin U-500
alternatives to, 109–113
avoiding medication errors, 99
dividing dosage, 100
glucolipotoxicity, 121–123
pregnant patient with T2D,
130–131
severe insulin resistance
syndromes, 98–101, 102–104
type B insulin resistance, 116
using via pump, 102–104,
105–108, 130–131
insulinomas, 307–308, 312, 321–322,
345–350
International Society for Pediatric and
Adolescent Diabetes (ISPAD)
guidelines for diagnosis and
management of monogenic
diabetes in children, 5
screening T1D patients for
thyroid and celiac disease, 146
intravenous immunoglobulin (IVIg),
171, 173, 351–353
IPF-1 (insulin promoter factor-1), 2–3,
10, 78
irbesarten, 376
islet autotransplantation, 332–334
ISPAD. *See* International Society for
Pediatric and Adolescent Diabetes
ITP (idiopathic thrombocytopenic
purpura), 151
IVIg (intravenous immunoglobulin),
171, 173, 351–353

K

ketosis-prone diabetes (KPD), 15–18,
24, 36–37, 39–42. *See also* diabetic
ketoacidosis
classification of, 33–34, 37, 40–42
defined, 32–33
with profound dyslipidemia,
156–159

provoked and unprovoked, 41
treatment for, 34

L

lanreotide, 191
late autoimmune diabetes in adults
(LADA), 133, 154
diagnosing, 53–56, 64–66, 67–69
in elderly patients, 83–84
presenting at varied ages, 61–63
type 1 diabetes versus, 58–60,
64–66, 67–69
type 2 diabetes versus, 64–66
LCD. *See* low-calorie diet
Lean, M., 273
Leprechaunism, 99, 102
Lim, E.L., 272
linagliptin, 79
lipodystrophy, 50, 99
lipoprotein lipase (LPL), 159, 279
lipotoxicity
glucolipotoxicity, 122–123
ketosis-prone diabetes, 36
liraglutide, 121–122, 258–260, 286
ketosis-prone diabetes, 157
type 1 diabetes, 113
type 2 diabetes, 244–246
lispro insulin
Addison's disease and T1D, 142
cardiac surgery in patient with
T2D, 198
factitious hypoglycemia, 314–315
insulin allergy, 255
LADA, 53, 60, 84
peritoneal dialysis and T1D,
250–251
persistent fasting hyperglycemia,
258–259
severe insulin resistance, 130–131,
209
subcutaneous delivery, 232–234
low-calorie (hypocaloric) diet (LCD)
insulin reduction and, 247–248
ketoacidosis in T1D patient on,
19–21
rapid weight loss following
introduction of, 19

reversal of T2D by, 271–273
LPL (lipoprotein lipase), 159, 279
lupus, 117, 118–120, 309

M

maturity-onset diabetes of the young
(MODY), 1–3
  albuminuria, 137–138
  coexistent with type 1 diabetes,
    5–7
  defined, 2, 5
  genetic mutations, 2, 6–7, 9–10,
    13, 78
  glucokinase, 80–82
  misdiagnosis of, 2–3
  newly diagnosed, asymptomatic
    hyperglycemia, 78–79
  probability calculator, 79
  unusual clinical presentation of,
    8–10
Mauriac, P., 176
6-mercaptopurine, 182
metabolic syndrome, 6, 17–18, 26–31,
  34
metaclopramide, 364
metformin
  ketosis-prone diabetes, 34
  lactic acidosis, 361
  LADA, 60, 68–69
  MODY, 79
  monogenic diabetes, 8–10
  neuropathy in T2D managed
    with, 354–356
  polycystic ovary disease, 372–374
  prevention of diabetes
    development, 285–286, 288
  prolonged insulin-free
    management of T1D, 265
  severe insulin resistance
    syndromes, 103
  type 1 diabetes, 61–62, 265
  type 2 diabetes, 109, 271, 276,
    339, 354–356
methocarbamol, 171
methyldopa, 376, 380
methylprednisone, 214–215
metoclopramide, 379–380

metronidazole, 364
microalbuminuria, 137, 376
mini mental state exam (MMSE),
  296–297, 299
MoCA (Montreal Cognitive
  Assessment), 297, 299
MODY. *See* maturity-onset diabetes of
  the young
monogenic diabetes
  IPSAD guidelines for diagnosis
    and management of, 5
  MODY, 1–3, 5–7, 8–10, 12–13
  unusual clinical presentation of,
    8–10
Montreal Cognitive Assessment
  (MoCA), 297, 299
mucocutaneous candidiasis, 143, 151
Munchausen-by-proxy, 332–334
Munchausen's syndrome, 321–323
myasthenia gravis, 150–151
myoglobinuria, 228

N

NAFLD (non-alcoholic fatty liver
  disease), 106, 177–178
NASH (non-alcoholic steatohepatitis),
  106
nateglinide, 284–287
nephronophthisis, 140
nephronophthisis-1 (NPHP-1) gene,
  140
nephropathy, 165, 375–376
nesidioblastosis, 312, 318, 330–331
neurogenic differentiation factor-1
  (neuroD1), 2–3, 10, 78
neuropathic cachexia, 83–84, 367–368
neuropathy
  acute sensory neuropathy in T1D,
    357–359
  chronic inflammatory
    demyelinating
    polyneuropathy, 351–353
  contrast between acute sensory
    and chronic sensorimotor
    painful neuropathies, 359
  diabetic amyotrophy and
    neuropathic cachexia, 367–368

high GAD antibody levels and
cerebellar atrophy, 369–370
metformin-treated T2D, 354–356
nondiabetic neuropathy in patient
with T2D, 361–362
severe distal symmetrical and
autonomic neuropathy in
patient with T1D, 364–365
neutral protamine Hagedorn (NPH)
insulin
complex enteral tube feedings,
201–203
delayed response to, 267–270
hemichorea-hemiballismus, 160,
162
insulin allergy, 255
peritoneal dialysis, 250–251
severe burns, 205–206
ventricular assist device
placement, 219
NIPHS (noninsulinoma
pancreatogenous hyperinsulinemic
syndrome), 307–308, 318
non-alcoholic fatty liver disease
(NAFLD), 106, 177–178
non-alcoholic steatohepatitis (NASH),
106
noninsulinoma pancreatogenous
hyperinsulinemic syndrome
(NIPHS), 307–308, 318
NPH insulin. *See* neutral protamine
Hagedorn insulin
NPHP-1 (nephronophthisis-1) gene,
140

O

obesity
insulin resistance in very obese
patients, 105–108
ketoacidosis in T1D patient on
low-calorie diet, 19–21
metabolic syndrome-related
comorbidities and
ketoacidosis, 26–31
Munchausen's syndrome, 321–323
reversal of T2D and development
of hypoglycemia, 329–331

reversal of T2D by weight loss,
271–273
obstructive sleep apnea (OSA), 258
octreotide, 51, 190–191

P

pancreatectomy
image-guided, minimally invasive,
345–350
islet autotransplantation,
330–332
pancreatitis, 278–279, 332
PCO (polycystic ovary disease), 99,
372–374
pens, poor injection techniques,
261–263
peritoneal dialysis (PD), 250–252
pernicious anemia, 64, 66, 69, 72,
150–151, 173, 369
phlebotomy therapy, 135
pioglitazone, 8, 109–110, 124–125,
265, 285–286, 288
plasmapharesis, 171
plasmapheresis, 307–310, 352
polycystic ovary disease (PCO), 99,
372–374
Porcellati, F., 344
pramlintide, 111
prediabetes
hereditary hemochromatosis,
135
prevention of diabetes
development, 284–288
prednisone, 118–119, 254, 309–310
autoimmune hepatitis, 182–183
following heart transplant, 215
pregabalin, 358–359
pregnancy
gastroparesis, 378–380
glucokinase MODY, 80–82
ketoacidosis during, 24
severe insulin resistance, 130–131
type 1 diabetes, 375–377
prochlorperazine, 378
propofol, 171
psychosocial stressors, 290–292
pumps. *See* insulin pumps

R

RA (rheumatoid arthritis), 150–151
Rabson-Mendenhall syndrome, 102
ranolazine, 194
RBP4 (retinol binding protein 4), 218,
220
refractory angina, 192–194
resistin, 219
retinol binding protein 4 (RBP4), 218,
220
retinopathy, 165, 375–376, 378
rhabdomyolysis, 46
    hyperglycemic hyperosmolar
        syndrome, 48
    patient in hyperglycemic
        hyperosmolar coma, 226–230
rheumatoid arthritis (RA), 150–151
rituximab
    stiff person syndrome, 171,
        173–174
    type B insulin resistance, 116–117
rosiglitazone, 345, 373
Rossing, K., 376

S

Schmidt syndrome. *See* autoimmune
    polyglandular syndrome type 2
self-monitored blood glucose
    (SMBG), discrepant results from,
    92–94
severe insulin resistance, 49–51
    alternatives to insulin U-500,
        109–113
    causes of, 99
    cosecreting adrenal tumor
        causing, 124–128
    following heart transplant,
        214–216
    glucolipotoxicity and concentrated
        insulin, 121–123
    intravenous and subcutaneous
        insulin, 208–210
    in patients with diabetes and
        cardiac arrest, 211–213
    pregnant patient with T2D,
        130–131

ruling out rare causes of, 102
    type A insulin resistance, 50
    type B insulin resistance, 50,
        115–117, 118–120
    type C insulin resistance, 50
    use of insulin U-500 in, 98–101,
        102–104, 105–108
SGLT-2 inhibitors. *See* sodium-
    glucose co-transporter-2
    inhibitors
sitagliptin, 6, 71, 92, 186, 220,
    247–248, 254, 287, 367
SLA (soluble liver antigen) antibody,
    180–182
SLC40A1 gene, 134
SLE (systemic lupus erythematosus),
    118–120, 309
sleep apnea, 184, 258, 302
sleepwalking (somnambulism),
    301–302
SMBG (self-monitored blood
    glucose), discrepant results from,
    92–94
sodium valproate, 171
sodium-glucose co-transporter
    (SGLT)-2 inhibitors
    combination therapy with GLP-1
        agonists, 244–245, 248–249
    LADA, 66
    type 2 diabetes, 109, 275–277
Solimena, M., 170
soluble liver antigen (SLA) antibody,
    180–182
somatostatin, 190–191
somnambulism (sleepwalking), 301–302
Somogyi effect, 59
SPS. *See* stiff person syndrome
statins, 272, 275, 279, 364–365, 376
Stener, B., 165
steroids
    CIDP, 352
    insulin allergy, 254–255
    severe insulin resistance, 99,
        127–128, 210
    steroid-induced hyperglycemia,
        24–25, 209, 254
    type B insulin resistance, 116–117,
        119–120

stiff person syndrome (SPS)
    characterization of, 169
    criteria for diagnosis of, 170
    in patient with multiple
        autoimmune diseases,
        172–174
    in patient with T1D, 169–171
    subtypes of, 174
sulfonylureas (SU), 67–68, 70, 194,
    288
    insulin antibody syndrome,
        307–308
    ketosis-prone diabetes, 37
    MODY, 3, 9–10, 13
    older adults, 276
    type 1 diabetes, 61–62
    type 2 diabetes, 245, 271, 276
systemic lupus erythematosus (SLE),
    118–120, 309

T

T1D. *See* type 1 diabetes
T2D. *See* type 2 diabetes
targeted temperature management
    (therapeutic hypothermia),
    211–213
TF. *See* enteral tube feedings
TFR2 (transferrin receptor 2) gene,
    134
therapeutic hypothermia (targeted
    temperature management),
    211–213
thiazolidinedione (TZD), 34
    polycystic ovary disease,
        373–374
    severe insulin resistance
        syndromes, 103
    type 2 diabetes, 109
thyroxine, 376–377
TNFα (tumor necrosis factor-α), 204,
    218–219
tramadol, 351–352
transferrin receptor 2 (*TFR2*) gene,
    134
tumor necrosis factor-α (TNFα), 204,
    218–219
Tuomi, T., 65

type 1 diabetes (T1D)
    acute sensory neuropathy in,
        357–359
    Addison's disease, 141–144,
        145–147
    albuminuria, 139–140
    APS-2, 149–152, 153–154
    autoimmune disorders in
        children with celiac disease
        and, 281–283
    autoimmune hepatitis, 180–183
    coexistent with MODY, 5–7
    defined, 2
    glycogenic hepatopathy in patient
        with, 175–178
    incidence of, 146
    ketoacidosis in patient on low-
        calorie diet, 19–21
    LADA versus, 58–60
    nonobese young people with,
        70–72
    peritoneal dialysis in patients
        with, 250–252
    pregnancy and diabetes
        complications, 375–377
    presenting at varied ages, 61–63
    prolonged insulin-free
        management of, 265–266
    severe distal symmetrical and
        autonomic neuropathy in
        patient with, 364–365
    stiff person syndrome in patient
        with, 169–171
    technologies for hypoglycemia
        reduction, 324–327
type 1.5 diabetes, 24. *See also* ketosis-
    prone diabetes
type 1a diabetes, 40
type 1b diabetes, 40
type 2 diabetes (T2D)
    combination therapy for, 244–246
    continuous monitoring for
        persistent fasting
        hyperglycemia, 257–260
    defined, 2
    development of hypoglycemia and
        reversal of insulin
        requirement, 329–331

dizziness, lightheadedness, and syncope, 184–188
factitious hypoglycemia, 314–316
ketoacidosis, 25
management with glargine insulin, 339–344
metabolic syndrome-related comorbidities and ketoacidosis, 26–31
metformin-treated, neuropathy in, 354–356
Munchausen's syndrome, 321–323
nondiabetic neuropathy in patient with, 361–362
in patient undergoing cardiac surgery, 196–198
postprandial hypoglycemia, 311–312
pregnant patient with, 130–131
prevalence of, 349
with profound dyslipidemia, 156–159
progressive hypoglycemia due to insulinoma, 345–350
psychosocial stressors, 290–292
recurrent hypoglycemia, 317–320
recurrent ketoacidosis, 15–18
refractory angina in patient with, 192–194
reversal of by weight loss, 271–273

SGLT-2 inhibitors, 275–277
stopping insulin in patients with, 247–249
use of insulin U-500 via pump, 102–104
ventricular assist device placement in patient with, 218–220
type A insulin resistance, 50
type B insulin resistance, 50, 115–117, 118–120
type C insulin resistance, 50
TZD. *See* thiazolidinedione

U

Umpierrez, G.E., 242

V

ventricular assist device (VAD) placement, 218–220
vigabatrin, 171
vitamin B_{12} malabsorption and deficiency, 356, 361–362
vitiligo, 118, 150–151, 173

W

Werner syndrome, 99
Whipple's triad, 74, 312
Wile, D.J., 362
Winter, W.E., 157

CPSIA information can be obtained
at www.ICGtesting.com
Printed in the USA
FFHW012014010519
52211623-57581FF